D1170764

USING SUPERHEROES IN COUNSELING AND PLAY THERAPY

About the Editor

Lawrence C. Rubin, PhD, LMHC, RPT-S, is a Professor of Counselor Education at St. Thomas University in Miami, Florida, where he also coordinates the Mental Health Counseling training program. He is a psychotherapist in private practice where he works with children, adolescents and families, providing assessment, counseling and play therapy. Rubin is a Registered Play Therapist Supervisor and current president of the Florida Association for Play Therapy. His research interests lie at the intersection of psychology and popular culture, in which context, he has recently edited a book titled "Psychotropic Drugs and Popular Culture: Essays on Medicine, Mental Health and the Media" as well as published several articles in the areas of professional ethics and play therapy.

Using Superheroes in Counseling and Play Therapy

Edited by

LAWRENCE C. RUBIN, PhD, LMHC, RPT-S

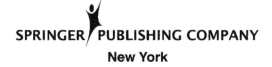

SPRINGER PUBLISHING COMPANY

New York

Springer Publishing Company, LLC
11 West 42nd Street
New York, NY 10036
www.springerpub.com

Acquisitions Editor: Sheri W. Sussman
Production Editor: Tenea D. Johnson
Cover Comic Art: Nicholas Gallo-Lopez
Cover Design: Mimi Flow
Composition: Techbooks

07 08 09 10/ 6 5 4 3 2 1

Library of Congress Cataloging-in-Publication Data

Using superheroes in counseling and play therapy/Lawrence C. Rubin, editor.
  p. ; cm.
  Includes bibliographical references and index.
  ISBN 0-8261-0269-7 (hardback)
  1. Play therapy. 2. Heroes. 3. Superhero films. 4. Fantasy. 5. Children—Counseling of.
I. Rubin, Lawrence C., 1955-
  [DNLM: 1. Play Therapy—methods. 2. Counseling—methods. 3. Child Psychology.
4. Adolescent Psychology. 5. Fantasy. 6. Imagination. WS 350.2 U85 2006]
RJ505.P6U85 2006
618.92'891653—dc22

                                                                    2006026582

Printed in the United States of America by Bang Printing.

For Randi, Zach, and Becca, my superfamily.

Contents

Contributors   xi
Foreword   xix
Preface   xxix
Acknowledgments   xxxi

SECTION I. Traditional Superheroes in Counseling and Play Therapy

1. **Introduction: Look, Up in the Sky! An Introduction to the Use of Superheroes in Psychotherapy**   3
   Lawrence C. Rubin

   Imagination, Fantasy, and Fantasy Play   4
   The Superhero Fantasy   7
   How Superheroes Can Help   15

2. **Superheroes in Therapy: Uncovering Children's Secret Identities**   23
   Robert J. Porter

   The Objective and Virtual Play Spaces   25
   Cases Studies   28
   Summary and Conclusion   44

3. **What Would Superman Do?**   49
   Cory A. Nelson

   Superheroes in Clinical Practice   50
   Adlerian Therapy—An Overview   52
   Superheroes and the Phases of Adlerian Therapy   52
   What Would Superman Do?   54

Case Study   60
Conclusion   66

4. Superheroes and Sandplay: Using the Archetype Through
    the Healing Journey   69
    William McNulty

    Sandplay Therapy   70
    Mythology and the Hero's Journey   76
    Case Studies   81

5. The Incredible Hulk and Emotional Literacy   89
    Jennifer Mendoza Sayers

    The Role of Emotions   90
    Emotional Literacy   91
    Neuroscience and Emotion   93
    Case Studies   96
    Conclusion   100

SECTION II. Superheroes and Unique Clinical Applications

6. Holy Franchise! Batman and Trauma   105
    Michael Brody

    Psychic Trauma   106
    Death Guilt   108
    The Solution   109
    Nonintegrated Personality   113
    Discussion   115
    Conclusion   119

7. Making a Place for the Angry Hero on the Team   121
    Harry Livesay

    The Angry Superhero   123
    The Appeal of the Angry Hero   126
    Anger, Aggression, and Boys   127
    Superhero Play   129
    The Angry Hero on the Team   131
    Case Studies   136
    Conclusion   138

8. A Super Milieu: Using Superheroes in the Residential
    Treatment of Adolescents With Sexual Behavior Problems   143
    *Karen Robertie, Ryan Weidenbenner,
    Leya Barrett, and Robert Poole*

Traditional Residential Treatment 144
Incorporating the Superhero and Supervillain 145
Cornerstone Superheroes 148
Integrating Superheroes Into the Residential Treatment
  Culture 161
Clothing 163
Conclusion 165
Postscript 166

9. **Superheroes Are Super Friends: Developing Social Skills
   and Emotional Reciprocity With Autism Spectrum Clients** 169
   Patty Scanlon

   The Appeal of Superheroes 171
   Autism Spectrum Disorders 172
   Play in Autism Spectrum Disorders 176
   Treatment 178
   Case Study 183
   Conclusion 187

10. **Superheroes in Play Therapy With an Attachment
    Disordered Child** 193
    Carmela Wenger

    The Role of Neuroscience 194
    The Therapeutic Appeal of Superheroes to the Child With
      Attachment Disorder 196
    An Orientation to Treatment 198
    Case Study 199

11. **Luke, I Am Your Father! A Clinical Application of the
    Star Wars Adoption Narrative** 213
    Lawrence C. Rubin

    Adoption, Superheroes, and Star Wars 213
    The Reality of Adoption 217
    The Case of Alex 218
    Conclusion 223

SECTION III. Nontraditional Therapeutic Applications of Superheroes

12. Becoming the Hero: The Use of Role-Playing Games
    in Psychotherapy 227
    George Enfield

Role-Playing the Superhero 228
Heroes and Their Journeys 229
Matching the RPG to the Client 230
Applying the RPG in Clinical Practice 231
Case Studies 232
Outcome and Reflections 240

13. **To Boldly Go! Star Trek Superheroes in Therapy** 243
Jeffrey Pickens

"Make it So!" The Positive Outlook of Star Trek 244
Crew Report: The Star Trek Characters 247
Ship Counselor's Log: The Case of Blake 252
Conclusions: Captain's Log—Beam Me Up! 264
Appendix A 268

14. **Hypnosis and Superheroes** 271
Jan M. Burte

About Hypnosis 272
A Legend in Their Own Minds 272
Managing Pain With Hypnosis 274
Trauma 278
Ego Strengthening and Self-Perception 282
Caveats 288
Conclusion 290

15. **Heroes Who Learn to Love Their Monsters: How Fantasy Film Characters Can Inspire the Journey of Individuation for Gay and Lesbian Clients in Psychotherapy** 293
Roger Kaufman

A Soulful, Archetypal Approach to Gay-Affirmative
Psychotherapy 295
The Gay Hero's Journey: Process of Individuation 298
Using Fantasy Films to Amplify Homosexual Archetypes
and the Journey of Individuation 302
Case Study: A Gay Man Finds Mirroring in *The Lord of
the Rings* 309
Conclusion: The Heroic Potential of Gay and
Lesbian Clients 315

Afterword 319
Appendix 321

Contributors

Leya Barrett, LSW, is a therapist in Program 1, "The Field of Dreams," at Onarga Academy in Illinois, where she has been employed for 7 years. The academy specializes in the treatment of adolescents with sexual behavior problems. She began her work with the academy as a case manager after obtaining her bachelor's degree in social work. She later advanced to the position of unit coordinator. After returning to school and obtaining her master's degree in social work, Leya started her journey as a family therapist. She enjoys using a variety of experiential therapeutic techniques with her clients. As a licensed therapist, she is always increasing her experience with expressive arts activities and finding new ways to bring treatment alive for her clients. The use of superheroes has been a natural fit with the adolescent male clients with whom she works. Although her knowledge of superheroes may be limited, avid interest and longtime acquaintance with comics have filled the void.

Michael Brody, MD, is a board certified child and adult psychiatrist in private practice. He was the CEO and creator of Psychiatric Center (2005), one the largest providers of outpatient care for the chronically mentally ill in the District of Columbia. He is chairman of the Television and Media Committee of the American Academy of Child and Adolescent Psychiatry. He is a professor of American Studies at the University of Maryland, where he teaches a course on Children and the Media. He has published widely on child media issues including superheroes from Batman to Spider-Man. He recently wrote and produced the film *Fifty Years of Children's Television, from Howdy Doody to Spongebob,* which focused on Batman, Superman, and the Power Rangers. He is also active in the Popular Culture Association, where he chairs the section on celebrity and posits that superheroes are true child celebrities. When he was 4 years old, he attempted to fly off his bed, like Superman, but learned to read while recovering, by understanding the words in the balloons over Robin's head in *Detective Comics*. Unlike Dr. Fredric Wertham (*Seduction of the Innocent*) who vilified comic books, he has given balanced testimony on violence on kid's TV to Congress, the Federal Trade Commission, the Federal Communications Commission, the Department of Commerce, and the White House.

Jan M. Burte, PhD, MSCP, is a clinical psychologist who has taught and lectured nationally and internationally on hypnosis for the past 20 years. He is a past director of the Milton H. Erickson Institute of Long Island, past president of the New York Society of Clinical Hypnosis, and a certified and approved consultant in clinical hypnosis (ASCH). Burte has been published in numerous journals and books, appeared on radio and television discussing the applicability of hypnosis for a wide range of patients and conditions. In addition, he is a certified sex therapist (American Association of Sex Educators, Counselors and Therapists), a diplomate in pain management (American Association of Pain Management), and holds a postdoctoral master's in clinical psychopharmacology. He is adjunct professor at Nova Southeastern University and is in private practice in Boca Raton, Florida.

George Enfield, MHR, MEd, NCC, PCC, is an Ohio licensed clinical counselor and president elect for the Ohio Play Therapy Association. He has master's degrees in human relations and education and has been working clinically with children since 1991. Over the past several years, Enfield has been a child therapist at Catholic Social Services, where he has also done group work with preadolescent and adolescent boys using tabletop and role-playing games to help develop problem-solving and predicting outcomes in social situations. Enfield grew up fascinated with heroes of all types, specifically Daredevil, the Mighty Thor, Hercules, Jason and the Argonauts, and Flash Gordon. Struggling early on to fit in socially and academically, he began to explore the world of the heroes, where he found both success and comfort. His growing fascination with heroes led him to miniatures, through which he formed connections with others. Enfield also struggled with learning difficulties and believes that his early experiences with these heroes gave him the skills and confidence to complete his education. It is his hope to use these experiences to help others to overcome their challenges.

Roger Kaufman, LMFT, is a licensed psychotherapist with a private practice in Hollywood, California, specializing in work with gay men and lesbians. He is also an instructor at the Institute for Contemporary Uranian Psychoanalysis, where he teaches classes on gay-affirmative psychotherapy and integrating Freudian psychoanalysis, as well as on object relations and Jungian psychology. He received his master's in clinical psychology from Antioch University and his bachelor's in history from Brown University. His personal fascination with symbolic depictions of the gay psyche in science fiction and fantasy films has lead to essays published in the *Los Angeles Times, White Crane Journal, Gay and Lesbian Review Worldwide,* and in the anthology, *Finding the Force of the Star Wars Franchise: Fans, Merchandise, and Critics.*

John Shelton Lawrence, PhD, showed early behavioral disorders stemming from encounters with fantasy superheroes. He had a kicking tantrum when the news of Franklin Roosevelt's death interrupted the Lone Ranger's radio show. As a second grader, he donned a home-made cape and broke a neighbor's telephone line while leaping from a shed. His understanding of superpowers matured, however, when he read *Mad Magazine*'s "Superduperman" in the early 1950s. That teenage skepticism grew into a philosophical teaching career, resulting in his current position as professor of philosophy, emeritus, at Morningside College in Iowa. With Robert Jewett, he developed the suspicion that America's righteous stance in the world often projects the story of the selfless crusader who can cleanly uses superpowers to rescue the innocent. They jointly authored *The American Monomyth* (1977, 1988), *The Myth of the American Superhero* (2002, winner of the John Cawelti Award for the Best Book on American Culture), and *Captain America and the Crusade Against Evil* (2003). He wrote "The 100 Million$ Men" on presidential action heroes and prepared a presidential filmography for *Hollywood's White House* (2003). For *Hollywood's West* (2005), he wrote "The Lone Ranger and the Adult Legacy of the Juvenile Western." He has teamed with Matthew W. Kapell to edit *Finding the Force of the Star Wars Franchise: Fans, Merchandise, and Critics* (2006). He lives in Berkeley, California.

Harry Livesay, LCSW, is a licensed clinical social worker in Rosenberg, Texas. He currently works for the Memorial Hermann Lamar School-Based Health Centers, where he provides individual and family counseling services to noninsured and underserved students of the Lamar Consolidated Independent School District. A clinical social worker and therapist since 1997, he developed an interest in therapeutic play with superheroes in the "Silver Age" of the 1960s as a first grader who was labeled as having severe learning difficulties and assigned to a low-level reading group. With the help of a worried, supportive, and innovative parent, Harry was introduced to the universe of comic books—a place of colorful covers showing powerful and confident women and men who live in a world of exciting adventures, vexing villains, and an infinite universe of new words and ideas. In his work as a therapist for a school-based clinic, Harry continues to share the benefits of superhero play with his clients by providing them a place to discover their own special powers and abilities and the opportunity to gain the same power and confidence through their interest in and enjoyment of superheroes.

William McNulty, LCSW-C, RPT-S, is a licensed clinical social worker and Registered Play Therapist Supervisor. He works in Rockville, Maryland, at the Reginald S. Lourie Center for Infants and Young Children as a therapist in the outpatient clinic and Therapeutic Nursery Programs. Superheroes have always been an important part of his life, first as a young child taking on the characteristics of superheroes while playing dress-up with friends and now professionally facilitating the play of clients who use superheroes in healing ways.

Cory A. Nelson, LPC, QMHP, is a licensed professional counselor in the state of South Dakota. He is currently working with adult males at the Mike Durfee State Prison in Springfield and doing contract work with children and adolescents for Lewis and Clark Behavioral Health in Yankton. Nelson got his first superhero action figures at age 3 and has been collecting comic books for more than 20 years. He first became interested in integrating comic books into therapy by using them as bibliotherapy with victims of abuse and neglect. As he continued to work with children, Nelson developed "What Would Superman Do?" as a way to help clients identify and incorporate superheroic traits into their own personalities and lives.

Jeffrey Pickens, PhD, is an associate professor of psychology in the Department of Social Sciences and Counseling at St. Thomas University in Miami, Florida. He received his BA and MA from the University of Florida, his PhD in Developmental Psychology from Florida International University, and his postdoctoral training at the University of Miami, School of Medicine, Mailman Center for Child Development. He received postgraduate training in attachment theory and evaluation as well as play therapy. Jeff is a lifelong Trekkie. He wishes to thank his wife, Frances, for her interest, support, and assistance in writing his chapter.

Robert Poole, BA, is the unit coordinator of Program 1, "The Field of Dreams," at the Onarga Academy in Illinois for 14 years where he started as a Case Manager. Robert holds a bachelor's degree in psychology from Eureka College, alma mater of President Ronald Reagan. Growing up in a small town, Robert cultivated an active imagination, as most young boys do, by playing army with neighbor kids and wanting to be a firefighter. Robert sees his superheroes as those who defend freedom, protect and help their neighbors in need, and instill healthy morals and values. His father is a former soldier and retired volunteer firefighter, his mother is the all-American stay-at-home mom, his sister is a nurse, and his wife works with Alzheimer's patients. Robert, too, is a volunteer firefighter. His superhero interests are of the human kind, and he strives to teach clients the value of real-life superheroes and role models.

Robert J. Porter, PhD, was involved in academic and clinical work at the University of New Orleans and the Louisiana State University Medical School for more than 25 years before moving to Tampa to pursue clinical interests in 1997. His clinical and research work has included speech and language, medical psychology, the relationship between psychological disorders, trauma, stress, and the body's physiology, and child and adolescent psychology. He was a principle architect of the Applied Biopsychology and Applied Developmental PhD programs at the University of New Orleans where he taught a wide variety of graduate and undergraduate courses. He currently teaches, on an occasional basis, at the University of Tampa and at Argosy University. Porter is internationally recognized for his work in psychology and brain function, biopsychology, and nonlinear chaos systems theory. "Dr. Bob," as his younger patients call him, has a private practice in Tampa where his primary responsibility is working with patients of all ages at Patients First Family Medicine. His interest in superheroes dates to his early childhood in rural New Hampshire where he would tie a towel around his neck and wonder whether he could fly off the barn roof. He says he still wonders.

Karen Robertie, MS, LCPC, is the clinical supervisor of Program 1, "The Field of Dreams," at Onarga Academy in Illinois. She has been employed by Nexus-Onarga Academy for more than 8 years. A licensed clinical therapist, she has almost 20 years experience working with survivors of trauma. She is currently working on her play therapy certification. When that is complete, she plans to begin working on her art therapy certification. Although her knowledge of superheroes is limited to her childhood desire to fly like Superman, and an adolescent crush on Robin, the Boy Wonder, Robertie later grew up to realize the power of creativity. Like her alter ego, "Create," she not only enjoys being creative, but she also enjoys assisting others in realizing their own creativity and expanding their horizons. Under her tutelage as clinical supervisor, the Field of Dreams has implemented and expanded the expressive arts treatment modality. Robertie is just a kid herself and is fond of saying, "Treatment can be fun!" and "Anything can be a treatment lesson!" She is thrilled to have found a profession that allows her to merge all of her favorite things.

Jennifer Mendoza Sayers, PhD, trained in behavioral psychology at the University of California—Los Angeles, in humanistic psychology at Saybrook Institute, and in neuropsychology at Fielding Institute. She has taught psychology courses at the University of Texas and Barry University in North Miami, Florida. She has published two home studies and other evaluation instruments. Sayers has served as president of the Broward County Psychological Association and is currently in private practice specializing in clinical neuropsychology with children and adults. Her interest in using superheroes in therapy stemmed from her sons' interests in comic books. Debating the premise that comic characters are literature, helped germinate the idea that these characters have depth applicable to therapy. She currently lives in Ellenton, Florida, with her family.

Patty Scanlon, LCSW, BCD, RPT-S, is in clinical practice in Indianapolis, Indiana. In 2003, she opened PlayJourneys, Inc., a private practice specializing in the use of play and sandplay therapy with children, adolescents, adults, and families. She specializes in the treatment of trauma and abuse, divorce, and autism spectrum disorders. Scanlon served on the board of the Indiana Association for Play Therapy from 1997 to 2001 and as InAPT President 1999–2000. Since then, she has been involved as chair of various committees of the Association for Play Therapy. She enjoys gardening and playing with her four dogs, Shiva, Erin, Kali, and Plato. As a young girl, she first attempted superhero flight off the side of the bathtub, using the shower curtain as a cape. She believes the curtain was too flimsy to fly. Her favorite superhero is the Cowardly Lion in the *Wizard of Oz*.

Ryan Weidenbenner, MS, LCPC, is the senior sexuality therapist working with children with sexual behavior problems at the Onarga Academy in Illinois; he has worked there for the past 9 years. He holds two master's degrees from Illinois State University, one in psychology and one in counseling, or as he likes to refer to them, theory and practice. He is also a graduate of Wabash College, one of the nation's few remaining all-male liberal arts colleges where he majored in psychology and English while minoring in speech and theater. These creative influences are readily apparent in his therapeutic work with the Onarga clients. A lifelong fan of comic books, role-playing games, and horror and science fiction film as well as other traditional adolescent interests, Weidenbenner has been instrumental in developing creative therapeutic interventions for a program milieu, which has become represented more and more by clients with significant deficits within their cognitive, emotional, and social development.

Carmela Wenger, LMFT, RPT-S, is a licensed marriage, family, and child therapist; a Registered Play Therapist Supervisor, and a California Association of Marriage and Family Approved Supervisor, who is currently in private practice. She has pursued a career-long interest in traumatized clients who are attachment challenged through her work with Children's Home Society, the Humboldt Family Service Center (HFSC), and the Headstart and TAPPEN programs in California. It was during her tenure at HFSC that she authored "The Suitcase Story: A Technique for Children in Out of Home Placement" published in the *American Journal of Orthopsychiatry.* Wenger authors the "Ask the Experts" column for the California Association of Play Therapy newsletter, teaches seminars in play therapy and attachment-based treatment of adults, and provides clinical consultation for Youth Services Bureau Shelter and Launch Pad. Through her work, she has come to appreciate that the most resilient children are those who identify with the rescuer rather than the victim role, and as a result, she has developed an appreciation for the diagnostic utility and healing powers of superheroes in therapeutic work.

Foreword

Finding Ourselves in Our Superheroes[1]

What is the social meaning of these supermen, superwomen, super-lovers, super-boys, supergirls, super-ducks, super-mice, super-magicians, super-safecrackers? How did Nietzsche get into the nursery?
—Dr. Fredric Wertham, *Seduction of the Innocent* (1954, p. 15)

In my early years ... at Bellevue Hospital when we were hard put to find techniques for exploring the child's emotional life, his mind, his ways of reacting, when the child was separated from the home and brought to us,... I found the comics early on one of the most valuable means of carrying on such examinations.
—Dr. Lauretta Bender, psychiatrist, and editorial board adviser to Superman comics (U.S. Senate, 1954, p. 152)

These contrary assertions by Drs. Bender and Wertham recall a time when superheroes had become public policy issues. Crime-themed comic books—even some featuring the perpetually beloved Batman, Superman, and Wonder Woman—were a national concern. J. Edgar Hoover for the FBI, the American Medical Association, the General Federation of Women's Clubs, the National Council of Juvenile Court Judges, the Catholic Legion of Decency, and the New York State legislature had all investigated comic books and at least partially condemned them (Beaty, 2005, p. 127; Nyberg, 1998, pp. 44–45). Cincinnati's Committee on the

---

[1] The author acknowledges valuable suggestions from Eric D. Lawrence, William Doty, Matthew Wilhelm Kapell, Roger Kaufmann, Carter Kelly, Marty Knepper, and Bernard Wittenberg.

Evaluation of Comic Books had reviewed 418 titles, finding the Lone Ranger, the Marvel Family, and Superman "objectionable" and Wonder Woman "very objectionable" (U.S. Senate, 1954, pp. 40–43).

Reflecting the grassroots fervor of the 1940s and 1950s, the *New York Times* reported comic book roundups and burnings instigated by the Catholic Legion of Decency and other groups (Catholic Students, p. 18; "Norwich Drive on Comic Books," p. 70). Public passions eventually took a national policy focus during 3 days of the 1954 Kefauver hearings on comic books and juvenile delinquency, a venue where psychiatrists delivered expert testimony for U.S. senators (Kihss, p. 29). Both Lauretta Bender and Fredric Wertham testified, disagreeing about every issue they were asked to address.

The engagement of clinical professions with the evolutionary content of children's consciousness then fit a pattern that has become far more recognizable now. Pulp novels, films, jazz, rock music, and girlie magazines had stimulated public anxieties before the 1950s; later cultural phenomena such as television, video games, rap music, electronic chat rooms, Internet surfing, and text messaging became new flashpoints for adult fear (Cohen, 1997). The great youth-focused cultural questions of the early 1950s were these: Are we, their elders, selling our next generation mind-poisoning fantasies? Are we granting access to technologies that will in turn endanger us—or even civilization itself? Psychiatrists, please tell us before it is too late!! At that time, the counseling professions lacked a unified, reassuring prescription, just as they do now.

Wertham shouted a resounding "yes" in response to these distressed questions, and for him responsible citizenship demanded an eradication of the superhero genre and, indeed, of all comic books from the lives of children. Because he did not believe in censorship for adults, he was willing to settle for age restrictions pegged at 15 years to keep the broadly defined "crime comics" from the hands of children.

Far more quietly and pragmatically, Bender said, "No, not at all" in response to questions about the alleged harms. She believed that therapy could not ignore what had increasingly become a part of the child's experience. With fellow child psychiatrist, Dr. Reginald S. Lourie, she had presciently remarked in 1941, "Anyone in contact with children of school age, and particularly those working closely with children, sooner or later becomes conscious of the extent to which the constant reading of comic books has invaded their daily activities, and play" (p. 541). Bender had accepted that "invasion" as a tool of therapy.

The conflict between Wertham and Bender, two of the best known practitioners and children's advocates of their period, is instructive in helping us frame the contributions of this fine book, one that advances the art of understanding the symptomatic expression of conflicts expressed by superhero fantasies. As Lawrence Rubin's introductory chapter makes clear, the contributors lean toward Bender as they chart a path for exploring the child consciousness of today.

FREDRIC WERTHAM AND LAURETTA BENDER

In the 1954 Kefauver hearings, Drs. Fredric Wertham and Lauretta Bender were the star psychiatric witnesses. Thinking superficially, one might have thought that they would agree about comic books and superheroes. After all, their careers show so many striking parallels, with a common mentor (Adolph Meyer) and appointments at identical facilities (Phipps Psychiatric Clinic at the Johns Hopkins University, Bellevue Hospital, and the medical faculty of New York University). They both committed themselves to children's psychiatry in New York City and the problems of juvenile delinquency.

Addressing children's superhero fantasies, Bender published her first professional article on children in 1941 and elaborated her understanding several times thereafter in journals and books. In addition to having scientific stature among her peers, she, like Wertham, had a flair for making her work known to public media. In the period between 1935 and 1988, the *New York Times* printed dozens of articles about her discoveries and innovative treatment methods. Just one example was her partnership with artist Bernard Sanders: they collaborated in teaching Bellevue children to express their emotions through drawing (Shultz, 1937, p. N6).[2]

Wertham, who also based his views about superheroes on encounters with clinical populations in New York City, began to publish his first articles on the subject in 1948, typically bypassing professional journals. Because of his level of personal anger, he preferred the role of "social psychiatrist" and directed his appeals directly to the public in popular periodicals such as *Saturday Review of Literature, Reader's Digest,* and *Ladies Home Journal.*[3] He sharply disagreed with Bender, often quoting her or like-minded colleagues in his writings without identifying the specific sources. He simply called her or anyone of similar opinion "an expert" or "one of the experts." This was quite unlike his practice of citing persons by name if they agreed with him. Aware that his deviation from the scientific style of attribution would be puzzling, Wertham created an elaborate explanation in his *Seduction of the Innocent,* a book published

---

[2] She was apparently a genial collaborator, her bibliography, by 1954, listed 11 coauthors for pieces on childhood symptom diagnosis and treatment (see Bender, 1954, pp. 261–262).

[3] See Beaty (2005, pp. 218–222) for a complete listing of Wertham's articles.

without source listings or footnotes. His words betray a conspiratorial mind-set in approaching anyone who disagreed with his interpretation of the superhero phenomenon.

> From magazines, newspapers and the radio, and from the endorsements on so many comic books, one may get the wrong impression that there are many scientific experts defending comic books. Actually the brunt of the defense is borne by a mere handful of experts. Their names occur over and over again. They are connected with well-known institutions, such as universities, hospitals, child-study associations or clinics. That carries enormous weight with professional people and, of course, even more so with casual lay readers and parents all over the country.
> In their actual effect the experts for the defense represent a team. This, of course, does not mean that they work as a team. They work individually. But their way of reasoning, their apologetic attitude for the industry and its products, their conclusions—and even their way of stating them— are much alike. So it is possible to do full justice to them by discussing them as a team rather than individually. There is little danger of quoting them out of context, for what they have to say is so cut and dried that one quotation from the writing of one expert fits just as well into that of another. (pp. 220–221)

But why was the conspiracy of this "mere handful of experts" opposing his views so pernicious? This takes us to the heart of Wertham's view of the superhero.

In his book *The Seduction of the Innocent* and in his other popular writings of the period, *everything* associated with superheroes was maligned, including the ads for bodybuilding, breast enhancers, BB guns, and knives. Wertham conceded no merit whatsoever to the comic book. "Comic books have nothing to do with drama, with art or literature" (p. 241); they are merely "temptation, corruption, and demoralization" (p. 55). Because he believed that comics were calculatingly designed to "seduce the innocent," he saw no evidence "that comic books come from the 'unconscious'" (p. 244); thus, they lacked any expressive value in the lives of children, as Bender and Lourie had contended (p. 46). Notwithstanding his reactionary laments, Wertham was a precursor to feminists who deplored the victim status of women in entertainment media and the persistent linkage of violence and eroticism (p. 32), yet he intensely disliked seeing women in comic books "placed on an equal footing with men" (p. 234) as Bender and Lourie had approvingly noted (p. 549). And like civil rights advocates who later deplored the racial and ethnic stereotypes pervading popular culture, he believed that the comics promoted "race hatred" because they presented a world of athletically heroic White men pitted against "inferior people: natives, primitives, savages, 'ape men,'

Negroes, Jews, Indians, Italians, Slavs, Chinese and Japanese" (p. 101). Adopting the language of Cold War patriotism to characterize comic book creators as reinforcers of America's racism, he told a legislative committee in New York that "the crime comic book industry is one of the most subversive groups in the country today ("Psychiatrist Asks," 1950, p. 50).

But it is the paradigmatic Superman that Wertham repeatedly denounced and used to define the subversive evil within U.S. culture: America's children "have been nourished (or rather poisoned) by the endless repetition of Superman stories." The toxicity stems from the fact that Superman is essentially "fascist" because he embodies "the Nietzsche-Nazi myth of the exceptional man who is beyond good and evil" (p. 97).

Here one can surely sympathize with Bender's complaint to the Kefauver committee about Wertham's ignorance. Not only was he culturally tone deaf to the portrayals of Superman's strength—labeling him, for example, as "a symbol of violent race superiority" (p. 381). Wertham was equally obtuse in his application of Nietzsche's Übermensch, accepting the Nazis' deceptive equation of Übermensch with the so-called master race. However, Nietzsche's icy ideal of self-transcendence is hardly a good marker because Superman so clearly stands within the pantheon of his own era's American superheroes. He acts as does the radio's Lone Ranger, selflessly restrained and precisely calibrating his often gentle strength, which he uses to bring evildoers to the doorways of the sheriff or police. And, above all, in his Clark Kent persona, Superman is depicted as lonely and insecure, as a teenage nerd who timidly craves his first date. It was because of his essentially Boy Scout demeanor and his iconic status as champion of "truth, justice, and the American way" that Superman could be used in World War II Bond drives. Wertham surely knew but did not acknowledge that Superman, Batman, and others had used their covers to promote the sale of war bonds during World War II ("War Bonds"). And speaking to the fascist themes in the superheroes, how could Wertham, a Jew, have failed to consider that comic artists such as Jacob Kurtzburg (aka Jack Kirby) had created a Captain America who presciently slugged Hitler's chin on the cover of *Captain America* in March 1941—before the United States had entered the war in Europe? And that Kirby had served as a combat infantryman of Patton's Third Army in France?

It is through such clear cultural identifications with America's causes and values that children are encouraged to feel a sense of social solidarity when they experience the superhero fantasy. Such identification explains why so many adults feel comfortable in allowing their children to consume fantasies that Wertham treated as merely fascist atrocities. The fantasies of selfless, perfectly calibrated power may become malignant when translated into stances for domestic crime or foreign policy challenges. But the notion of benevolent, overwhelming force is certainly less a contamination than it is a continuation of the "redeemer nation" ideal.[4]

One way of measuring Wertham's ignorance of American mythology is to remind ourselves about the lives of some of the comics creators. In his *Men of Tomorrow* book dealing with the birth of the superheroes in the Golden Age of comics, Gerard Jones (2004) described several principals of the industry who had fought fascism in Europe and given to Jewish philanthropies. They, of all people, felt betrayed and wounded by Dr. Wertham (p. 274). The grievance is still felt in the comics community today, which often displays the kind of visceral contempt for him that he expressed toward superheroes, comic books, and their creators.

Anyone who reads Wertham's anecdotes about his clinical sessions with comics-addicted children may get the sense that he is looking past their experience to locate the evil that he must destroy through social reform. He did in fact conceive of himself foremost as a "social psychiatrist," who refused to locate pathological causes in patients themselves (Beaty, 2005, pp. 18–47). He saw himself as having clean hands because neither he nor his associates in fighting comics "got any money, ever" (Wertham, p. 82). It must have been difficult for him to contain his rage against producers in those clinical sessions where children confessed their corruption by comics and the ways in which their crimes merely copied the scripts they had learned (Wertham, p. 275).

BENDER AND THE SUPERHERO

By contrast, Lauretta Bender presented herself in the Kefauver hearings as a paragon of therapeutic calmness. Rather than making one unitary judgment about the value and effect of superhero comics, she saw highly variable realities for different children. She volunteered that "the less intelligent children and those who have ... less reading capacity collect the most comics" (U.S. Senate, 1954, p. 152). On the issue of destructive imitations of behavior, she testified that a few children might be provoked to acts of delinquency as a result of encountering fantasies (p. 159). She also related that children in her ward at Bellevue had made Superman capes for themselves in occupational therapy—followed by an epidemic of "bumps" as children wore them and leaped from radiators or bookcases. It was this clinical experience that led her to advise National Comics Publications *not* to market uniforms for children (U.S. Senate, 1954, pp. 157–158). As for children's worried reactions to fantasy in

---

[4] See Jewett and Lawrence, *Captain America and the Crusade Against Evil* (2003, pp. 55–78).

popular culture more generally, she reported that the Frankenstein monster films and Disney's "disturbing mother figures" proved far more troublesome. "The mothers were always killed or sent to the insane asylums in Walt Disney's movies" (p. 153). Because children identified with the characters who lost their mothers, the consequence could be nightmarish fears.

Bender believed that negative effects in superhero materials could sometimes be moderated by appropriate adult decisions, and, even if not, were outweighed, in her estimation, by the benefits of superhero fantasies. She felt that many children could resonate with "the concept of the body image and what can happen to it under different emotional circumstances," directing admiration to "the uncanny capacity for the script writers to delve down into their own unconscious and dig up these problems and depict them" (U.S. Senate, 1954, p. 160). She believed that the materials fulfilled many "psychological needs of the child," dealing experimentally as they did with "problems of the relationship of the self to physical and social reality," offering "continuity by a central character who ... invites identification," and fantasies of conflict "with good ultimately triumphing over evil" (Bender, 1944, p. 226). In identifying with figures such as Clark Kent/Superman, the child's ego could expand, becoming "strong, brave, good" (p. 230). In the "girl characters," Bender saw an engagement "with the problem of passivity-activity, femininity-masculinity, or aggression and submission, and have dealt with these in as modern a way as the latest psychoanalytic studies." Although she did not find Wonder Woman's all-purpose lariat convincing as a symbol of power, she thought her "a good try at solving the very timely problems of the girl's concept of herself as a woman and her relationship to the world" (pp. 230–231).

Apart from questions about superhero representations and their effects, she found access to the superhero contents in children's minds a valuable part of therapeutic practice. In her article with Reginald Lourie (1941), she presented four clinical cases with children aged 10, 11, and 12 who constructively played with superhero themes in dealing with issues of personal boundaries, wavering superegos, and the transcendence of personal fears. One case involving a girl named Helen, age 11, is a concession that a comic book plot—amid many other stress factors, including grand mal seizures and her first menstrual period—precipitated a "state of great agitation" (pp. 543–544). In that case, the comic book plot helped the therapist understand the circumstances of family life that had produced such severe pressure for the child. In these cases, one gets a sense of a flexible, caring intelligence that recognizes the role of superhero themes and seizes them as opportunities to understand, and to perhaps help, in healing.

WHERE AMERICAN CULTURE WENT THEREAFTER

Every observer knows that Dr. Wertham lost his battle against the superheroes. He understood neither his adopted culture nor his own limitations in trying to change it. Although he did succeed in shaming the "true-crime" horror comics out of business, the superheroes that he loathed thrived and survived. The Congress that invited Wertham's expert opinion took no legislative action, ultimately leaning in Dr. Bender's direction when its posthearings Interim Report of 1955 stated, under its summary heading "Excessive reading of crime and horror comics is considered symptomatic of emotional pathology," reached this psychiatric conclusion: "it appears to be the consensus of the experts that comic-book reading is not the cause of emotional maladjustment in children" (Senate Report, 1955, p. 16). Rather than legislating, Congress relied instead on the industry's self-regulating Comics Code Authority, an outcome that Wertham called a betrayal of American families by Senator Kefauver (Beaty, pp. 163–64).

The superheroes themselves, like other market commodities, have had since that period their ups and downs and perpetually reinvent themselves to renew their appeal. But in recent decades they have become a dominant presence in American entertainment. Blockbuster films such as the Christopher Reeve Superman series, the *Spider-Man, The Hulk, Star Wars,* and *The Fantastic Four,* as well as television series such as *Buffy the Vampire Slayer* and *Xena: Warrior Princess,* all play on the big screen or on television and then are replayed in personal DVD players that are now common in children's bedrooms. And in ways that Wertham could not imagine at the time, the superheroes evolved culturally, psychologically, and politically. Superheroes of assorted ethnicities entered a landscape that had been dominated by Caucasian men. DC, Marvel Comics, and smaller companies have developed an assortment of black superheroes.[5] The young Powerpuff Girls "save the world before bedtime."[6] Darth Vader, one of the most widely known figures in history, is a morally dual figure who wavers between impulses to dominate or destroy and his willingness to be loved. The Hulk character, especially in Ang Lee's film rendition of 2003, depicts the tragic consequence of great physical power in someone who becomes emotionally and socially isolated. With the introduction of Spider-Man in 1962, the superhero became more introspective

---

[5] Like so many other superhero phenomena, they are well displayed on the Internet in the Museum of Black Superheroes: http:\\www.blacksuperhero.com.

[6] "Saving the world before bedtime" was the tagline for the 2002 movie, *The Powerpuff Girls.* There is also a board game produced by Milton Bradley called *Saving the World Before Bedtime.*

and neurotically beset by normal problems—poverty, unemployment, and a sense of guilt about his uncle's death among these issues.

These figures, and their ever-proliferating companions, who represent so many different ethnicities and statuses in our society, are surely subtle enough in their escapades to engage the minds and emotions of children. The larger cultural questions about whether our culture needs so many savior figures and how their symbolic values collide with or augment democracy are worth debating. But for the therapeutic, I vote with Dr. Bender, as do the contributors to this volume. Because superheroes are on our mind, let's talk about them and see where the discussion takes us. There is also something democratic about a therapy that can respond empathically to the experiences that patients enjoy and feel that they understand emotionally. Healthful insights may lie on the horizon.

John Shelton Lawrence
Morningside College, Emeritus

REFERENCES

Beaty, B. (2005). *Fredric Wertham and the critique of mass culture*. Jackson: University Press of Mississippi.

Bender, L. (1944). The psychology of children's reading and the comics. *Journal of Educational Sociology, 18*, 223–231.

Bender, L. (1954). *A dynamic psychopathology of childhood*. Springfield, IL: Charles C. Thomas.

Bender, L., & Lourie, R. (1941). The effect of comic books on the ideology of children. *American Journal of Orthopsychiatry, 11*, 540–550.

Catholic students burn up comic books. (1948, December 18). *New York Times*, 18.

Cohen, R. (1997). The delinquents: Censorship and youth culture in recent U.S. history. *History of Education Quarterly, 37*, 251–270.

Jewett, R., & Lawrence, J. S. (2003). *Captain America and the crusade against evil: The dilemma of zealous nationalism*. Grand Rapids, MI: Eerdmans

Jones, G. (2004). *Men of tomorrow: Geeks, gangsters, and the birth of the comic book*. New York: Basic Books.

Kihss, P. (1954, April 23). Senator charges "deceit" on comics. *New York Times*, 29.

Norwich drive on comic books a success as children rush to trade 10 for a classic. (1955, February 27). *New York Times*, 70.

Nyberg, A. K. (1998). *Seal of approval: The history of the comics code*. Jackson: University Press of Mississippi.

Psychiatrist asks crime comics ban. (1950, December 14). *New York Times*, 50.

Shultz, G. (1937, May 2). Drawings aid in curing children. *New York Times*, N6.

U.S. Senate. (1954). *Juvenile delinquency (comic books). U.S. Congressional Senate hearings before the Subcommittee to Investigate Juvenile Delinquency. Committee on the Judiciary, United States Senate, Eighty-third Congress, Second session pursuant to Senate Resolution 190. Investigations of Juvenile Delinquency in the United States. April 21, 22, and June 4, 1954.* Washington, DC: U.S. Government Printing Office.

U.S. Senate. (1955). Committee on the Judiciary. Report No. 62. Comic Books and Juvenile Delinquency. Interim Report of the Committee on the Judiciary pursuant to S. Res. 89 and S. Res. 190.

War bonds (83d Cong. 1st Sess.; 83d Cong. 2d Sess.). (2000). In T. Pendergast & S. Pendergast (Eds.), *St. James Encyclopedia of Popular Culture* (Vol. 5). Detroit, MI: St. James Press.

Wertham, F. (1954). *Seduction of the innocent.* New York: Rinehart.

Preface

Like scores of children, I spent countless hours following the exploits of a legion of colorful superheroes. Each had powers and abilities far beyond those of anyone I knew. Many nights, while concealed beneath my blankets, flashlight in one hand and comic book in the other, I was mesmerized and wondered silently and privately. What would it be like to have X-ray vision, to retreat to a secret cave in my own basement, to ensnare villains in a powerful web of my own making, to fly? And if somehow I did manage to obtain such powers, how ever would I conceal them from parents, teachers, and friends while confronting the daily rigors of childhood—all in a single bound?

Although I was to travel the long and treacherous road to adulthood, science fiction, fantasy, and outer space, with all of its strange inhabitants, was always a friendly rest stop for me. I journeyed with James Kirk and the crew of the U.S.S. *Enterprise,* eagerly anticipated each installment of the Star Wars saga, and ravenously consumed every new superhero television show and movie. Now that I am grown with children, I can relive my passion for all of it.

I am reminded of an old *MAD Magazine* cartoon strip that chronicled a boy's academic journey. Inspired by an encounter with his grandfather's pigs whose nasty smell and beady eyes upset him, it began with a second grade "What I did on my summer vacation" report. Although his spelling and grammar improved over the years, the boy's fascination with that early childhood experience lead him to revisit the topic in evolving venues from a high school term paper tie-in to a *Tale of Two Cities,* to a college introduction to psychology analysis of the long-term effects of childhood trauma (being stared at by smelly pigs). The crowning jewel in his academic crown was a PhD dissertation relating swine vision to behavioral disturbances in rural residents. You get the idea!

Was the little boy in the above scenario attempting to sublimate and thus overcome his childhood pig-related trauma through scholarly and professional pursuits? Am I somehow guilty of a similar intellectual opportunism—at the reader's expense? Perhaps, perhaps not! As an academician and clinician, I have always found ways to integrate my passion for popular culture into my work, and it seemed natural to turn my attention to superheroes. Am I, just like this little boy, trying to work through, make up for, overcome, or resolve as yet unfinished childhood business? Is this why I have become a therapist—and for that matter, and of all things, a play therapist. Perhaps, perhaps not!

Far more interesting than my career motivation is the reason behind this book. I believe, as did Joseph Campbell, in the power of myth. I believe, as did Rollo May, that cultures cry for myth. I believe that today's children need heroes, not only their parents but also heroes with powers and abilities far beyond those of mortals that stretch into the very recesses of their imaginations and the worlds of possibility—and impossibility. I believe that adults who value myths and legends of heroes and superheroes are the carriers of those stories. And finally, I believe in childhood!

Lawrence C. Rubin

Acknowledgments

This book is dedicated to my children, Zachary and Rebecca, who are beginning to sense their own powers and who bring out the superhero in me. This book is also dedicated to Randi, my wife, who has drawn me from my fortress of solitude. And finally, this book is dedicated to my parents, Esther and Herb, who bought me superhero comics when I was a child and had the good sense to save them for me over the years.

I thank Sheri W. Sussman of Springer Publishing Company, LLC who was willing to take a chance with this volume, one very different from those she has previously edited. I also thank John Shelton Lawrence for our fascinating muses on the subjects of superheroes and culture, as well as Sandi Frick-Helms who supported me in writing on the topic of superheroes in psychotherapy. I am, of course, indebted to the clinicians who have contributed to this volume as well as to all of the clients whose stories made it possible.

USING SUPERHEROES IN COUNSELING AND PLAY THERAPY

Traditional Superheroes in Counseling and Play Therapy

Introduction: Look, Up in the Sky! An Introduction to the Use of Superheroes in Psychotherapy

Lawrence C. Rubin

In the safety of the playroom, a 5-year-old carefully divides superheroes by color into the forces of good and evil, their impending clash once again dramatizing the tension and confusion left in the wake of her parent's divorce.

An 8-year-old expresses powerful and aggressive fantasies in the form of an all-powerful "psycho-monster," whose efforts to destroy the universe are vanquished by a legion of benevolent and nurturing superheroines.

A reflective 11-year-old, fascinated by the relationship between Darth Vader and Luke Skywalker, carefully composes a new episode in the Star Wars saga, attempting to rewrite the history and outcome of his own adoption.

A depressed, substance-abusing 24-year-old law student labors to add another detail to the costume of his ever-evolving, alter-ego superhero, Courageous Cal, a cross between the Incredible Hulk and the Michelin Man.

—Excerpted from author's clinical casework (2000–2005)

Of the various theories, tools, and techniques available to the therapist, one of the most powerful resources for self-understanding, growth, and healing may well be fantasy. It is the metaphoric place where problems of the past and present meet the possibilities of the future, in conflicts both minor and epic. It is the place in which children and adults escape from but also make sense of their worlds by creating and then living their stories—their own personal mythologies. As is often the case with the world around them, this inner place is typically populated by villains who hurt and heroes who help. Most special among the latter is the superhero—the unique, larger-than-life figure who by virtue of gift, accident, calling, or legacy possesses powers and abilities far beyond those of mortals. With the advent of mass media and technology in the early 20th century, superheroes have become a mainstay in popular and American culture. Given their endurance, ubiquity, popularity, and appeal, it is not surprising that superheroes have found their way into the fantasies and metaphoric stories of children, adolescents, and adults as well as the therapist's office. This book is written for those interested in how these superhero fantasies inhabit the minds of our clients, both the young and the youthful, and the accommodations that therapists need to make in recognizing and incorporating them into their clinical work with a broad range of clients.

IMAGINATION, FANTASY, AND FANTASY PLAY

With the exception of fantasies that isolate rather than aid socialization, impair rather than strengthen reality functioning, or arrest rather than enhance development, fantasy and imaginal activities have long been regarded as windows into and contributing forces in cognitive, social, and emotional growth.

From a cognitive perspective, fantasy play, with its reliance on internal representation and symbolism, has been linked to the growing child's ability to assimilate experience and in so doing to develop a sense of understanding and mastery (Piaget, 1962). For Piaget symbolic play "provides the child with the live, dynamic, individual language indispensable for the expression of his subjective feelings for which collective language alone is inadequate" (p. 167). Along similar lines, Erikson (1963) suggested that fantasy allows the child, freed from the constraints of reality, to alter and experiment with otherwise unalterable constructs such as bodily limits, gravity time, causality, and even identity. In keeping with Piaget's and Erikson's cognitive–developmental views, Sawyer and Horm-Wingerd (1993) suggested that whereas object-dependent (sensorimotor) play allows children to explore the properties of their physical world, object-independent (symbolic–representational) play, allows for social interaction and problem solving.

Vygotsky (1978) regarded fantasy play as a window into children's burgeoning understanding of their current reality, the limitations of their abilities within that reality, and as a stage on which they can experiment with competencies and understandings beyond the constraints of their intellect and experience. For Vygotsky, although imagination, fantasy, and symbolic play liberate a child from the constraints of objects, experience, and the immediate perceptual field, they also create a "zone of proximal development" in which a "child always behaves beyond his average age, above his daily behavior . . . as though he were a head taller than himself" (p. 102). In the context of superhero fantasy play, which is addressed in detail later, Vygotsky would likely argue that the child was exploring complex and as yet incomprehensible roles, rules, and concepts such as strength, power, justice, and morality.

Exploring the similarities between fairy tales and fantasy, Bettleheim (1975) noted that "fantasy fills a huge gap in a child's understanding which [is] due to immaturity of his thinking and lack of pertinent information" (p. 61). Bruner (1986) went one step further than these other cognitivists by studying the relations among imaginary play, language, and social development. For him, play was intimately connected to (social) problem solving, with the added distinction of being enjoyable, particularly when a partner or caring observer was present. He noted,

> thought and imagination begin in the form of dialogue with a partner . . . the development of thought may be in large measure determined by the opportunity for dialogue, with the dialogue becoming internal and capable of running off inside one's head on its own. (p. 82)

Fantasy and imaginal activity are as profound in their adaptive impact in the social and emotional domains as they are on intellectual development. After observing a toddler engage in the creative enactment of the separation experience, Sigmund Freud (1920/1955) noted that "in their play, children repeat everything that has made a great impression on them in real life, and that in doing so, they abstract the strength of the impression and make themselves a master of the situation" (p. 17). Later, his daughter Anna Freud (1965, 1966) suggested that fantasy play could be considered both a means of working through intrapsychic (sexual and aggressive) conflicts and a form of regression in the service of psychic development. For her, fantasy play was also a tool, no less important than dream interpretation and free association for understanding how the child made sense of parents and family. Fantasies and fantasy play are, in a sense, externalized, action-based dramas that, although anchored in the present, provide the child with an opportunity to revisit past situations and problems, as well as venture into the future of possibilities (Miller, 1974). They are time machines for exploring inner and outer worlds.

Fantasy and imaginal play also provide the child with tension reduction that is often associated with conflict resolution. By structuring and restructuring social, moral, and emotional dilemmas in the imagination, children gain relief that comes with mastery, even though that mastery may be fleeting. For Landreth (2002), fantasy play is a safe and controlled way to express emotions, to assimilate novel experiences, and to distance oneself from otherwise painful events. Along similar lines, Irwin (1983) argued that children's symbolic play provides a means with which to understand better how they view themselves and others and express their worries, wishes, defenses, and worldview. In his treatise on the importance of fairy tales in child development, Bettleheim (1975) suggested that fantasy "provides a favorable solution to present predicaments because with hope for the future established, the present difficulty is no longer insufferable" (p. 125). He further noted that "while the fantasy is unreal, the good feelings it gives us about ourselves and our future are real, and these real good feelings are what we need to sustain us" (p. 126). Even violent fantasies and aggressive fantasy play have been regarded as important outlets for anxiety, a means of feeling stronger, and a way of moving children to new levels of cognitive and emotional development (Brody, 2005; Jones, 2002).

As this discussion of fantasy and imaginal play suggests, there is no one consistent function of fantasy and imagination. They serve the developing person on many levels and for many years, even beyond the point in life when fantasy is subordinated to so-called mature logic and more rational problem-solving processes. Vygotsky nicely summed up the issue by stating that "the old adage that a [preschool] child's play is imagination in action must be reversed: we can [also] say that imagination in adolescence and school children is play without action" (p. 93).

The Relationship Between Fantasy and Metaphor

Taking Vygotsky's notion on the relation between play and imagination one step further and into the realm of adulthood, it can be argued that metaphor accomplishes for the adult what fantasy does for the child. A metaphor, simply described, is one thing expressed as another. This is analogous to the symbol in fantasy play. During play, the child's block becomes a train, a pet morphs into a jungle beast, and, with outstretched arms, a bicycle ride is magically transformed into a jet-propelled adventure. For the adult fighting a progressive illness, searching for identity, trapped in an unsatisfying relationship, or attempting to balance priorities, a metaphor can communicate rich insights and generate possible solutions.

In the literature, metaphor has been described as a form of symbolic language that "allows more abstract ideas (like relationships) [to be] understood in terms of more concrete experiences (like journeys)," (Wickman et al., 1999, p. 389), as a tool that allows us to "explore and expand current experience into previously unrecognized possibilities" (Lyddon et al., 2001, p. 270), and as a "small unit in the narrative mode of thinking [that] helps us discover not only what happened but also the cognitive and affective significance those events have to the person" (Sims, 2003, p. 530). Taken together, these conceptualizations suggest that, like fantasy play and imagination for children, metaphor for adults is a potential resource through which they can connect with inner processes as well as with an attentive audience; travel between past, present, and future; and express and possibly alter their self-perceptions and worldviews. Furthermore, as play has been regarded the language of childhood and toys its words (Ginott, 1961; Landreth, 2002), metaphor has been considered an important mode of communication for adults that makes use of symbols, stories, and ceremonies to facilitate new patterns of thoughts and feelings (Combs & Freedman, 1990). Suffice it to say that as a potential vehicle for communication, insight, transformation, and growth, metaphor is as limitless as a child's imagination.

THE SUPERHERO FANTASY

The superhero has captured the American imagination for nearly three-quarters of a century. A mere 3 years after the introduction of Superman, psychoanalysts Lauretta Bender and Reginald Lourie (1941) explored the appeal and constructive therapeutic applications of superheroes in clinical work with children. They argued that as a mythological and folkloric icon, the superhero had a definite place in the playroom by helping children to deal with the real dangers of the world. Their young clients used Superman-based fantasy play for a variety of purposes, including for personal protection, as a barrier against antisocial behavior, as an ego ideal and a problem solver. A few years later, Bender, who had been monitoring the impact of comics on her clients, came to appreciate the power of the symbol of the superhero to "provide a step toward the final mastery of reality" (Bender, 1954, p. 233). Over the next 75 years, children, teens, and adults followed the exploits of a veritable galaxy of superheroes through comics, radio, television, film, video games, and mass-marketed action figures. Although it is difficult to determine exactly how many superheroes have come and gone over the decades, experts in the field suggest that the number is more than likely in the thousands (Lawrence, 2005, personal communication; McDermott, 2005, personal communication). What exactly is the appeal of these do-gooders and their heroic adventures, and exactly why are they so perennially interesting to children, adolescents, and adults—and, as we shall see later, so very useful as therapeutic allies.

To answer this question, it is important to define sufficiently the concept of the modern superhero. Although several authors have provided important defining features (Fingeroth, 2002; Reynolds, 1992; Simpson, Rodiss, & Bushell, 2004), it is Lawrence and Jewett's (2002) integrated conceptualization, based on the notion that the genre is the modern-day variant of classical mythology, that is most informative. According to them,

> The [American] monomythic superhero is distinguished by disguised origins, pure motivations, a redemptive task and extraordinary powers. He originates outside of the community he is called to save, and in those exceptional instances when he resides therein, the superhero plays the role of the idealistic loner. His identity is secret, either by virtue of his unknown origins or his alter ego: his motivation is a selfless zeal for justice. By elaborate conventions of restraint, his desire for revenge is purified. Patient in the face of provocations, he seeks nothing for himself and withstands all temptations. He renounces sexual fulfillment for the duration of the mission, and the purity of his motivation ensures his moral infallibility in judging persons and situations. When he is threatened by violent adversaries, he finds answers in vigilantism, restoring justice and thus lifting the siege of paradise. In order to accomplish this mission without incurring blame or causing undue injury to others, he requires superhuman powers. The superhero's aim is unerring, his fists irresistible, and his body incapable of suffering fatal injury. (p. 47)

This scenario is quite different from the paradigm of so-called classical mythology, in which the hero, arising from a besieged society undertakes a transformative and typically perilous adventure, after which he returns to reestablish harmony to that society. Unlike the classical hero, the modern superhero never fully integrates back into society and is continually confronted with irreconcilable tensions both within him or herself or the society. Lawrence and Jewett noted that whereas the adventures of the classical hero center on initiation, those of the modern superhero focus on redemption. They continued:

> He unites a consuming love of impartial justice with a mission of personal vengeance that eliminates due process of law. He offers a form of leadership without paying the process of political relationships or responding to the preferences of the majority. In denying the ambivalence and complexity of real life, where the moral landscape offers choices in various shades of gray rather than in black and white [the superhero myth] gives Americans a fantasy land without ambiguities

to cloud moral vision, where the evil empire of enemies is readily discernible, and where they can vicariously (through identification with the superhero) smite evil before it overtakes them. (p. 48)

Lawrence and Jewett's (2002) insightful depiction of the nature and purpose of the superhero as well as his or her place in society is highly informative, both validating and expanding on Bender and Lourie's early therapeutic experience of and with the genre. As such, it quite neatly establishes a framework, or foundation for using superheroes in psychotherapy. Key aspects of the superhero motif are now discussed, and readers are asked to consider how each of these may have clinical utility in their own practices.

Origins

The traditional superhero has alien origins, as in the case of Superman's infant arrival from the doomed planet of Krypton and subsequent adoption; violent early childhood traumatization, as in the case of the murder of Batman's (Bruce Wayne's) parents; or is orphaned, as in the case of Spider-Man, who is subsequently adopted and raised by his aunt and uncle. Other superheroes, such as the X-Men, each born a mutant, are raised in a group foster home, where they learn to harness their mutant abilities, or are removed from their parents at birth to protect them, such as Luke Skywalker of the Star Wars saga. Still others, such as the underwater superheroes Aquaman and the Submariner, are born of fantastical unions—human fathers and Atlantian mothers. Finally, some superheroes lose their parents to seemingly natural disasters. Storm, one of the female X-Men, lost both of her parents in a hotel collapse, and in the spirit of Joseph Campbell's notion of the "call to adventure," sets out on a quest to understand and harness her ability to control the weather.

Regardless of origins, each of the various superheroes grows up without his or her biological parents in some variant of the traditional nuclear family. They rarely enjoy uncomplicated relationships with subsequent parent substitutes or surrogates. According to Reynolds (1992), "the [super] hero is [one way or another] marked out from society. He often reaches maturity without having a relationship with his parents" (p. 16). These unfortunate circumstances in the early lives of various superheroes are the first of many adversities they will face on the road to superheroism, laying the foundations for both their greatest failures and most glorious triumphs. Whether alone or as part of a superhero "family," they survive and ultimately rise above their early family disruptions.

Costume

As the mission of the superhero is typically driven by these early childhood experiences, so, too, is the formation of their superidentity. This identity is brought into bold relief by the super-costume—their trademark in the eyes of others—but, more important, the external signifier of their evolving internal experience of super-personhood. Whereas Superman came to Earth fully swaddled in the brightly colored material that would eventually become his costume, Peter Parker labored over the design for his Spider-Man outfit. Tony Stark wraps himself in super-strong armor in order to express his Iron Man invulnerability in the face of congenital heart disease; Batman's mysterious costume reflects the dark depths of his personal struggles, and Wonder Woman's scant yet patriotic costume, complete with lasso, is commentary on the fusing of sexuality and power. Reynolds (1992) further explicated the role of the costume by suggesting that it demarcates the superhero from ordinary people and from other superheroes and villains; symbolizes inner struggles; either accentuates or conceals sexuality; and, most relevant for therapeutic use, establishes the duality of the particular superhero.

Dual or Secret Identity

The issue of duality represented by a secret identity undergirds many of the superhero fantasies, often highlighting Jungian archetypical conflicts. The secret identity of the superhero ostensibly allows her or him to function at an everyday level—to blend into the crowd, so to speak—while also doing the difficult work of saving humanity. Who is not familiar with the image of Clark Kent dashing into the corner phone booth, emerging moments later as the Man of Steel? However, and at a much deeper level, dual identity allows the superhero to conceal and thus rise above vulnerabilities, to express her or his most primal longings and needs, and ultimately to provide a means with which to integrate otherwise irreconcilable oppositions in the superhero's (and our own) human nature. Through their dual natures, superheroes are also able to wrestle with, and at times break free from both societal and historic conflicts between good and evil, justice and power, strength and weakness, male and female, human and divine, science and faith, prosocial and antisocial, individual and collective. For Reynolds (1992), the dual nature of the superhero temporarily, albeit artificially, establishes neat boundaries or restraints around inherently gray and thus irreconcilable tensions.

By virtue of movies, action figures, and video games, and to a lesser extent comic books, most children and adults are familiar with the dual nature of blockbuster superheroes. The meek and passive Clark Kent becomes the mighty humanist Superman, the philanthropic Bruce Wayne transforms into the vigilante Dark Knight known as Batman, meek Bruce Banner explodes through his clothing when angered to become the Hulk, and Amazon-princess-turned-commoner Diana Prince becomes powerful Wonder Woman. Equally powerful in their symbolic duality, although not as popular beyond comic book audiences, are civil engineer Alan Scott, who wields a object-changing ring as the Green Lantern; Norrin Radd, who as the Silver Surfer can rearrange molecules; teenager Serena, aka Meatball Head, who along with the Sailor Scouts battles evil as Sailor Moon; and finally every-guy Donald Blake, who, with his Uru Hammer, can control the weather, fly, and travel through dimensions as Thor. Each of these characters offers endless therapeutic opportunities.

Superhero Families—Ties That Bind

The superhero genre owes as much of its popularity and appeal to the superhero family as it does to the singular sensations, that is, Superman, Wonder Woman, and the Hulk. What consumer of comic or popular culture is unfamiliar with the Fantastic Four, the X-Men, the Avengers, the Justice League, Femforce, and even the Teenage Mutant Ninja Turtles, Mighty Morphin Power Rangers, and Powerpuff Girls. If it is indeed true that there is strength in unity, the universe of possibilities opens wide when we add superabilities to the unity. Paraphrasing Aristotle's conceptualization of partnership and friendship in the context of a prototypic superhero family, the Fantastic Four, Ryall and Tipton (2005) noted that

> the superhero team [is] a vibrant family unit made up of friends who really care about each other, despite their differences and disagreements [and as family members] support each other (utility), enjoy each other (pleasure) and care about each other's good (virtue). (p. 126)

The superhero "families" unite under a variety of outlandish circumstances. The Fantastic Four (the Human Torch, the Thing, Invisible Woman, and Mr. Fantastic) accidentally acquire their superpowers following exposure to cosmic radiation, whereas the X-Men (Rogue, Storm, Mystique, Wolverine, Iceman, Phoenix, and Dr. Xavier), after experiencing an inexplicable leap in evolution, are born with latent superhuman abilities, which manifest at puberty. Members of the Justice League (Martian Manhunter, Green Lantern, Batman, Superman, Wonder Woman, Aquaman, and the Flash) and the Avengers (Thor, the Hulk, Ant Man, the Wasp, and Iron Man), each have their own unique transformation legends. The Powerpuff Girls are, in essence, test-tube babies.

Regardless of their origins, each of these "families" is united for the purpose of serving the greater good, typically by fending off villains. As discussed later, the ties that bind members of these various supergroups also impose on them struggles and conflicts readily encountered by everyday, run-of-the-mill, nonsuperheroic families. When they are not united against a world threat, they squabble, argue, and compete with and express love, anger, and jealousy toward each other. They continually struggle to balance individual and group needs and to reconcile their calling with the desire to blend back into the citizenry and escape the demands of their superheroic callings. They can be as dysfunctional as families can be, struggling with boundaries, betrayals, and threatened disintegration, and they can rise to the Aristotelian heights of utility, virtue, and pleasure—all the while saving humanity.

Superpowers and Fatal Flaws

The most defining and recognizable feature of the superhero is his or her unique gift and commitment to using it for the greater good—whether present at birth, acquired through accident, or learned through arduous training. The superhero "understands that we have our talents and powers in order to use them, and to use them for the good of others as well as ourselves is the highest use we can make of them" (Loeb & Morris, 2005, p. 15). To name just a few, these superpowers include flight, speed, invulnerability, acute sensory capacity, telepathy, invisibility, shape shifting, and genius. Conversely, each of the famous superheroes also possesses an Achilles' heel, a vulnerability that imposes a limit on them and, in certain ways, infuses humility into their otherwise godlike persona. This juxtaposition of superpower and fatal flaw is the essence of the superhero's (and our) basic conflicts, that is, between hurting and helping, connecting and isolating, self-indulgence and self-denial, persevering and giving up.

These Achilles' heels reveal much about how superheroes balance mortality and immortality. Some superheroes are susceptible to the same natural threats that challenge mortals. Super-sleuth Batman, supersensitive Daredevil, lightning-fast Flash, brilliant and powerful Iron Man, the talented Huntress, and submariner Aquaman are vulnerable to such things as bullets, arrows, fires, heart disease, and alcohol. Other superheroes are threatened only by forces beyond those of our world, if at all, such as the mighty Superman, who is weakened only by Kryptonite, fragments of his destroyed home planet, and Wonder Woman, who as an Olympian goddess is virtually indestructible. Others superheroes who are otherwise magnificently gifted, can be defeated by forces that wouldn't even scratch mere mortals. Green Lantern, who is able to change objects with the aid of his Lantern ring, is powerless in the face of wood and the color yellow; the strong and quick Blade can be weakened by exposure to direct sunlight, and Submariner, who can breath and vanquish enemies underwater, doesn't do well in a waterless environment. Finally, several of the superheroes simply do not hold up well in the face of emotion. The Hulk, although exceptionally strong, cannot handle anger. Captain Marvel, who possessed a litany of mythological attributes, can be undone by his naiveté. Sailor Moon, who is a master of disguise, can be defeated by her crybaby alter ego Serena. The Silver Surfer, who can rearrange his molecules, could just as easily face defeat because of a loss of will.

Transformation

Most superheroes dedicate their powers and their lives to a calling, often sacrificing material pursuits, family bonds, and romantic ties to fight villains or uphold the greater good. Although many of them become aware of their superaptitudes (and superflaws) early on and slowly grow into them, others undergo a later transformation—either in adolescence or early adulthood. For some, the transformation is abrupt—the consequence of a scientific experiment gone awry, an accident or hubris. For others, the transformation follows a perilous journey to either the inner depths of the psyche or the far reaches of distant lands. Regardless of the scenario, the individual is forever changed. For Fingeroth (2004), "the hero can be said to be someone who rises above his or her fears or limitations to achieve the extraordinary" (p. 14). In his depiction of the hero of antiquity, Campbell (1956) described the calling, the journey away from the familiar through perils and otherworldly challenges followed by the enlightened return and redemptive acts. Reintegration into society is at the discretion of the transformed hero. For modern (super)heroes, the transformation leaves them isolated forever with reintegration possible only through renunciation of their super powers or concealment of those powers beneath a secret identity. In both scenarios, transformation is the heart of the mythology.

As noted earlier, the transformation may be abrupt and of scientific (or pseudo-scientific) origin. College biology major Jay Garrick was transformed into the lightning-fast Flash after accidentally inhaling fumes from spilled from chemical bottles; his successor, police scientist Barry Allen, was endowed with super speed when a lightning bolt hit chemicals with which he was working. Shy, self-effacing high school student Peter Parker developed the strength, agility, and sensory prowess of Spider-Man after being bitten by a radioactive spider. The Fantastic Four were instantly transformed when their test rocket ship was bombarded by cosmic radiation. Other abrupt transformations follow otherwise mundane circumstances. While saving a bystander from an oncoming truck, athletic bookworm Matt Murdock was doused with radioactive materials, later becoming Daredevil. In contrast, other superheroes embark on transformative journeys. Following a severely traumatic early family life, Elektra Nachios studied exotic martial arts, through which she both fought villains and continued to struggle with good and bad as Elektra. Similarly, Ororo Munroe of the incredible X-Men, followed a calling to return to South Africa and trek across the Sahara desert, an adventure during which she became Storm. In the context of their use in psychotherapy, and regardless of the nature of their transformations, the various superheroes had to learn to harness their newly acquired super powers or fatal flaws.

Science and Magic

Technology lays the fruits of science at our feet. We routinely and quite unthinkingly use gizmos and gadgets in every facet of our lives, without questioning their underlying scientific principles. In the superhero universe, science is routinely "used as an alibi for magic" (Reynolds, 1992, p. 53). Rockets, robots, interplanetary and time travel, mutatagenic cosmic radiation, not to mention a dazzling—albeit highly improbable—array of super powers including shrinkability, stretchability, combustibility, and invulnerability, are the norm. The superhero fan is asked to accept as possible all of these, just as scientists ask us to accept as fact their wondrous speculations. And we do! Koontz (1992) urged us to consider that

> every time a superhero lifts a building into the air, why don't all the bricks, held together by cement and pressure suddenly start falling apart? Those are the types of ordinary problems that seem never to occur in any superhero adventures. Basically, superheroes perform super acts and the logic squad cleans up afterwards. (p. 3)

Clearly then, the price of admission into the superhero universe is suspension, or perhaps willingness to expand belief into the world of possibility, impossibility, and magic.

Technomythic has been offered by Lawrence and Jewett (2002) as a term to describe this incorporation of technology into the superhero genre. For them, "the technomythic mode in stories of superheroic redemption arose in conjunction with evolving technologies of presentation that functions to preserve their currency and aura of credibility" (p. 8). For superheroes to do what they do—fly, move planets, rearrange molecules, that sort of thing—we are asked to consider that today's realities are little more than yesterday's dreams. And dreams are the place where magic abounds. They are the place where the boundaries between reality and fantasy, past and present, inner and outer merge, often endowing the dreamer with powers and abilities much like those of superheroes.

The Villain

What would the world of superheroes be without the villains? From Beowulf to Batman, the forces of light and good have derived their meaning and importance only by virtue of the presence of darkness and evil. Both superheroes and super-villains, besides having traumatic origins and dual identities, are smart, resourceful, and powerful, not to mention colorfully clad. However, the heightened sense of morality and singular focus on the common good that characterize the superhero are brought into bold relief by the sadistic, megalomaniacal, and antisocial ways of their nemeses. Their bios and job descriptions are clearly quite different. Fingeroth (2004) drew a tongue-in-cheek analogy between the fireman and the superhero, noting, "The superhero's role is to get the cat out of the tree, not to prune the tree or discipline the cat" (p. 162). Aligning the superhero with the fireman in this way, Fingeroth and others, most notably Reynolds (1992), have seen the superhero as reactive, or not out to change the world, whereas the villain is very much proactive and interested in change—almost exclusively to their benefit. Whether it is a need for revenge, power, display, or world domination, the villain exists to shake things up and in doing so gives meaning to the superhero's quest. In the Jungian sense, the epic battles between superheroes and supervillains represent the battles within each of us. Whether the villains take the form of tricksters or shadows, they offer a vivid glimpse into the often-irreconcilable tensions in both the personal and collective unconscious. For Fingeroth (2004), "In confronting super villains, therefore, superheroes enact our own inner and societal dialectics about issues of life and death ... they are very much the dream life—including the nightmares of our society" (p. 166).

To summarize, the superhero genre is a rich platform from which to explore a broad array of both personal and collective issues. Origins, dual identities, superpowers, fatal flaws, and stories of transformation are elements, among others, of the genre that enhance its richness. How can this richness be harnessed by clinicians working with children, adolescents, and adults? Superheroes and their adventures clearly entertain, but how can they help?

HOW SUPERHEROES CAN HELP

Undergirding the realm of children's fantasy, fantasy play, and superheroes is myth and myth making. Whether we are talking of the "classical" hero's right of initiation (Hercules, Prometheus, Odysseus) or the contemporary hero/superhero trials of redemption (Superman, X-Men, Wonder Woman), cultures "cry for myth" (May, 1991). May speculated that through the collective storytelling that is mythology, people make sense in and of a senseless world, narrate patterns that give significance to their experience, and help to self-interpret in relation to others and society. Within these collective dreams and fantasies, the hero— or superhero in our case—helps us to focus and express ideals, carry hopes and aspirations for the future, and anchor us to history (Campbell, 1956). Myths do for society what fantasies and metaphor do for the individual.

Fantasy, play, and imagination function as a developmental time machine of sorts, transporting its occupant between past, present, and future in attempts to construct meaning, express emotion, find meaning, and explore identity. Much in the same light, myth for Rollo May, can be either regressive, by expressing archetypal struggles between primitive forces, or progressive, by revealing new social insights and possibilities. If we look at children's fantasy play in general, and superhero play in particular, we see the great potential for the same process at work. Through superhero fantasy play or the use of superheroes as metaphor, children and adults can work on and resolve past crises (regressive), express current issues and struggles and experience catharsis around them, or relate desires for the way they would like things to work out for them (progressive). Within this broader context, superhero fantasy play and metaphoric storytelling are, in essence, personal myth making, no less epic or important to the individual as they are to the culture in which he or she lives. This is consistent with Campbell's notion that dreams (fantasies) are personal myths, whereas myths are collective dreams (fantasies).

Facilitating personal myth making through superhero fantasy play may be a productive means to counter the ravages of contemporary society on childhood, which include consumerism, strained family ties, poverty, media saturation, and overstimulation (Steinberg & Kincheloe, 1997). Driven to produce, conform, adapt, and grow up quickly, children more than ever need heroes (not to be confused with celebrities) who are distinct from parents. In this regard, "as children shape their behavior and values, they may look to heroes and role models for guidance ... and media [television, movies, comics, action figures] depict a variety of additional possible heroes" (Anderson & Cavallaro, 2002, p. 181). On this latter point, it is not superhero fantasy play per se that will save the culture of childhood. Instead, this volume advocates that superhero fantasy play and its use in metaphor development are forms of personal myth making that can be a means for growth and change in the individual, just as it is an impetus on a larger scale for cultural self-expression and development.

Consider the following:

The best superhero comics, in addition to being tremendously entertaining, introduce and treat in vivid ways some of the most interesting
and important questions facing all human beings—questions regarding
ethics, personal and social responsibility, justice, crime and punishment,
the mind and human emotions, personal identity, the soul, the notion
of destiny, the meaning of our lives, how we think about science and
nature, the role of faith in the rough and tumble of this world, the
importance of friendship, what love really means, the nature of family,
the classic virtues like courage . . . determination, persistence, teamwork
and creativity. (Morris & Morris, 2005, pp. xi, 17)

How then, can the therapist harness the power of superheroes and
their mythology to serve clients? In numerous ways! Just as superheroes
have origin and transformation myths, clients both young and old continually attempt to understand their own origins, whether linked to violent betrayal or a seemingly uneventful adoption. Just as superheroes are
transformed by circumstances beyond their control, so, too, are clients
altered by adversities and vicissitudes that include abuse, divorce, illness, loss, and relocation. Their ability to adapt to these transformative
experiences lays the groundwork for the struggles and triumphs to follow. Although clients do not have superpowers or fatal flaws, identifying
with the physical and moral strengths of a superhero can be transformative and aid in overcoming disability and deficiency, whether real or
perceived.

As is true for superheroes, clients have their arch enemies, either in the
form of classroom bullies, abusive parents, toxic teachers, or labyrinthine
legal systems. For the superhero, concealed and dual identities set the stage
for externalization of inner conflicts, just as clients continually struggle
to reconcile opposing inner forces and powerful conflicting emotions.
Whereas the superhero takes up causes such as world peace, disarma-
ment, and justice, clients struggle no less with their own personal battles
for equality, esteem, and connection. Whether transformed by science
or magic, superheroes rarely fit in, just as clients wrestle with gender,
racial, and cultural disenfranchisement in the course of finding inner and
outer peace. As children and adolescents begin to understand the abilities
and limitations of their developing bodies and minds, they begin to ask
questions about strength, mortality, gravity, consciousness, and morality
(Bender, 1954). Superheroes are seemingly tailor-made vehicles for exploring these complex, often abstract issues. Finally, there are those amazingly
colorful costumes that provide clients an opportunity either to identify
with their favorite superhero or to establish the parameters of their own
burgeoning identity.

In the chapters that follow, therapists from diverse theoretical orientations, who work with an array of challenging clients in various clinical settings will demonstrate how clients of all ages utilize the stories and adventures of the modern superheroes to create their own effective personal mythologies. While the cases are based on real clients or clinical amalgams, their identities have been protected.

Section 1 of the book, *Traditional Superheroes in Counseling and Play Therapy*, establishes the foundation for the use of some of the more popular superheroes in psychotherapy and play therapy. The current chapter has established the foundation for the relevance of superheroes in the treatment of children, adolescents, and adults. In chapter 2, "Superheroes in Therapy: Uncovering Children's Secret Identities," Robert Porter demonstrates how three superhero myth elements—fear of exposure, restrained hidden powers, and separation from true family—parallel common core elements of therapy with children and adolescents and, in so doing, point the way to meaningful and successful interventions. In chapter 3, "What Would Superman Do?" Cory A. Nelson introduces and illustrates a technique that helps clients reframe events and "act as if" they are either a superhero of their own making or one from a comic book. Through this process, they create their own healing and problem-solving metaphors. Chapter 4, "Superheroes and Sandplay: Using the Archetype Through the Healing Journey" by Bill McNulty, is based on the premise that (child) clients' work in the sand tray parallels their journey, both in therapy and in life. Drawing on Campbell's hero and Jung's archetypes, it demonstrates how clients, just like prominent superheroes, can be transformed by their challenges and struggles. In chapter 5, "The Incredible Hulk and Emotional Literacy," Jennifer Mendoza Sayers explores the concept of emotional literacy in children and teens, with particular therapeutic applications using various superheroes

Section 2, "Superheroes and Unique Clinical Applications," focuses on using superheroes with unique clinical populations and issues. In chapter 6, "Holy Franchise! Batman and Trauma," Michael Brody argues that the Batman myth brings together Freud's trauma theory and Erickson's thoughts on personality development, thus serving as a tailor-made vehicle to help therapists communicate with and initiate the healing process with traumatized and sexually abused children. In chapter 7, "Making a Place for the Angry Hero on the Team," Harry Livesay discusses the "angry" superhero, who, like many children, experienced early trauma and societal alienation resulting in anger and isolation. He demonstrates that just as the Justice League and the X-Men accept, heal, and assimilate their angry members, so can the angry child become a valued member of the team—at home, in school, and within the larger community. Chapter 8, "A Super Milieu: Using Superheroes in the Residential

Treatment of Adolescents With Sexual Behavior Problems," Karen Robertie, Ryan Weidenbenner, Leya Barrett, and Robert Poole explore and demonstrate the appeal and practical applications of hero and superhero mythology in the residential treatment of sexual offenders. They discuss the relationship between the "super" and the "everyday" hero as it applies to treatment of this challenging population through the use of storytelling, music therapy, role-playing, and comic-book drawing. Chapter 9, "Superheroes Are Super Friends: Developing Social Skills and Emotional Reciprocity With Autistic Spectrum Clients" by Patty Scanlon, explores the role of superhero-based play therapy with young clients manifesting symptoms along the autistic spectrum. In chapter 10, "Superheroes in Play Therapy With an Attachment Disordered Child," Carmela Wenger explores and demonstrates the usefulness of superheroes and the superhero metaphor in the assessment, diagnosis, and treatment of a young client with attachment difficulties. Chapter 11, "Luke, I Am Your Father! A Clinical Application of the Star Wars Adoption Narrative," I discuss the case of Alex, and 11-year-old child, whose identification with Luke Skywalker helped him compose a new episode in the Star Wars saga to cope with the circumstances of his adoption.

Section 3, "Nontraditional Therapeutic Applications of Superheroes," explores several unique applications of superheroes and their mythologies in counseling with clients of all ages. In chapter 12, "Becoming the Hero: The Use of Role-Playing Games in Psychotherapy," George Enfield demonstrates how this unique genre, specifically applied to superheroes, can provide the therapist with a springboard for problem exploration, metaphor development, and treatment. In chapter 13, "To Boldly Go! *Star Trek* Superheroes in Therapy," Jeff Pickens examines the allure of the *Star Trek* universe and its heroes and then outlines clinical applications as well as related topics of racism, addiction, gender roles, and prejudice. In chapter 14, "Hypnosis and Superheroes," Jan Burte demonstrates how superhero traits and abilities can be incorporated into the hypnotherapeutic treatment of individuals experiencing pain, trauma, and medical conditions. Finally, chapter 15 is titled "Heroes Who Learn to Love Their Monsters: How Fantasy Film Characters Can Inspire the Journey of Individuation for Gay and Lesbian Clients in Psychotherapy." There, Roger Kaufman explores how the heroes in films such as *E. T.,* *Lord of the Rings,* and *Star Wars* can be understood in a way that is potentially meaningful for any client coming to terms with the significance of his or her gay desire.

The Appendix provides the reader with a thumbnail guide to the potential use of superheroes in psychotherapy with children, adolescents, and adults. Enter now, the realm of fantasy, imagination, and the superhero.

REFERENCES

Anderson, K., & Cavallaro, D. (2002). Parents or pop culture?: Heroes and role models. *Childhood Education, 78,* 181–189.

Bender, L. (1954). *A dynamic psychopatholgy of childhood.* Springfield, IL: Thomas Books.

Bender, L., & Lourie, R. (1941). The effects of comic books on the ideology of children. *American Journal of Orthopsychiatry, 11,* 540–550.

Bettleheim, B. (1975). *The uses of enchantment: The meaning and importance of fairy tales.* New York: Vintage Books.

Brody, M. (1995). Batman: Psychic trauma and its solution. *Journal of Popular Culture, 28,* 171–178.

Bruner, J. (1986). Play, thought and language. *Prospects: Quarterly Review of Education, 16,* 77–83.

Campbell, J. (1956). *The hero with a thousand faces.* New York: Meridian Press.

Combs, G., & Freedman, J. (1990). *Symbol, story and ceremony: Using metaphor in individual and family therapy.* New York: Norton.

Erikson, E. (1963). *Childhood and society.* New York: Norton.

Fingeroth, D. (2004). *Superman on the couch: What superheroes really tell us about ourselves and our culture.* New York: Continuum Books.

Freud, A. (1965). *Normality and pathology in childhood: Assessments of development.* New York: International Universities Press.

Freud, A. (1966). *The ego and its mechanisms of defence.* New York: International Universities Press.

Freud, S. (1955). Beyond the pleasure principle. In J. Strachey (Ed. & Trans.), *The standard edition of the complete psychological works of Sigmund Freud* (Vol. 18, 1st ed.). London: Hogarth. (Original work published 1920)

Ginott, H. (1961). *Group psychotherapy with children: The theory and practice of play therapy.* New York: McGraw-Hill.

Irwin, E. (1983). The diagnostic and therapeutic use of pretend play. In C. E. Schaefer and K. J. O'Connor (Eds.), *The handbook of play therapy* (pp. 148–173). New York: Wiley.

Jones, G. (2002). *Killing monsters: Why children need fantasy, super-heroes and make-believe violence.* New York: Basic Books.

Koontz, D. (2002). Men of steel, feathers of fury. In L. Gresh & R. Weinberg (Ed.), *The science of superheroes* (pp. xxi–xxiii). Hoboken: Wiley.

Landreth, G. (2002). *Play therapy: The art of the relationship* (2nd ed.). New York: Brunner Routledge.

Lawrence, J. S., & Jewett, R. (2002). *The myth of the American superhero.* Cambridge, England: Erdmans.

Loeb, J., & Morris, T. (2005). Heroes and superheroes. In T. Morris & M. Morris (Eds.), *Superheroes and philosophy: Truth, justice, and the Socratic way* (pp. 11–20). LaSalle, IL: Open Court Press.

Lyddon, W. J., Clay, A. L., & Sparks, C. L. (2001). Metaphor and change in counseling. *Journal of Counseling and Development, 79*(3), 269–274.

May, R. (1991). *The cry for myth*. New York: Delta.

Miller, S. (1974). *The psychology of play*. New York: Aronson.

Morris, T. & Morris, M. (Eds.). (2005). *Superheroes and philosophy: Truth, justice, and the Socratic Way*. La Salle, IL: Open Court Press.

Piaget, J. (1962). *Play, dreams and imitation in childhood*. New York: Norton.

Reynolds, R. (1992). *Super heroes: A modern mythology*. Jackson: University of Mississippi Press.

Ryall, C., & Tipton, S. (2005). The Fantastic Four as a family: The strongest bond of all. In T. Morris & M. Morris (Eds.), *Superheroes and philosophy: Truth, justice, and the Socratic way* (pp. 118–129). LaSalle, IL: Open Court Press.

Sawyer, J. K., & Horm-Wingerd, D. M. (1993). Creative problem solving. In C. Schaefer (Ed.), *The therapeutic powers of play* (1st ed; pp. 81–105). Northvale, New Jersey: Aronson.

Simpson, P., Rodiss, H., & Bushell, M. (Eds.). (2004). *The rough guide to superheroes: The comics, the costumes, the creators, the catchphrases*. London: Haymarket Customer.

Sims, P. (2003). Working with metaphor. *American Journal of Psychotherapy, 57*(4), 528–536.

Steinberg, S., & Kincheloe, J. (1997). No more secrets: Kinderculture, information saturation and the post modern child. In S. Steinberg & J. Kincheloe (Ed.), *Kinderculture: The corporate construction of childhood* (pp. 22–35). Boulder, CO: Westview Press.

Vygotsky, L. S. (1978). *Mind in society*. Cambridge, MA: Harvard University Press.

Wickman, S. A., Daniels, M. H., White, L. J., & Fesmire, S. A. (1999). A primer in conceptual metaphor for counselors. *Journal of Counseling and Development, 77*(4), 389–394.

CHAPTER TWO

Superheroes in Therapy: Uncovering Children's Secret Identities

Robert J. Porter

> Play permits the child to resolve in symbolic form unsolved problems of the past and to cope directly or symbolically with present concerns. It is also his most significant tool for preparing himself for the future and its tasks.
>
> —(Bettelheim, 1976)

Play is integral to psychotherapy (Winnicott, 1996)—not only in the case of children but with adults as well. This view of play is consistent with the broader view that psychotherapy involves the exploration of a creative space defined jointly by the therapist and patient (Winnicott & Winnicott, 1982). In therapy, the process of creative play provides a bridge from inadequate or maladaptive behaviors to more adequate and adapted ones (Piaget, 1945). Play, therefore, can also serve to mark progress in therapy and expose the changes that are occurring in patients' thinking and emotional life (Kaduson & Schaefer, 2000).

For children, play provides a safe place to problem solve, a place in which hidden needs can emerge and the challenges of meeting needs, or of having them denied, can be explored. An important aspect of this problem solving is that the child can explore how needs can be met in various roles, identities, and social relationships (Bettelheim, 1976). It is in this sense that the role of superheroes in play can be of particular interest.

Children use superheroes as a way to work through their feelings of strength or weakness and as a way to compare superheroes' qualities with those of their ideal selves or of their ideal parental figures. In addition to facilitating exploration of qualities of self and family, play also helps to clarify the self vis-à-vis community values. In play and stories, the ultimate triumph of superheroes over villains teaches lessons of community and culture and provides reassurance to children who may choose good acts instead of the antisocial ones that are suggested by their troubling thoughts (Russ, 2003). Superhero play thus supports exploration of personal, family, and cultural values and contributes to the development of an internal sense of self and self-regulation in a social context.

Superhero play is particularly valuable to children who experience feelings of inadequacy or abandonment or who fear punishment or ridicule because of their secret thoughts, desires, and anxieties. Sometimes, these fears are based in overt rejection by others because of differences in appearance or ability. Of course, most children have these feelings at one time or another, which explains the nearly universal appeal of superhero stories and fantasies. One important part of this appeal is that superheroes often have secret identities.

The classic storybook, comic, and television superheroes have secret identities that allow them to lead lives independent from judgment of and interference by others. Story lines frequently involve the superhero's struggle to avoid exposure and his or her struggle with the lonely burden of a secret life. Children can use the vehicle of secret identity in two ways: either to cloak their weaknesses psychologically or to imagine (future) transformation into more powerful figures.

Particularly empowering to a child who is overwhelmed with feelings of helplessness and negative judgment by others are superheroes' confidence that they have the power to control their fate regardless of circumstances. Super-confidence emerges from the knowledge that in their "secret identities," they are more powerful than their tormentors and detractors and that even if they have to restrain their powers and must allow themselves to be intimidated or discounted, they will eventually be both victorious and admired. In these ways, superhero play in therapy safely allows children to have secret identities.

Another characteristic of many superheroes and mythic figures is their alienation or separation from their true families. Regardless of the adequacy or inadequacy of the foster parenting of the orphaned, neglected, or abandoned superhero, the superhero maintains hope that someday he or she will be restored to a family of truly loving and understanding parents. This characteristic of the superhero myth is a particularly strong one when working with neglected, abused, or abandoned children and enables them to work through the possibility that they can be powerful without the desired parenting and that absent parents do care about them.

Each of the cases in this chapter reflect the themes just outlined. I use the stories of three children to illustrate how a therapeutic setting that includes superhero elements (in addition to ordinary ones) can be helpful in pointing the way toward interventions, as well as to monitor therapeutic progress.

THE OBJECTIVE AND VIRTUAL PLAY SPACES

It is in playing, and perhaps only in playing, that the child is free to be creative.

—(Winnicott, 1996)

Toys, dolls, and other instruments of play are common components of the offices of therapists who work with young clients. More recently, electronic materials and computer programs have appeared as part of play therapy (Rieber, 1996). My office includes both traditional and computer-based play opportunities.

Physical toys include a variety of superhero and nonsuperhero action figures and related paraphernalia (vehicles, weapons, enclosures, a sand-tray, etc.). I try to keep the collection updated, noting changes in afternoon and Saturday morning cartoon contents and themes and monitoring the individual interests of the children with whom I work. Superheroes include wrestlers, soldiers, doctors, police officers, firefighters, and other everyday heroes in our culture, as well as more abstract figures such as angels, wizards, or good witches. The toys include figures of both genders, a variety of skin colors, and some child superheroes (e. g., from the *Dragon Ball Z* collection based on the television series). I also have a comparable collection of supervillains or generic "bad guys," including representations from comics, movies, and television and abstract elements such as demons, evil witches and sorcerers, and black knights.

Play—superhero and otherwise—may also include paper and pencil, colored crayons and markers, a whiteboard and markers, scissors, tape, glue sticks, staplers, and decorative elements such as colored pipe cleaners, string, and stickers. I have developed some simple drawing skills and use them frequently in play. Fortunately, children are very forgiving of nonexpert drawings, as long as they feel that the essential elements are represented.

I have found three contexts to be particularly useful in encouraging the visual, constructive play of children while maintaining a free, creative space. These include Winnicott's Squiggle Game (Winnicott, 1989), the Story Maker, version 2.1 (Spa Software, 2005) and Hero Machine

(Hebert, 2001/2004) computer programs. Links to detailed information on the computer programs are provided in the references to this chapter. Brief explanations are provided here, and examples of children's work are shown in the case discussions.

The Squiggle Game

Winnicott's Squiggle Game is a simple one. I use a modified version of his original task (Winnicott, 1989). I begin by folding a piece of ordinary, unlined paper into quarters. Each quarter is used once, with drawings on one side only. I usually start with, and use three quarter-folded sheets, but any number may be used. After a brief explanation, we play the game, with the child and I taking turns. First the child takes his or her turn, then the therapist, and so forth, until 12 quarter panels have been completed. I then tear the panels apart and place the child's drawings in front of him or her and ask the child to arrange them to make a story "like a comic book." When the story arrangement is completed, I ask the child to tell the story, which I write down. I then ask open-ended questions about elements and themes.

The creation of the panel drawings is straightforward process. The person whose turn it is gives the paper and pencil to the other player. The other player places the pencil on the paper and, with eyes closed, rapidly makes a "squiggle" on the blank panel. There are no restrictions on the squiggles; they can be simple or complex, meaningful or not. I model "random," moderately complex squiggles. The first player then retrieves the paper and, looking carefully at the squiggle mark, "makes it into" a picture or object. All or part of the mark may be used; the paper may be rotated to any orientation, and as many elements as desired can be added. If the child desires, squiggle parts may be erased, although I encourage the child simply to ignore unwanted elements.

The child is not told that the end result is to be a story, nor is the number of squiggles to be done announced. (This cannot be done, of course, if the game is repeated at a later date.)

I have used the squiggle game successfully with children as young as 4 years, although for the youngest and least skilled children, I may simply complete the squiggle for them in terms of what they say they see.

The Story Maker

The Story Maker program was developed by an English company (Spa Software, 2005) and is part of a suite of educational programs. The short description that follows does not do it justice. Interested readers are encouraged to visit the Web site to appreciate the scope of the program.

The Story Maker allows the creation of a series of story pages, each one of which starts as a blank slate. The user can select a background picture from a large gallery of settings (forests, fields, town squares, construction sites, underwater scenes, and so forth); one's own pictures can also be imported. The backgrounds are simple and stylized. Once the background is selected, the user can select from a large number of story elements that are conveniently grouped in several dozen categories such as Adults, Children, Animals, Fairy Tales, Vikings, Space, Beach, Spooky, Zoo, and so forth. There are human figures, animals, and fanciful creatures, as well as story elements such as vehicles, furniture, toys, and theme-specific elements such as pirate treasure, farm equipment, or circus components. Each figure can be selected and placed anywhere on the page and changed in size or orientation. Elements may be arranged over or behind other elements, and groups of elements can be combined and moved together or duplicated across pages.

One captivating characteristic of the program is that the elements can be dynamically and automatically made to move about the page. The elements themselves are not animated, but each one can be programmed to move about the page in any pattern desired. For example, elements can appear or disappear, and the movement of one object can be linked to movements of other elements so, for example, a dog could be made to appear from behind a tree and chase a cat off the screen.

Hundreds of sounds and noises are available to be linked to objects and their movements (motors starting and running, footsteps moving away, running water, screams, ray-gun fire, sound effects, animal sounds, and so forth). In addition, page captions and balloons for thought or characters speaking can be added and filled in, and synthetic voices of men, women, and children (with English accents!) can be selected to read the balloon-text aloud.

The Story Maker program has been revised many times over the years. It is sophisticated yet easy for children (and adults) to use. It appeals to even the most computer-game-experienced of my patients, and it is devised to provide more opportunity for creative expression than I have seen in other similar programs. An important feature is that the picture library can be easily expanded with one's own pictures. Mine has superheroes added. Although only one example using the Story Maker is included in this chapter, it is a frequent component of my work with children.

The HeroMachine

The HeroMachine is another program that has evolved over the years. Developed by Jeff Hebert (2004), it is a Macromedia file that is played in a browser (like Internet Explorer or FireFox). This clever program is easy to use but allows for a wide variety of creative design.

The purpose of the HeroMachine is to create a "hero," male or female. The child begins by selecting a blank body type of a man or woman. Both muscular and more ordinary body types are available, as are shorter and taller versions. The selected body appears as a faceless, naked mannequin in a fixed pose. A menu allows the child then to pick facial features and clothing for the hero.

There are literally thousands of possible combinations of elements. For example, there are a dozen or more each of eyes, noses, mouths, ears, skin colors, and hairstyles. There are undershirts, overshirts, long- and short-sleeved shirts, jackets, coats, underpants, overpants, boots and shoes, masks, helmets and hats, various decorative elements (e. g., belts and sashes), and a large collection of weapons, shields, lightning bolts, magic wands, and other objects that the figure can hold. The figure can be accompanied by any one of a large selection of animal companions (spiders, lions, birds, dragons, etc.). Colors of every element in the creation can be chosen from a wide selection of color chips.

A completed figure can be named, saved, printed in color or gray scale, and reloaded for later modification if desired. The use of the program is "point and click." The hardest part (but also the most enjoyable and creative) is choosing from the vast array of possible elements and their combination.

CASES STUDIES[1]

Jacob

At only 4 years old, Jacob was left by himself while his mother went to meet men and use drugs. By the time he was 5, authorities had been called several times to investigate neighbors' concerns about physical abuse and reports of hearing him crying alone in the apartment. The last time they investigated, they found him semiconscious and bleeding from the head. His mother admitted jumping on top of him and banging his head on the concrete floor when he would not stop "whining." Jacob fought the police as they took his mother away.

---

[1] The cases presented as examples in this chapter are based on the therapeutic progression of actual cases. The identifying details of the cases have been changed, and, in some instances, aspects of different cases have been combined to provide an illustrative narrative. All creative work is that of the children. Additional pictures can be found at http://www.drbobtampa.com.

Jacob found the mother he needed when placed in foster care. Doris was an attentive but firm mother. She and her husband had two other foster children. They had all the children in school and after-school care on workdays.

Doris brought Jacob to the clinic when he was 6 years old because he was becoming increasingly difficult to deal with at home, school, and in after-school care. Jacob was expected to do chores at home, follow the home bedtime routine, and complete his school and after-school activities with less supervision than when he was younger. Jacob was, however, hyperactive and impulsive. He seemed to avoid or forget tasks, and he would wander about the classroom when he was supposed to be seated. Jacob would sometimes become angry when denied some activity or toy, or when he was asked, for example, to comply with after-school care rules or to clean his room. On those occasions, he lost control and threw things or pushed or hit other children.

Jacob's schoolteacher, the woman who was his after-school care teacher, and his mother, were all becoming frustrated with him. Their frustration was appearing in increased frequency and intensity of verbal criticism of him and in more severe punishments. Their approach was not working, and things had become worse during the last several months. My introducing Doris and her husband to some parenting skills, including behavioral contracting helped, but Jacob continued to frustrate his caregivers.

After intake and several weeks of sessions, I referred Jacob for evaluation for attention-deficit/hyperactivity disorder (ADHD) and he was prescribed Ritalin. This reduced his hyperactive and impulsive behaviors almost immediately, but his angry outbursts continued (although with less frequency) and he began to show increasing signs of anxiety, including compulsive behaviors and nightmares.

My initial work with Jacob, which included sand play, drawings, and action-figure play, tended to revolve around issues of control. Jacob would draw people and animals or place actors during sand play within enclosures or surrounded by walls, trees, or other barriers. When he drew or spoke of interactions among actors, the interactions frequently involved one participant attempting to contain or restrain the behavior of another.

Jacob especially enjoyed my superhero–supervillain collection of action figures. He engaged "Good" and "Bad" forces in battles in the sand-tray, and bad guys were repeatedly vanquished. The superhero action figures were usually frustrated, however, because the bad guys would not stay dead or vanquished. The defeated and dead would arise again to present new challenges to Jacob's superheroes. Jacob's battle stories never ended. There was never a final heroic victory; there was never peace in Jacob's world.

A key conceptualization in the treatment of Jacob was his experience of an abandoning and abusive mother. Those experiences contrasted
dramatically with those of his loving but firm foster mother. One important consequence of this contrast was Jacob's anxiety symptoms. He
was open and sometimes desperately sincere about his desire to comply with his teachers' and mother's requests, but he nonetheless found
himself frequently failing to meet their expectations. As a result, he was
very anxious about his misbehavior. In some cases, Jacob's inability to
conform his behavior seemed to be related to his ADHD and the related
attention and memory problems. In other cases, his emotional responses
might be attributed to persistent posttraumatic stress disorder (PTSD)
anxiety related to his traumatic treatment. Working with Jacob in therapy suggested, however, that his primary problem was his strong desire
to please the women who where involved in his care, his fear of incurring
their anger, and his internal experience of not being able to comply with
their expectations. This was a vicious cycle, of course, because his failure to behave led to more displeasure and anger in his caregivers, which,
in turn, led to higher anxiety, an increase in his internal need to control
his behavior to please them, an even greater anxiety when he could not
and, consequently, a progressively greater and greater disruption of his
thoughts and behavior.

A turning point in Jacob's therapy occurred one day when his mother
commented that Jacob was beginning to talk a lot about God and Jesus,
sometimes in angry ways. Doris and her husband took Jacob to a main-
stream Protestant church that included Sunday school experiences. Jacob
had enjoyed Sunday school in the past. However, he had recently startled
several teachers there by rejecting some activities having to do with Jesus;
they were especially concerned that he had expressed feelings of hating
Jesus.

Talking with Jacob over the next two sessions, it became apparent
that the source of his anger at Jesus was his experience at the after-school
care, which was provided by a Christian fundamentalist church that provided low-cost, well-run care near the family home. During the period of
Jacob's increased behavioral problems and shortly after his being brought
to the clinic, the after-school teacher had elected to use Jacob's interest
in God and Jesus to facilitate behavior control. She explained to Jacob
that God wanted him to be good in school, after school, and home and
that God would be angry if he did not behave. She was quite clear that
Jacob's bad behavior was the work of the Devil inside of him. Jacob's
interpretation of the teacher's comments was that God did not want
him to be angry or mad and that the Devil was the source of angry
and mad feelings. When Jacob was angry, therefore, or acted in ways
he later regretted, the Devil, he understood, was the source. Jacob was,

therefore, very pleased when the teacher explained that Jesus could drive the Devil out and help him to behave. All he had to do, she explained, was pray to Jesus for help, and both the Devil and the bad behavior would go away. He was told to say to himself, "What would Jesus do?" and Jesus would help him. Jesus became Jacob's superheroic ideal (and parental figure).

Jacob did pray, and to his delight, his prayers were answered, for this was at the time he was prescribed Ritalin, and his attention and focus increased and problems in school and after-school care decreased. Jacob found, however, that the results of prayer were inconsistent. In some cases, and despite his deepest and most sincere prayers, he was frequently unable to meet the expectations at school, after-school care, and home. He had "bad," angry thoughts, which he understood to come from the Devil. The thoughts persisted even when he prayed to Jesus to help him, and he would lose control and act out in angry ways. Jacob literally perceived himself as beset by the Devil and abandoned by Jesus. Ironically, Jesus, the superheroic King of Peace, was not bringing Jacob peace.

The interventions for Jacob took place over two sessions and were designed to (a) use his faith and his church and family resources to help him deal with anger and control issues; (b) help him distinguish between feelings and actions; and (c) help him accept his own angry feelings as acceptable and his angry behavior as also being acceptable under some circumstances. The intervention plan was reviewed with Doris, and she was present during the sessions.

Because it appeared that Jacob had identified Jesus as an example, and a source, of self-control, I asked him to think about what Jesus was like as a boy. I gave an example of Jesus going to the temple as a child and talking to the priests. But, I pointed out, Jesus had not told his parents where he was going, and they were afraid something bad had happened to him. They were angry and upset with him. No matter what, however, his parents loved him and forgave him. Jacob was intrigued.

I asked Jacob to tell me if he thought Jesus was ever angry or acted angry. Jacob was not sure. I spoke with him of an older Jesus going to a temple and being angry with the people there because they were selling things at tables and doing dishonest things in the holy temple. Using drawings, we explored the events of Jesus entering the temple, seeing the problems, yelling at the people, and overturning the tables. Jacob was amazed.

I encouraged Jacob to think about how Jesus must have been as a boy. I had Jacob draw Jesus' house and bedroom. He was careful and thoughtful as he drew Jesus' bed, window, bookshelf, and a number of small stick figures. When I asked him about those, he said that they were "Jesus' superhero action figures." I pointed out that they were all over the floor. He described how Jesus had been playing out a battle of good guys and bad guys (just as Jacob did in therapy). I asked Jacob what Jesus' mother might say about the action figures, and he agreed she might tell Jesus to "Pick them up!" We developed a story with additional drawings of Jesus forgetting to pick up his action figures because he got interested in another game. Jesus' mother got angry, raised her voice, and told him to pick them up. Jesus did, and he and his mother then enjoyed some happy time doing something together.

Subsequent sessions' therapeutic play continued to involve conflicts between superheroes and supervillains, and good continued to triumph, sometimes by vanquishing the enemies and other times by converting them to friends. Now, and in contrast to the past, when the bad guys were eliminated, they stayed eliminated. In Jacob's new world, his superhero army always won, and he could finally be a prince of peace.

Carl

Carl's grandmother, Bev, brought him to therapy because the school was concerned about his frequent anger and loss of control, sometimes coming on with little warning. Eight-year-old Carl would sometimes yell violent threats at other children, and he frequently drew pictures of elaborate battles between a lone, heroic figure and hordes of stick figures who were "chopping up good guys" or killing and mauling them with guns, cannons, fighter planes, tanks, and other weapons (see Figure 2.1).

Carl had come to live with his grandmother the previous year when his bipolar, drug-addicted mother had been arrested and convicted of various offenses. She was scheduled to be released in several months but was having difficulty following prison rules. Carl's addict father had disappeared before Carl was 3 years old, and his location was unknown. Carl had lived with his grandparents as in infant and toddler but went to live with his mother, on and off, during the 2 years before her arrest.

An extensive clinical evaluation of Carl revealed a history of irritable mood, conflict with his younger sister Dorothy (6 years old), cyclic mood changes of a 1- or 2-week duration, expansive mood periods but with irritability, hypersensitivity to some sounds (loud whispering, sharp sounds such as falling coins, etc.), as well as the previously noted elaborate, violent drawings or verbally described scenes of mayhem.

Most recently, Carl's teacher had given the class an assignment to write sentences using their spelling words. Carl, who had been in trouble with his teacher for angry outbursts that morning, wrote a series of sentences, using the spelling words but describing scenes of hurting a cat. When confronted, Carl was defiant. When the teacher said it was OK, in

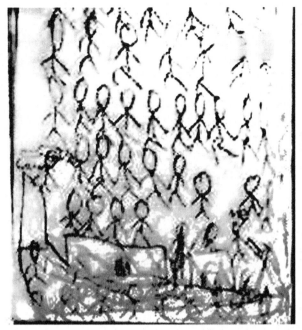

Figure 2.1 An example of one of Carl's drawings, produced early in therapy, of a superhero, bottom center, fighting off hordes of "bad guys" who are trying to invade his fortress.

this case, because it was a school assignment, she was surprised when Carl became angry and agitated, ripped up his paper, and refused to complete the sentence assignment.

Carl was a slight child, somewhat shy, and moderately hyperactive. I observed that his flow of thought was sometimes loose but logically ordered. When alone with me, he was generally relaxed and engaged in sessions. If his grandmother was present, however, he tended to be less engaged and sometimes passively resistant to doing play.

Carl admitted to thoughts of violent conflicts, like those he drew, but said, "I would never hurt anybody." He said he had both good and bad dreams. He also said, "I fall a lot in my dreams," but could not remember any of these dreams. He referred to his little sister as a "kindergartener" and as "Dorothy the dope, who's a pest."

When asked to draw a happy scene, he drew a beach. When asked to tell a story about the beach, he talked about fishing and how he liked it a lot and said that his grandfather would take him. "I like it, but I feel sorry for the fish being hooked." Carl elaborated by supposing that hooked, dead fish went to heaven with God. Carl explained that heaven had some good–bad people in it (i.e., people who were *simultaneously* good and bad) and that if he, Carl, were in heaven, he would "sneak in a pistol and kill the good–bad people." He supposed he could kill God, too, "but not with a pistol, I would need a nuclear bomb. And then I'd be God! And I would say 'No homework!' "

I referred Carl to a university testing center for evaluation with a suggested differential diagnosis of bipolar, PTSD, and anxiety disorder, with symptoms of ADHD, and asked for an evaluation for psychotropic medication. The appointment, however, was set for more than 2 months away. Carl's primary care doctor decided to begin the antidepressant, Zoloft, at Bev's request, and Carl began therapy with me.

Carl's first HeroMachine picture was "Grave Man." He explicitly chose the largest male figure, the largest gun, and the most protective of armor, a large tail, and broad wings (see Figure 2.2). He also used my superhero–supervillain set of toys to act out battles like those he drew. Carl's grandmother reported little noticeable change with Zoloft after

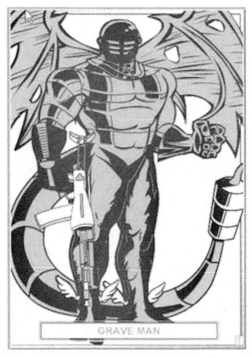

Figure 2.2 Carl's first HeroMachine figure. Note the choice of massive body, heavy armor, and large weapon.

4 weeks. I thought I noted some increase in loose association but improved containment of affect. The medication was subsequently stopped.

A recurrent theme of Carl's play and commentary was an avoidance of anything feminine (e. g., he was annoyed that an older, fatherly man referred to him as "dear" and mentioned that one of his mother's boyfriends was "cool, but he wore earrings"). He was particularly disparaging of his sister and her "girl things" When evaluated by a female at the university, he expressed annoyance with her strong negative reaction to his telling his violent stories and drawing pictures of mayhem. (She told Bev to put away all knives and weapons in their apartment). When describing the encounter, he referred to her as "a wussy. She doesn't understand me. I am not going back!"

Carl's grandfather was asked to bring him to a session. He expressed a feeling that Carl was not understood. He said that he understood that Carl's thoughts were based in anger, and he felt the teacher and university evaluator were overreacting. Interaction between Carl and his grandfather was positive, although grandfather was sometimes stern and mildly intimidating. The grandfather admitted to using corporal punishment (spanking, on the bottom, with his hand, "when absolutely necessary"). Carl's grandfather's demeanor was in clear contrast to that of his grandmother who was matter-of-fact, breezy, and more permissive. During this session, Carl listened while his grandfather and I talked about him, and he drew a series of pictures on the whiteboard I have on my office wall. First he drew a battle scene as usual, and then he erased that and drew a single scary "alien face"; he replaced the alien with a simple, rather mild "mad face." As the session drew to a close, Carl erased the board and carefully drew a detailed rose, thorns and all, and colored the delicate flower carefully. He did not erase the rose when he left.[2]

Carl's therapy work revealed a complex emotional life. As noted earlier, he spoke of fishing and fish dying, but he expressed sadness that the fish were hurt when hooked. In later therapy sessions, he reported exhilarating dreams of "flying over everything" but some fear of falling "even in the good dreams." Carl referred to the good–bad people on several occasions and once referred to God as "good but mean." During play with Power Ranger action figures, the conflict was between good and bad guys, but Carl had the bad guys "turn into good guys," rather than die, when they were defeated by the good guys. Conflicts frequently

---

[2] The photo of Carl's rose was not reproducible. The drawing was remarkably detailed, with careful attention to the overlapping red petals, with delicate leaves and with clearly constructed, and threatening thorns. It is easy to conclude that Carl was representing himself as valued, vulnerable, but prickly. The interested reader is referred to the web site www.drbobtampa.com for links to an image of Carl's rose.

involved a weak figure fighting overwhelming evil hordes, with the weaker figure's eventual victory being due to some special weapon or magic force.

Carl liked the Squiggle Game and asked to play it often. He was creative and elaborate in his creations. On one occasion, he turned my squiggles into a man smoking a cigar, a rare fish with a light that hung over its head (a real fish, actually), a jack-o'-lantern, an alligator-dragon, and a pig with big legs. When asked to create a story, he spoke of Halloween and placed me in the story in an alligator-dragon costume (scary and wise?), and himself in a pig costume (weak and insignificant?). Context suggested his grandfather was represented as the cigar-smoking man (who gave out Halloween candy), and that the fish was related to his love of fishing and dead fishes in heaven (with halos).

Carl produced a new hero during this period. This hero was of more ordinary physical build than the first, and was armed with a less imposing sword instead of a large gun. The new hero (Figure 2.3) also had a yin–yang symbol on his chest and an eagle companion. Carl explained that

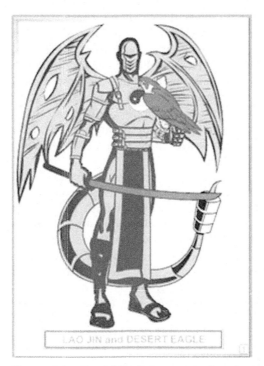

Figure 2.3 One of Carl's heroes, produced sometime in middle of therapy. Note lighter armor, smaller weapon, and yin–yang symbol. Carl said the name was from "a TV show."

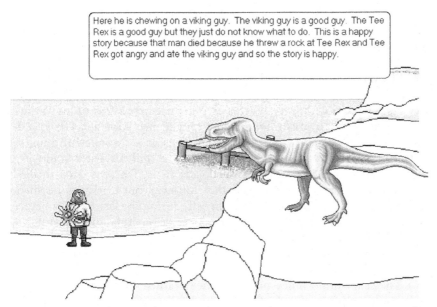

Here he is chewing on a viking guy. The viking guy is a good guy. The Tee Rex is a good guy but they just do not know what to do. This is a happy story because that man died because he threw a rock at Tee Rex and Tee Rex got angry and ate the viking guy and so the story is happy.

Figure 2.4 Page from Carl's "Tee Rex" StoryMaker story. Caption at top is also quotes in the text. When activated Tee Rex moves over to Viking and devours him. Text describes events in Carl's own words, transcribed by the therapist.

this hero was based on the "Lao Jin" character on a television show who was powerful because he could make things "turn out right."[3]

Carl was introduced to the Story Maker program and enjoyed creating several stories. Most were loose amalgams of elements with simple themes. One, however, involved a *Tyrannosaurus Rex* confronting an attacking Viking on the beach (see Figure 2.4). Carl explained (via dictation to me) the interaction as follows:

> Here he is chewing on a Viking guy. The Viking guy is a good guy. The T. Rex is a good guy, but they just do not know what to do. This is a happy story because the man died because he threw a rock at T. Rex, and T. Rex got angry and ate the Viking guy, and so the story is happy.

The conceptualization of Carl's case included addressing thought control and mood elements of his apparent bipolar mood disorder, his anxiety and possible PTSD symptoms, and some ADHD symptoms of

---

[3] The television show may have been *Double Dragon*, a show (and also a set of video games) in which two brothers, separated from each other early in life, are raised by enemy martial arts experts. They are set in battle against each other but eventually figure out who the real bad guys are and unite against them.

inattention and forgetting that Carl displayed when trying to complete tasks such as working the controls of computer programs. The clearest component of Carl's emotional picture, however, was his intense anger, especially when dealing with female figures (e. g., Carl refused to create a female hero figure) and his persistent feelings of vulnerability and weakness.

As I worked with Carl, he was able to articulate a fear of his mother coming home from prison and taking him to live with her. His grandmother would present this possibility to Carl as a "wonderful thing to look forward to" and would explain how he and his sister could live with their mother when she returned. His sister, Dorothy, was thrilled with this idea (see Dorothy's case that follows), but Carl was terrified. Carl had lived with his mother, by himself, during the last months before she was arrested and convicted of drug possession and domestic violence charges (violent attack on her paramour). He was happy living with his grandmother, and especially his grandfather. He did not want to leave and live with his good–bad mother.

The scary importance of his mother's return was clearly evident in a dramatic improvement in Carl's mood following the report from the prison that his mother would not be released for at least another year because of "failure to follow rules." This event gave me more time to work with Carl on the issue of his mother's return and to help him understand that his grandmother had permanent custody of him. He was helped to understand that he would be able to visit with his mother but always have grandmother's house to go to. His mood improved.

During the last three or four sessions I had with Carl, before he began therapy at a nonprofit community resource, he produced two more male heroes. The first, produced early in the period, is similar to his earlier one, but the hero no longer has his weapon; he is protected, however, like the first hero, by an eagle who appears as a gryphon. The hero's chest symbol has changed to a blue shark, perhaps reflecting hidden danger below the surface (see Figure 2.5).

The final hero (Figure 2.6) had a face that was still shielded like before, but he was nonetheless noticeably more exposed and vulnerable. The sword returned as a weapon, but the companion appeared as a rat (named Stuart, like the lovable cartoon mouse) who had scary, sharp teeth but who was also loving and sweet, like a rose.

Dorothy

(*Note: Dorothy is the younger sister of Carl, from the previous case example. They have the same mother but different fathers.*)

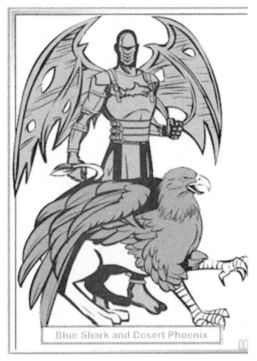

Blue Shark and Desert Phoenix

Figure 2.5 One of Carl's heroes from late in the middle of therapy. Note there is no weapon and the transformation of the companion into a gryphon from an eagle (compare with Figure 2.2). The insignia is a shark.

Dorothy, 6 years old, was initially seen because her grandmother, Bev, was concerned about sibling conflict with her brother, Carl. Bev was also concerned because the school was reporting that Dorothy was often irritable, becoming passive–aggressive when asked to do something (one teacher reported, for example, that Dorothy "rolled on the classroom floor and screamed 'Nooooo!' when denied something she wanted). Bev expressed the opinion that Dorothy might be acting up because her mother had been recently contacting her from prison and had told Dorothy that she would be home in about 3 months. Bev was unclear what the living arrangements might be at that time, but Dorothy said she wanted to live with her mother. On the other hand, Bev said she had also recently been asked by Dorothy's father to have more time with the girl, perhaps even take custody of her. When visits with the father were arranged, however, Dorothy said she did not want to go and argued and "misbehaved" when with her father.

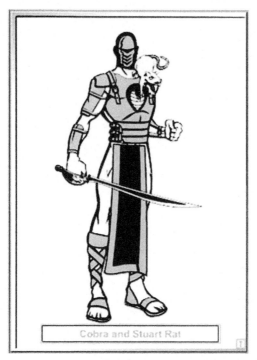

Cobra and Stuart Rat

Figure 2.6   Carl's last hero. The light weapon returns, the chest insignia is a cobra, and the companion is "Stuart" (like Stuart Little the mouse character) but with sharp teeth.

My first few meetings were with Dorothy and her grandmother. Dorothy was shy and somewhat reluctant to talk. After the first session, however, Dorothy was willing to meet with me alone. She spontaneously constructed an elaborate picture when given crayons and paper. She drew a castle with small windows. She spoke of a princess in the castle and said that it is sad the princess could not come out. The connection with her imprisoned mother seemed obvious. Dorothy clearly idealized the princess and expressed the belief that all would be well and the princess would be freed. In other respects, Dorothy's play was superficial and light. She avoided topics with emotional content. Between sessions, Bev reported that the problems with her father were getting worse. I encouraged Bev to invite the father to come and see me with Dorothy.

Dorothy's father, John, came to the first session by himself. He was engaging, but shy, appearing embarrassed about his unskilled job and his difficulty making ends meet and not being able to provide Dorothy with more. He expressed hope that he would soon earn more. He expressed a strong desire to be more involved with Dorothy but said that Bev was sometimes reluctant and that she allowed Dorothy to determine when John could see her.

John explained that when he first began to take Dorothy on visits, she was very avoidant. She would hide under the table and not come out, for example. He tried both yelling and pleading but found that waiting worked best. He admitted to being manipulated somewhat by Dorothy and to sometimes "bribing" her, but he also expressed frustration that she did not follow his directions. The interpersonal dynamic between Dorothy and John in later sessions revealed the frustrating and manipulative pattern reported by the father.

Parenting skills training, based in my own *Almost-Perfect Parenting* program (Porter, 2005) and on *123 Magic* (Phelan, 1995) were implemented. John was quick to catch on and Dorothy was resistant, but eventually she adapted positively to a structured routine and boundaries. *Almost-Perfect Parenting* techniques of "Let's have a do-over" and "I made a mistake," as well as "Dr. Bob Time" (a mutual time-out followed by problem solving) were also successfully implemented. Dorothy nevertheless continued to be unpredictably angry and restless with her father.

During this series of sessions, Dorothy generated two "heroes" (seen in Figure 2.7). One was a female "Cat Woman." This hero was masked, her body covered and protected; she had a cat face and a cat companion. The second was a "Cat Man" who has similar features to Cat Woman but held a shield and had a eagle companion. The figure is mildly threatening but had no weapon.

Dorothy explained that the woman had the power to change things from bad to good ("stones into snakes," for example, snakes being "good"), could transport "a little girl" to "any place she wants to be, like a park," and could magically change the moods of people from sad to happy with a "magic word like 'abracadabra.'" The Cat Man, on the other hand, had the power to "get the bad man that has taken over the castle and throw him in a dungeon, so the castle can be happy again."

Dorothy further elaborated the story of the Cat Man: "He can capture the bad, angry man who shot and killed the little girl, put him in jail, bury the little girl and go home to bed and dream of being loved as a friend by everyone." These features of the male story were interpreted as reflecting Dorothy's hope to reunite the family, her desire for her father to make things right for her mother, and a masked desire to have a prior and possibly abusive, paramour of her mother's punished. (This latter theme could not be confirmed by the time therapy ended.)

The circumstances of Dorothy's unpredictable anger with her father became clearer in a later session where John said that Dorothy had become

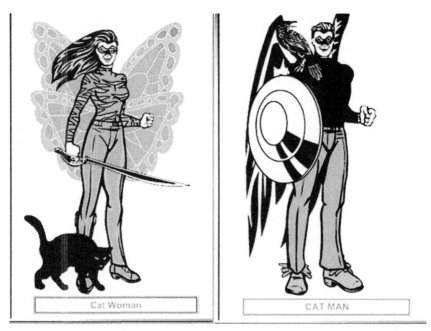

Figure 2.7 Dorothy's first female and male hero figures. For the female, note the complete protection of the body, the cat face and mask, the weapon, and the hissing cat. In its original form, the figure's costume is intense shades of red. For the male, note the absence of weapon, with the appearance of man hiding behind the shield. The man has a cat face, a mask, and a bird-eagle companion.

angry when he had mentioned that he would like to have her live with him, even after her mother was released from prison. When I met with Dorothy alone, she explicitly expressed a fear that her father would keep her from living with her mother, once her mother was released from prison. She fantasized that her father and mother might reunite but was especially concerned that her father would not do so and would also not let her see or live with her mother.

Dorothy and her father were brought together to discuss her fears. John was helped to articulate a vision of the future in which Dorothy could visit or live with either parent whenever she wished and however a judge would determine. Dorothy then expressed some concern about this and appeared worried about hurting her father's feelings. John was able, based on prior *Almost-Perfect Parenting* coaching, to recognize this concern of Dorothy's and to clearly state that he would love Dorothy forever, regardless of where she lived. Upon hearing this, Dorothy was visibly relieved.

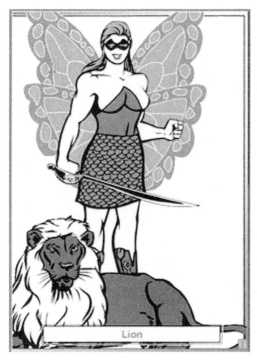

Figure 2.8 A female hero of Dorothy's during the middle of therapy. Note there is less body coverage, a stronger body type, a human face, and a lion companion instead of black cat (compare with Figure 2.4).

In later sessions, Dorothy produced two new female heroes and one new male one. The first female figure was distinctly different from the earlier one (see Figure 2.8). The figure was less shielded by clothing, had no wings, and was no longer a "Cat Woman," although she was more muscular and continued to be masked and to brandish a sword. Dorothy also added a bigger cat companion, a male lion.

The last male figure of Dorothy's was weaponless (see Figure 2.9), as was the first, but was nonthreatening (although still masked) and handsome and heroic in dress and pose. A final female figure, Buckbeak and Owner (Figure 2.10), included an unarmed, unmasked, confident female figure and a companion and gryphon-like protector, combining the earlier male hero's eagle companion with the later female hero's male lion protector.

Subsequent sessions involved problem solving of father–daughter conflicts. Dorothy would sit on the floor at her father's feet and play with a dollhouse. In one session, she explained that the house was arranged

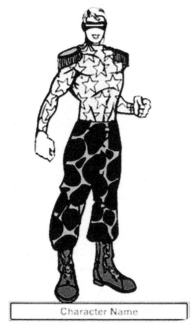

Character Name

Figure 2.9 Dorothy's last male hero. Note the human face and heroic, powerful stance (not hidden by shield). Dorothy did not name the figure.

to keep occupants safe from outside "snakes and mountain lions." In the second session, the house was carefully divided into mother and father parts with separate bedrooms.

By the last therapy session, Bev reported that Dorothy's fights with her brother had decreased, that negative reports from school had decreased, and that Dorothy was doing "what we tell her, with fewer complaints." John happily reported getting a promotion at work. It appeared that John and Dorothy, together, might be able to make the castle happy again.

SUMMARY AND CONCLUSION

All three children had experienced abuse or neglect at the hands of a parent. It is not surprising, then, that many of the themes of idealized parents, or a return to real, loving (and powerful) parents, were present in the children's therapy. An important key for the children is that real foster parents were available to embody elements, and provide the love and attention of the idealized images. From a family dynamics perspective,

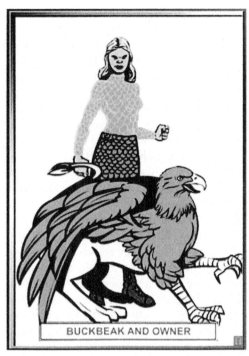

BUCKBEAK AND OWNER

Figure 2.10 Dorothy's last female hero. Note the human face, the lack of a weapon, and the companion that is both the bird-eagle seen in the earlier male figure (Figure 2.7) and the lion from a later female figure (in Figure 2.8).

it appears important to make sure that the play therapy involves both the exploration of the superhero idealizations as well as an attempt to integrate these idealizations with the best qualities of the child's custodial parent figures.

In each case, a transformation of the child's views of herself or himself occurred. These changes were evidenced in a number of ways. In Jacob's case, the well-meaning after-school care custodian undermined his view of himself as responsible for his behavior. As a result, Jacob placed himself in the care of an idealized superhero, whom he believed could do (and appeared to have actually done) miracles to control Jacob's thoughts and behaviors. Jacob's joyful dependence on an external locus of control crumbled, however, when his superhero appeared to forsake him. In Jacob's case, the idealized parent could be made more real, and Jacob himself could gain "superpowers" to control himself by facilitating an identification of Jacob with his superpower (Jesus), in addition to the identification of Jesus as a superparent.

Carl's abuse history was not much different from Jacob's. In both cases, a biological parent failed to live up to minimal levels of care. Carl, however, internally struggled with the good–bad images of himself and of his mother. No matter how valiantly fought, Carl's fears always returned, and his mother had a persistently negative image, even as he suffered the deprivation of her good side. Important, and easily missed by some around him, was Carl's essentially positive and sensitive view of himself that conflicted with the strong negative feelings of potential loss of control of his rage and his feelings of helplessness. For Carl, superhero play represented a transformation, a process in which an integrated image of strength and gentleness replaced the fearful image of weakness armored by protective but distancing rage. This transformation promised to allow Carl to close the distance between himself and his female caretakers, and perhaps even be able to deal with his good–bad mother directly.

Unlike the two boys, Dorothy's root problem was her rarely returned love of her idealized mother and her fear of further rejection from her. Also unlike the boys, Dorothy had a father who was capable of providing the love she needed as well as a safe context for her to explore her feelings and problem solve. To approach her father, however, appeared to her to threaten further rejection from her mother. The therapeutic task was one of facilitating a productive development of a father–daughter relationship while affirming Dorothy's feelings about her mother. It was also necessary to build Dorothy's resilience by fostering a healthier self-image, which inoculated her against the rejections that are likely to follow the return of her mother.

All three children represent the ways in which creative play, and particularly superhero play, can facilitate therapeutic work and can mark progress in therapy. The play of these "superhero" children allows both the child and the therapist to see and strengthen the child's secret identity.

It's never too late to have a happy childhood.
—Tom Robbins, *Still Life With Woodpecker*

REFERENCES

Bettelheim, B. (1976). *The uses of enchantment: The meaning and importance of fairy tales*. New York: Random House.

Hebert, J. (2001/2004) *HeroMachine*. Bertram, TX: AFD Studios (jhebert@texas.net). Retrieved July 26, 2006, from http://www.heromachine.com

Kaduson, H. G., & Schaefer, C. E. (Eds.). (2000). *Short-term play therapy for children*. New York: Guilford Press.

Phelan, T. W. (1995). *1-2-3 magic: Effective discipline for children 2–12* (2nd ed.). Glen Ellyn, IL: Child Management.

Piaget, J. (1945). *Play, dreams and imitation in childhood*. London: Heinemann.

Porter, R. J. (2005). *Almost-perfect parenting*. Unpublished workshop materials. Contact author via http://www.drbobtampa.com

Rieber, L. P. (1996). Seriously considering play: Designing interactive learning environments based on the blending of microworlds, simulations, and games. *Educational Technology Research and Development, 44*(2), 43–58.

Russ, S. W. (2003). *Play in child development and psychotherapy: Toward empirically supported practice*. New York: Erlbaum.

Spa Software (2005). StoryMaker v2.1. Retrieved July 25, 2006, from http://www.spasoft.co.uk

Winnicott, D. W. (1989) The Squiggle Game (Chapter 40, pp, 299–317) in *Psychoanalytic Explorations*. London: Karnac Books; Cambridge, MA: Harvard University Press.

Winnicott, D. W. (1996). *Thinking about children*. London: Karnac Books.

Winnicott, D. W., & Winnicott, C. (1982). *Playing and reality*. London: Routledge.

C H A P T E R   T H R E E

What Would Superman Do?

Cory A. Nelson

Every good superhero story and every superhero has an origin. So, too, does the What Would Superman Do? (WWSD) technique. Although my personal interest in superheroes dates to early childhood, my professional interest stems from a unique early clinical experience. Soon after beginning employment as a home-based therapist, I began treatment with an 8-year-old boy and his family. I was to be the third therapist from the same agency to work with the family, the others being shifted to different portions of our seven-county coverage area. This boy and his family are discussed in greater detail in the case study that follows. Suffice to say that on the day before a breakthrough session with him, this boy had seen the movie *Steel*, named for the protagonist who was one of the characters that replaced Superman following his death in the early 1990s. Steel, who wears a suit of armor of his own design, is a good man with a great deal of love for his family and community. Surprisingly, the client was drawn to this character, because he seemingly did everything in his power to provoke chaos in his family. Together we wondered what Steel might do in particularly difficult or challenging situations and would later use the character to help bring about change in this child—and ultimately in his family.

Around that time, his sister, who was involved in a church youth group, began wearing a "WWJD" (What Would Jesus Do?) bracelet. Intrigued by this notion, I similarly wondered what Superman might do in difficult situations and was particularly interested in Superman because of his goodness, strength, and infallibility, as well as the fact that he is probably the closest character to Jesus in superhero mythology. From this line of reasoning was born the technique I call "What Would

Superman Do?" that has been used with a number of children diagnosed with attention-deficit/hyperactivity disorder (ADHD), oppositional defiant disorder (ODD), and anxiety issues. Although Superman may at first seem too familiar and his plotlines too scripted to be useful as a therapeutic resource, quite the opposite is true. It is because of limited recent exposure in video games and movies, compared with blockbuster heroes such as Spiderman and the X-Men, that he is less likely to be chosen by my clients as their favorite.

SUPERHEROES IN CLINICAL PRACTICE

Since their inception in the early part of the 20th century, comic books were children's primary source of access to superheroes. That has changed a great deal in the past few decades and has been reflected in fewer comic book retailers. There have, however, been some signs that the comic book industry is attempting to reverse this trend (Dean, 2002).

In the so-called silver age of comics, they could be purchased anywhere—from grocery to book stores. Now it is difficult to find comic books for sale outside of a specialty comic or bookstore or at a comics convention. The escalating cost of an average comic book may also have contributed to children and teens choosing to spend their money on more dynamic, stimulating, and interactive forms of media such as action figures, video and role-playing games, or movies, or they may choose simply to watch television.

Cartoons now appear to be the venue through which most of my clients come into contact with superheroes. Cartoon Network has popularized many of the traditional superheroes including Batman, Superman, the Justice League, Teen Titans, and Static. Additionally, recent blockbuster movies such as *Batman Begins, The Fantastic Four, X-Men I–III and Superman Returns* have greatly expanded the penetration of superheroes into popular culture. Before the first *Spiderman* movie, it was not uncommon for a young client to be unfamiliar with this superhero.

As the only male therapist at an agency covering seven counties in a Midwestern state, my caseload comprises primarily boys. As a result, WWSD has been used most often in the treatment of boys ranging in age from 7 to 13 years. Although the technique has also been applied with female clients—most recently with a girl experiencing anxiety related to her parent's divorce—the larger readership among my clients is male. Additionally, although superheroines have been featured in increasing numbers in comic books and movies, there still appear to be more male than female superheroes, and males are usually depicted as more powerful. Female superheroes have been described as being more intelligent (Young, 1993) than their male counterparts, but they are simply not as physically powerful and for this reason may not appeal as much to boys. Many well-known female superheroes such as She-Hulk and Cat Woman either debuted as sidekicks to or spin-offs of their male counterparts (Fingeroth, 2004). Additionally, although several female superheroes work alone, most of the more popular ones, such as Storm and Invisible Girl, work with a team, and even fewer have a comic book dedicated to their solo adventures. An easy way to illustrate that superheroes such as Superman are geared more toward male readers is to visit the toy aisle in any department or superstore in search of action figures. On a given day, and depending on what movie is in vogue, it can be difficult to find female action figures.

In the past, virtually every square inch of my office was filled with comic books, *Star Wars* posters, comic book posters, and action figures— a virtual sensory overload! Concerned that this might overly influence my client's choice of play material, I have scaled back so that every hero is represented only once, rather than three or four times. Some of my clients will freely look around the office, not saying much or simply asking questions about what they see. Some will spot a superhero or two with whom they are familiar and begin to ask questions about the ones they do not know. Consistently, and whether or not they are familiar with the various superheroes, they want to know about the heroes' powers, weaknesses, and origins. In the rare instance of not being able to find their favorite superhero, they tell me all about the hero and why he or she is important.

It is the children who spontaneously express or demonstrate an interest in the superheroes to whom I introduce WWSD. Because these particular children are already both familiar and comfortable with superheroes, they are also receptive to the idea of using them in treatment.

WWSD is not a technique that I expect to work with all clients in all situations. It is simply one, albeit a favorite, resource in my therapeutic toolbox. In the past, colleagues have asked me if hundreds of dollars are required to purchase action figures and comic books for therapeutic display and use. The answer that I offer is, "Not at all!" I have done therapeutic home visits with as few as two or three superhero action figures, with which I was easily able to gauge the client's receptivity and comfort level. It is certainly important, although not crucial, that the therapist have at least some familiarity with the superheroes that he or she brings into the playroom. Before discussing how I have used the WWSD technique in clinical practice, it is important to first present a brief overview of Adlerian theory, as it forms the basis of my application of the technique.

ADLERIAN THERAPY—AN OVERVIEW

One of the central elements of Adlerian theory is the notion of social interest—that we are socially embedded (Ansbacher & Ansbacher, 1956; Dinkmeyer, Dinkmeyer, & Sperry, 1987). This is consistent with the story line of many superheroes, who, although possessed with extraordinary powers, do not typically perceive themselves to be better than anyone else. They do acknowledge, however, that their unique gifts can benefit others, and as a result, they set forth to make the world a better place, although always struggling to fit into the society they serve.

The family is the first social group to which a child belongs. If unable to establish a positive connection to the family, the child may turn to negative ways of fitting into it. The manner in which the child ultimately establishes a place and role in the family determines his or her "lifestyle," which comprises self-perception, a worldview, and an interpersonal style (Kottman, 1995). As the child begins to engage in social relationships outside of the family, they apply this lifestyle; sometimes in an adaptive fashion and other times in a maladaptive way.

Many families develop a set of expectations about who a child is and what they can expect behaviorally from her. These expectations can isolate the child in a psychological "box," which then sets additional limits on his or her lifestyle and is, more often than not, psychologically confining (Kottman, 1995).

From an Adlerian perspective, behavior is goal-directed. Rudolf Dreikurs identified four primary motivations for children's misbehavior—attention, power, revenge, and proving inadequacy (Dreikurs & Soltz, 1964). Several years later, Dinkmeyer and McKay (1989) identified four goals that motivate positive behaviors. These included attention, involvement, and contribution; autonomy and self-responsibility; justice and fairness; and the avoidance of conflict and acceptance of other people's opinions. According to these Adlerian-based authors, the majority of children referred to work toward improving their behavior. The goal of the Adlerian psychotherapist is to assist clients in moving from the maladaptive to healthy goals and behaviors.

SUPERHEROES AND THE PHASES
OF ADLERIAN THERAPY

Adlerian therapy is comprised of four phases. The first phases centers around establishing the therapeutic relationship, which forms the foundation for all future interactions. The development of a relationship between the client and therapist is considered integral to a successful outcome. When beginning to work with a client, it is only after I believe that a relationship is being established that I begin to consider whether the WWSD technique would be effective. One of the considerations in this decision is the extent to which I have developed a sufficient appreciation for and understanding of the client's needs and interests. A client without any interest in superheroes would not likely benefit from pretending to be a superhero when faced with a challenge.

The second phase of Adlerian therapy involves exploring the client's lifestyle. In her book *Partners in Play,* Terry Kottman (1995) offered a list of lifestyle questions for both parent and child. These questions focus on such issues as family atmosphere and constellation, school functioning, social interactions, feelings, and both the child's and parent's goals for each other. During the course of the lifestyle interview, clients who are interested in superheroes might be asked what super power they might want to possess, what they would do with those powers, and how those powers might change their or someone else's life.

The third phase of Adlerian therapy involves helping the client to gain insight into his or her lifestyle. According to Kottman (1995, p. 149), "the counselor's goal is to help children better understand the goals of their behavior; their basic convictions about themselves, others, and the world; and the behaviors they use to gain significance and a sense of belonging." Through role-playing and a discussion of the client's perceived traits and those of the superhero that he discussed earlier, the client's maladaptive perceptions and interactions can be explored. It is also during this phase of therapy that bibliotherapy is used to help a child develop insight, consider a different perspective, or learn alternate ways of interacting (Muro & Kottman, 1995). In using bibliotherapy, it is important to choose books that are developmentally appropriate, engaging, relevant to, and relate directly to their life situation (Hynes & Hynes-Berry, 1986; Shrank, 1982).

A number of comic books specifically address sexual and physical abuse, but it may be particularly helpful to use specific comic books to showcase superhero traits and the lifestyles that they lead. Certain superheroes lend themselves well to particular types of clients. *Impulse* is relevant to the psychological issues experienced by clients with ADHD, *The Incredible Hulk* can assist with anger management, and the issue of the *Amazing Spider-Man* in which he sifts through the rubble of the World Trade Center after September 11 can be used to understand the ugliness behind fears related to terrorism. It is helpful to have copies of comics relevant to a broad range of clinical issues in the office at any given time.

The use of superheroes in assisting clients to gain insight is similar to the cartoon interventions described by Crowley and Mills (1989). In the cartoon intervention, a child is asked to draw cartoon helpers who can help them with their problems. The cartoon then becomes a vehicle or metaphor for suggesting various ways to perceive self, others, and the world. Children can then use the cartoons to find their own ways to deal with their problems.

The final phase of Adlerian therapy is to reorient and reeducate the client. According to Kottman (1995), "The main goals of therapy during the reorientation/reeducation phase of Adlerian play therapy are for children to learn and practice new ways of (a) viewing themselves, others, and the world; (b) behaving in various situations; and (c) relating to other people" (p. 181).

It is during this phase that clients are aided in generating alternative thoughts, feelings, and actions; are taught new skills and behaviors; and are encouraged to practice their new skills and behaviors both inside and outside of the therapy session. It is in this phase that clients are asked to begin to act like a favorite hero or a hero that they have created. Using the persona of the hero aids the client in coming up with alternative behaviors, feelings, and thoughts.

Reorientation and reeducation also leads to termination of therapy as clients demonstrate evidence that they have changed their lifestyle, and their goals for behavior have shifted from negative to positive.

WHAT WOULD SUPERMAN DO?

Heroes and Antiheroes

Once a therapeutic relationship has been established, the therapist can consider whether the WWSD technique is appealing to the client. In this context, clients are first asked to identify a favorite superhero and to explain why that character is important to them. I have had several clients who do not identify with superheroes; rather, they choose villains or a group I refer to as "antiheroes." The villains speak for themselves; they are usually egomaniacs bent on world domination, or at very least, on destroying their nemesis—a superhero. The antihero is more difficult to define. In the black and white, good and evil world of superheroes, the antihero blurs the boundaries between right and wrong. These are heroes for whom the end justifies the means—at any cost. Often, the antihero has no qualms about killing if it helps achieve his or her mission.

In my clinical work, some of the more common antiheroes include the *Punisher*, a man fighting a war on crime by killing those he judges to be guilty; the *Crow*, a man resurrected from the grave to avenge his and his fiancée's deaths, and *Spawn*, a trained killer who is murdered and strikes a deal with the Devil, allowing his return to Earth in exchange for the promise to lead the armies of hell against those of heaven. In using several of these antiheroes, I have found that many parents have been disturbed by Spawn because of his hellish origins. Although some of the other, more traditional and commonly known superheroes such as Batman did experience a vengeance-driven phase, this motif is more consistent with the antihero.

When clients choose a villain or antihero rather than a superhero, they are then engaged in a discussion of the attractiveness of the villain. Quite commonly, these particular clients' choice reflects identification with the villain that is rooted in the so-called box, or negative identity, that their family has ascribed to them. Once this process of identification is accomplished, the client can step out of that box within the safe confines of the therapy session, and they often then choose a superhero. In the event that clients remain steadfast in their choice of a villain, that character's positive traits can be identified. With most villains, positive attributes are few and far between, in which case, the WWSD may not be appropriate.

When a client does choose to work with an antihero, the next step is to fully discuss the character and the client's identification with the need and desire for vengeance. I describe the antihero's mission and ask the client what he anticipates happening to the antihero once the mission is completed. With some of these antiheroes, clients comes to realize that the mission will never be completed (the *Punisher* will never eliminate all crime in the world), and the antihero will go through the remainder of life perpetually angry and unhappy. Clients can then be engaged in a discussion of what their life would be like if their own needs for vengeance against the people in their world who have wronged them were satisfied. As an example, with one such client, I used a comic book in which a boy was abused and picked on by his teachers, peers, and father. The character awakens one morning with super strength. Although he successfully slaughters all of these villains, he is apprehended and comes to realize what he has done. He then experiences a great deal of guilt and remorse. Use of such a technique, allows for a therapeutic discussion about how vengeance does not always make a person's world better—just the opposite. If such a client chooses to retain the antihero, we proceed in a similar fashion.

Choosing the Hero

Once the client chooses a superhero, a list of personality traits is created by addressing a number of questions including but not limited to the following:

- Is the hero honest?
- How does the hero treat other people?

- Does the hero do things for personal gain or because they are the right things to do?
- What are the hero's weaknesses?
- What are the hero's superpowers and abilities? Is the hero reliable?
- Does the hero appear brave?
- Is the hero fair?
- Does the hero make the community better?
- Does the hero help those in need?
- Why does the hero do what he or she does?

If a client has difficulty deciding on the qualities of a particular hero, the therapist may introduce movie clips, cartoons, and selected comic books that demonstrate the hero not only using his or her powers, but also exhibiting the heroic morals code and character.

After the list of heroic qualities is completed, clients are asked to identify their own personality traits, reflected in how they treat others, their motivation for some of the ways they act in different situations, whether they are reliable, and the extent to which they do or do not help others. In doing so, clients begin to conceptualize themselves through the lens of the superhero with whom they identify. When processing clients' lists, it may also be helpful to elicit perceived strengths and weaknesses from family members, school personnel, and others involved in their treatment. This allows clients, who may perceive themselves only in negative terms, to appreciate that they also possess positive attributes. After the two lists have been completed, clients and therapists compare their own and the hero's traits. It is around this time that clients are asked to discuss what they would change in their own self-description, so that they could be more like the superhero with whom they identify.

An Example—Impulse

I have successfully used the superhero Impulse in my work with clients diagnosed with ADHD. Impulse, grandson of the second Flash, was born with super speed and an absence of helpful caregivers. Raised in a virtual-reality environment, he did not learn that there were consequences for any of his actions. When something went wrong, the computer program simply reset itself. Ultimately, Impulse was transported back in time to the present and raised by another person with super speed, who helped him to think before he acted.

The *Impulse* comic book has been particularly effective with middle-school-age children. Despite his great speed, Impulse's alter ego, Bart Allen, must perform daily activities at regular speed and sit through seemingly endless and boring classes. He is ultimately cast as a day-dreamer. His lack of focus and attention result in numerous school-based problems, including frequent trips to the principal's office and being terrorized by class and schoolmates. As the comic book series progresses, Bart begins to learn from his mentor Impulse, how to formulate a plan before rushing into action. In one of the story lines, Bart is confronted by several difficult decisions and must deliberate on each while considering both consequences and possible solutions. Clients with ADHD identify with these particular scenes and discuss how they have the ability to do what Impulse ultimately learns to do—plan ahead.

Who Was That Masked Man?

Once traits of the hero are compared and contrasted with those of the client, the discussion shifts to the alter egos of the hero. The therapist may address why many heroes choose not to have their identity known by the general public and how having a secret identity allows them to live normal lives when not acting as a hero and keeps their loved ones safe from reprisal.

It may also be pointed out that the hero continues to act heroically even when not in costume. Peter Parker would never shove an old lady in front of an oncoming subway train, Bruce Wayne would never rob a bank, and Clark Kent would not fight with a friend over a baseball game. In this vein, it may be useful to review some of the origin stories to appreciate how the heroes acted before they got their powers or before they put on their costume for the first time. It is important to stress to the client that these heroes were heroic long before they put on colorful costumes, that they received gifts and decided to do something to help others, and, to do that, they needed the hero identity.

Introducing the Most Daring Hero of All

The next step in the process is helping clients to design superheroes of their own making. Although existing superheroes are appealing in their own right, creation of an individualized and personalized character increases clients' investment in the process. This process is initiated by creating a name for the superhero, along with an origin story and an alter ego. Many times, clients pick a name that is similar to that of an existing hero, but then they choose additional unique characteristics. In designing the hero, a considerable amount of time should be spent discussing the heroes' powers and their purposes. Some heroes, such as Batman, have no super powers per se; however, they typically possess an array of gadgets that they use in fighting the forces of evil. If a client designs a hero who has no superpowers, they can be encouraged to create a number of these gadgets that contain unique characteristics.

Over the course of creating supercostumes with clients, I have encountered some very talented young artists who develop intricate designs. Some of these particularly creative and artistic clients have had difficulty committing their ideas to paper because they are unsure of their artistic abilities, as well as concerned how their work will be judged. When this occurs, I have used a boyhood toy called the Mighty Men and Monster Maker, which was produced by Tomy Toys in 1978. This toy contains tiles depicting legs, torsos, and heads that can be mixed and matched. Once the desired combination is found, the person using the toy puts in a piece of paper, rubs a crayon broadside over the paper that sits atop the tiles, and ends up with a picture of a mighty man, a monster, or some combination of both. This toy has allowed even the most artistically challenged client to create a colorful representation of their superhero (see Figure 3.1-The Mighty Men and Monster Maker kit).

The next step in the process is identification of the superhero's strengths and weaknesses. At this point, it is helpful to revisit the list of both clients' positive traits and those characteristics that clients would

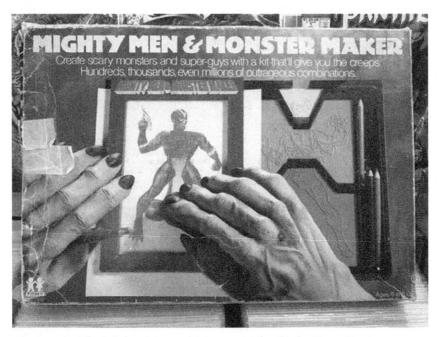

Figure 3.1   The Mighty Men and Monster Maker kit by Tomy Toys.

like to improve. The therapist may point out how clients' traits affect their life and how the proposed improvements can be implemented. Clients may be reminded that Superman's greatest weakness is kryptonite, the result of which is that he neither seeks it out nor stays around it by choice. He gets away and tries to stay away from it. In a similar way, if a client has a sibling who can become particularly agitating, the therapist can suggest that he or she simply treat the annoying sibling as Superman would treat kryptonite—by staying away until the annoying part is over. If it comes out again, it is time to leave before the annoying behavior elicits an aggressive response.

Role-playing is then used to help clients re-create and act out a life experience that was difficult for them and caused problems. For example, if a client regularly fights with a sibling(s), the therapist could portray that brother or sister while the client is encouraged to act like the superhero he created. He is then asked to reenact the scenario from the vantage point of his superhero. Once the client perceives some mastery over that situation, other problematic scenarios from his life can be role-played in a similar fashion, each time from the vantage point of their created superhero.

At the end of the role-playing for a particular session, clients are directed to try to act in superhero mode the next time that they are faced with a challenge at home, school, or elsewhere. I also discuss their secret identity and leave it up to them to decide whether they would like to tell others about their heroic alter ego. The session is ended by reminding the client how the heroes act when they are out of costume and how they acted before they became heroes. They are further reminded that no superhero was perfect when he or she first discovered their superpowers and that superheroes continue to improve themselves even after they begin their superheroic adventures. An excellent example of this point is a scene in the first *Spider-Man* movie in which he labors to perfect his web-casting ability.

In the sessions that follow, the client and therapist process how the WWSD technique was implemented and what changes, if any, they noticed in their interactions with others. Some of the more challenging moments from the week are then discussed, as is how the client's superhero alter ego handled the situation and how he might approach both similar and different situations in the future. Role-playing around those anticipated situations is then practiced. The entire process is then looped (reviewed) back a few steps while continuing to move it forward. As therapy progresses, challenging situations become less intense, less frequent, and a less disturbing experience for clients. Over the course of my own work with WWSD, I have observed that clients come to rely less and less on the superhero and increasingly on the secret identity. At this point, the therapeutic goal is for clients to understand that it is not only superheroes who possess the capacity for good deeds, the clients themselves do as well. It is important that clients begin to perceive themselves as agents for positive change and healthy relationships.

As clients continue to develop insight and skills, it is useful to revisit their superhero powers and gadgets. This allows them to revise their superheroes by either adding or deleting gadgets from their arsenal. With most clients, I have observed reduced reliance on gadgets, although some continue to augment their arsenal by adding superpowers. For example, after the death of his grandfather, one particular client added the superpower of being able to speak to the dead. Conversely, I have also had clients identify several weaknesses in their superhero and then eliminate them as therapy progressed. For example, one of my clients who regularly battled with his younger sibling described the annoyance as having the same effect on him that kryptonite has on Superman. As therapy progressed, this client's superhero was able to resist the urge to engage in these battles, and as a result, he was no longer weakened by his brother.

Precautions and Consultation

I am very conservative in considering whether to use WWSD when working with victims of trauma, particularly if there is evidence of dissociative symptoms. Under these circumstances, I may use comic books, but only as bibliotherapeutic resources. When I begin my therapeutic work with the technique, I routinely consult with the client's parents and school personnel to help them understand how he will be working with the superhero theme. It is important for these individuals to understand the WWSD so that they can be prepared for any behavioral changes that may occur, such as a boy wearing a towel on his head in attempts to emulate a particular superhero. I also stress to the parents and school staff that they may only acknowledge the client's superidentity if he reveals it to them. I do not reveal the name of the superhero because the client will do so when he deems it appropriate, or safe, to do so.

CASE STUDY

Background

Billy was an 8-year-old boy living in a small Midwestern town with his mother, stepfather, older and younger biological sisters, and two older stepsiblings. Billy had been placed at a regional children's hospital on two occasions when his behaviors became too much for his mother and other family members to handle. Billy was prone to anger outbursts in which he become physically assaultive toward whomever had triggered his rage or anyone who attempted to intervene. The only person Billy did not engage during such outbursts was his stepfather, who was very emotionally detached and who worked long hours to support the family. Billy's anger was directed primarily toward his younger sister, an older stepbrother, and his mother. These seemed to be the people who could instigate an anger response from Billy in the least amount of time. As part of his rages, Billy soiled himself and smeared the fecal material on the walls of the bathroom and his bedroom. This behavior worsened in direct relation to the intensity of his anger.

Before initiating his therapeutic contact with me, Billy had been prescribed several medications. When he began treatment with me, he was taking Adderall (amphetamine mixed salts) to control the symptoms of ADHD. His diagnosis was ADHD, ODD, encopresis, and a rule-out for bipolar disorder. Billy was seen every 8 weeks by his psychiatrist, whose office was 2 hours away.

Treatment Engagement and Early Obstacles

In the beginning phases of treatment, I worked individually with Billy twice weekly, visiting with him both at home and at school. Relatively few behavioral problems had been reported at the school; however, the personnel there knew he was having significant problems at home and therefore excused him from class for treatment. Although Billy had worked with other therapists before me, been hospitalized on two occasions, and frequently been threatened with additional hospitalization when he misbehaved, he warmed up to me surprisingly quickly. In retrospect, this quick attachment suggested a correspondingly weak bond with his family members.

Billy demonstrated good insight, reflected in his ability to identify the things that angered him and to generate alternatives to acting out. However, his ability to implement these strategies was limited. For example, when asked why he would remain in the living room when his sister was being mean to him instead of leaving as we had previously discussed, Billy would claim that he had forgotten our discussion. Therefore, we worked together to identify signals that alerted him to his developing anger so that he could avoid losing control of it. Approximately a month after therapy began, Billy had become more physical with and aggressive toward his siblings. To help him, I brought a bag of old magazines and told Billy to shred them as he felt his anger begin to build. This was not effective in the home because he refused to remove himself to the designated "shredding room." He had difficulty sufficiently containing the anger to redirect himself into the activity, let alone leave the room to do so. Role-playing and play therapy did not bring forth any more consistent of a response.

As I approached exhausting everything I could think of to help Billy and his family, he told me of a movie he had seen the day before called *Steel*. Billy, who was described by his mother as being incapable of concentrating for more than a few minutes—on anything—was able to provide me with a scene-by-scene recitation of the movie. His retelling of the movie was so detailed that it took up almost three-quarters of our scheduled session. I noted how excited he was when describing the movie and the superhero it portrayed.

"What Would Superman Do?" to the Rescue!

Billy and I continued our previous discussion of *Steel* and what he liked about the main character. Billy was particularly engaged by John Henry Irons, who upon witnessing injustice suffered by his family and neighbors, designed a supersuit and proceeded to protect those he cared for and eliminate threats to the neighborhood. Remembering that Billy's sister had shown me her WWJD (What Would Jesus Do?) bracelet before the beginning of the session, I asked Billy what he would do if he were Steel to protect his family. I then encouraged him to think about what Steel would do if his own sister was teasing him or if his stepbrother took something without asking. We then speculated on what Steel might act like when not wearing his supersuit, and came to the conclusion that superheroism comes from the inside, not from the costume. I ended the session by asking Billy to consider the question, "What would Steel do?" whenever he felt anger during the upcoming week.

Before the next meeting, I received a favorable report from Billy's mother, who indicated that although he had had a few instances of yelling and screaming, he did not become assaultive. Billy reported that he had tried to imagine what Steel might do and, as a result, had an easier time controlling his anger than he had experienced with previous interventions we attempted. Although Billy was able to make some different choices when he felt himself becoming angry, he did not know exactly what to do when it escalated. Therefore, we practiced relaxation exercises and decided that this was probably something Steel would do if he needed to protect loved ones.

Only the Shadow Knows

Fine-tuning of the process continued over the next several sessions until, finally, Billy reported that he wanted to create a superhero of his own. He had settled on a name—Shadow. Unlike Steel, this superhero wore no armor. Furthermore, Shadow did not have any superpowers to speak of. Instead, he had a number of gadgets that allowed him to fight crime and help those he cared about. As we talked about the hero Billy was creating, I focused on the gadgets and what those things meant to him. Shadow had a gadget that allowed him to fly and provided him with superstrength and invisibility, as well as the ability to breath underwater. Shadow also had a force field that protected him from all except his "inner circle" of family and friends. As Billy described the shield, it seemed as though his inner circle included much of the town. He soon realized that although the shield might indeed keep him safe, it would also prevent him from meeting anyone new. Billy decided to drop the force field from the Shadow's repertoire of gadgets and abilities.

The time came for Billy to design the Shadow. Neither he nor I were very artistic, and as previously mentioned, I drew on my childhood Mighty Men and Monster Maker that I had brought with me for that session. Billy chose a few looks for Shadow and used the toy to create a likeness of his hero. With that done, we discussed Shadow's origin story, what type of person he was, what his life had been like, and how he came to find or create his gadgets.

The origins of Shadow reflected Billy's own life and carried his name. Like Billy, Shadow lived in a blended family and struggled with anger. Shadow had found his first gadget in an old shed on the family property, where he fled after a fight with his mother. When turned on, the small box turned him into a shadow. In this state, he traveled throughout the town to discover what people thought of him. What Shadow found was that people seemed to like him but not his angry outbursts. As he was preparing to return to the shed, Shadow saw a group of older boys picking on a small child. Shadow intervened and frightened away the older boys. He returned to the shed and took the shadow box apart to find out how it worked. Once he saw the inner workings, he could visualize what he would need to do to create his own gadget. As Shadow's anger diminished, he became closer to family members, and they with each other. As a result, Shadow and his family moved from their small town to a small city nearby, where he continued to fight crime and stand up for the "little guy."

Billy and I discussed what Shadow was like when he was not being a hero. Like Steel, we decided that Shadow acted like a hero even when not in costume. Shadow put his family first. He was honest, brave, and smart. He only hurt people if there were no other way to deal with them, creating a gadget that would detain rather than hurt them until the police arrived. Shadow did not swear, was respectful of others, and worked hard in school to make his family proud of him. His family did not know about the superhero in their midst but did approve of what they had heard about the hero known as Shadow.

As we continued to work on Shadow, I asked Billy to put himself in the shoes of the hero he had created whenever faced with a challenge at home or school. By the time we had completely developed the character, Billy's behavior at home had greatly improved. He was catching himself before acting out and was more respectful in his interactions with everyone in the family. Because of this, the assaults on his family decreased to the point of a few minor episodes of retaliation against his sister for hitting him first. Interestingly, this sister began aggressing more toward Billy and others in the family, and as a result, his mother asked that I provide treatment to her after I finished with her son. The role of "identified patient" had apparently shifted to Billy's sister.

Transitions

Several things happened in quick succession following this series of events. Billy's mother and stepfather separated, with Billy, his sisters, and mother moving into a smaller house in the same town. His stepfather and stepsiblings moved a few hours away. Billy was initially abusive toward his sisters and mother; however, this was short-lived, and he otherwise handled the transition well. During this period, I initiated family therapy with those remaining in the household, focusing on communication and working through their feelings related to the separation.

As family treatment progressed in conjunction with Billy's individual therapy, his mother informed me that she and her husband had reconciled. The family would be reunited and would relocate to the town in which the stepfather and his children lived. This meant that Billy and his family would be moving out of our catchment area, and I had two remaining sessions to process termination. Although this was not the ideal way to end treatment, I did manage to sum up the work we had done together and how far Billy had come in just over a year by playacting a hero that he had created. By the last session, Billy's family reported that he was no longer disrespectful toward anyone in his family and no longer expressed his anger through aggression. We ended by bringing Shadow's story to an end; he was to move to a different home and city. I reminded Billy that he would be Shadow as long as he wanted and could continue to be what he wanted to be rather than what others expected him to be.

Billy did show substantial improvements in behaviors, remaining on his medications throughout therapy. During the year that Billy worked in therapy as Shadow, few adjustments were made to his medication.

Billy and Phases of Adlerian Therapy

Before implementing WWSD with Billy, I had been working with him for about 4 months. That allowed us to establish a therapeutic relationship, which is the first phase of Adlerian therapy. Billy trusted me as his therapist. If I had rushed through the first phase and not established a bond of trust, it is unlikely that therapy would have progressed. A large part of building that trust likely came from my talking with his mother about treatment options other than placing him back in a regional psychiatric hospital.

Much of the second phase of Adlerian therapy—exploration of the client's lifestyle—was also done in the first 4 months of therapy. Through interviews with Billy, his mother, and others in the family, I gained a better understanding of his patterns of thoughts and actions (his lifestyle) and was able to solidify progress before transitioning into the third phase of therapy.

It is in the third phase of therapy, during which the child gains insight into his lifestyle, that the WWSD technique was implemented. In Billy's case, his choice of Steel as a character gave me a glimpse of someone who was very concerned about being dedicated to his family. This insight into Billy's worldview had not been previously available. By going through and listing the traits of the hero Billy chose and a list of traits that he saw himself possessing, he gained a deeper awareness of the relation between his behavior and perceived role in the family. From that point, he was able to use what he knew about himself to begin to interact with the family in different ways.

The fourth phase of therapy, reorientation and reeducation, progressed as Billy created his own hero. The gadgets that Billy chose reflected some of the resources he felt he needed to function within his family. The gadgets that provided Billy with superstrength and protection were those resources needed to interact better with his family. Steel's ability to fly metaphorically reflected Billy's new real-life ability to leave a situation when he became angry and before he flew into a rage. As Billy's skills in dealing with the people in his life grew, his need for hero's gadgets diminished. He learned to rely on himself more and on his superhero less. In a sense, Billy was able to give up his transitional identity as his own matured.

Postscript

Billy was the first client with whom I used the WWSD technique. There have been some modifications in the process since that time. I now solicit more information about the client's interpretation of the hero and ask him to begin the creation process before considering what the hero would do in a similar situation. In Billy's case, the process was new, and I was eager to effect change for him and his family as quickly as possible. I have since come to learn that change does not always move at the speed of a superhero.

CONCLUSION

Superheroes are a part of our culture. Each time I speak about the "What Would Superman Do" technique, I begin the presentation by asking the audience to identify either their favorite superhero or a superpower they would like to have. I have yet to have someone be unable to come up with answers to either question.

We get to know these heroes when we are children. We marvel at their exploits, and some part of us identifies with their problems and sees a bit of ourselves in the hero. For most, this fades as we age, but the fondness often remains. I have had adult clients in their 60s spy an action figure in my office and talk about a time they followed that hero's exploits and what the hero meant to them.

In a society where we seem to have fewer and fewer people in the public spotlight whom our children can look up to, fictional heroes can bridge the gap between what is and what could be if every person were honest, brave, giving, dedicated, trustworthy, and kind. Seeing things and filtering them through a hero's moral code can allow a child to begin to work toward the goals of positive behavior and to view his or her life and circumstances in a different way.

REFERENCES

Ansbacher, H., & Ansbacher, R. (Eds.). (1956). *The individual psychology of Alfred Adler: A systematic presentation in selections from his writings*. San Francisco: Harper & Row.

Crowley, R., & Mills, J. (1989). *Cartoon magic: How to help children discover their rainbows within*. New York: Magination.

Dean, M. (2002). State of the comics industry 2002: Recovery of decline? *Comics Journal, 245*, 6–14.

Dinkmeyer, D., Dinkmeyer, D., & Sperry, L. (1987). *Adlerian counseling and psychotherapy* (2nd ed.). Columbus, OH: Merrill.

Dinkmeyer, D., & McKay, G. (1989). *The parent's handbook: Systematic training for effective parenting (STEP)* (3rd ed.). Circle Pines, MN: American Guidance Service.

Dreikurs, R., & Soltz, V. (1964). *Children: The challenge*. New York: Hawthorne/Dutton.

Fingeroth, D. (2004). *Superman on the couch: What superheroes really tell us about ourselves and our culture*. New York: Continuum Books.

Hynes, A., & Hynes-Berry, M. (1986). *Bibliotherapy: The interactive process*. Boulder, CO: Westview Press.

Kottman, T. (1995). *Partners in play: An Adlerian approach to play therapy*. Alexandria, VA: American Counseling Association.

Muro, J., & Kottman, T. (1995). *Guidance and counseling in elementary and middle schools: A practical approach.* Dubuque, IA: Brown & Benchmark.

Shrank, F. (1982). Bibliotherapy as an elementary school counseling tool. *Elementary School Guidance and Counseling, 16,* 218–227.

Young, T. (1993). Women as comic book super-heroes: The "weaker sex" in the Marvel universe. *Psychology: A Journal of Human Behavior, 30,* 49–50.

CHAPTER FOUR

Superheroes and Sandplay: Using the Archetype Through the Healing Journey

William McNulty

Fantasy play is a developmentally appropriate and natural form of communication for children. Children are able to displace and project feelings and behaviors that are too difficult to express or too frightening to confront in reality. Within the therapeutic relationship, fantasy play takes on a number of functions that support the development of the child. These include exploration of reality and social roles, mastery of stress and anxiety, and expression of wishes and fears (Davies, 2004). Fantasy play also represents the child's attempt to organize their experiences and may very well be one of the few times they feel more in control and thus more secure (Landreth, 2002).

Winnicott (1992) described play as a transitional activity that takes place in a zone between the individual's subjective and external realities. This subjective reality is a safer place for the children to explore the aspects of their external reality that are too painful or too difficult to confront directly. Play helps the child to create a bridge between the content of fantasy and what is experienced in real life. Within fantasy play, objects are used to embody various aspects of the child's personality that are too complex, unacceptable, and contradictory for them to handle. This permits the child's ego to gain mastery over these elements (Bettelheim, 1975).

Through fantasy play, the child develops and retains her fantasy world, her capacity for imagination, and learns to move comfortably between her inner life and her current reality (Chethik, 2000). This parallels the process that occurs in the sandtray between the client's unconscious inner world and the conscious world of the sandtray and reality.

SANDPLAY THERAPY

Margaret Lowenfeld, a British child psychiatrist, is credited with the development of the use of miniatures in a tray with sand. She based this idea on an H. G. Wells book *Floor Games*. In this book, Wells described a type of play that he and his two sons engaged in with a few wooden blocks and miniatures of people and animals. With these materials, they would play games and build cities and islands on the floor. Lowenfeld called this the World Technique. Dora Kalff, a Swiss analyst, began to study Lowenfeld's technique at the encouragement of Carl Jung, her teacher. She adapted this technique to her own analytic training with a major difference being that, unlike Lowenfeld, she did not interpret the trays. She called her technique sandplay therapy. Sandplay is a nonverbal form of therapy that is said to reach the preverbal level of the psyche through the use of active imagination (Weinrib, 1983). Sandplay therapy is different from sandtray therapy in that sandtray therapy is a more generic term referring to a variety of effective ways of using sand, figures, and a container from different theoretical perspectives (Cunningham, 2005).

The tools of the sandplay process include a tray, sand, and several miniatures representing various categories including people, animals, buildings, vehicles, natural objects, fantasy, and furniture. Each sandplay miniature collection is unique, and personal, communicating the psyche and unconscious of the therapist to the sandplayer (Hegen, 2005). This collection will grow and change as the therapist evolves both as a person and as a clinician. The collection is said to be a living extension of the container (therapist) and the environment (Turner, 2005). The collection is arranged on shelves depending upon the personal taste of the therapist. Some use groupings according to categories such as animals and people, and others group according to developmental level with easy access to certain types of figures according to the age of the client.

The traditional sandtray, as originally described by Kalff is 28.5 inches long by 19.5 inches wide by 3 inches deep. It is meant to hold a person's steady gaze, which may encourage concentration and intensification of the psyche's energies and pull it toward centering (Cunningham, 2005). The size of the tray also facilitates a relaxation of the hold on conscious awareness and allows access to less conscious perceptions, which emanate from the central archetype of the self (Turner, 2005). By having the client focus on the experience of working in the tray, they may be more able to tap into unconscious materials. This "in-between space" of the tray, a term coined by Ruth Ammann (1991), is where the client's inner and outer life can develop and reveal itself, which makes the tray therapeutic. The sides and bottom of the tray are blue to represent the sky or water. The blue is a natural and neutral color so that it does not influence the client in either a positive or a negative way.

The sand is probably the most important component of the process. It is seen as cleansing, healing, sacred, and grounding (Turner, 2005). The sand can be used by the client in either dry or wet form. The client can choose to solely work with the sand in the tray instead of utilizing the objects. Using wet sand is an invitation by the ego to engage in unconscious materials in a more intimate way (Turner, 2005). The symbolic meaning of adding water is that the water is absorbed into the sand and thus goes physically deeper into the tray. Clients decide when they are ready to engage in this deepening process. With these objects, the client and therapist work together through the relationship to explore unconscious processes by creating a concrete manifestation of their inner world.

Kalff (1991) suggested that within the unconscious, there is, given the proper conditions, an autonomous tendency for the psyche to heal itself and grow toward fullness and balance (Weinrib, 1983). These proper conditions that are needed are present in the atmosphere that the therapist creates through the relationship with the client. This is called a "free and protected space" and is defined as an atmosphere of letting clients know that they are free to do what they want to do within the frame of the tray without being punished or criticized by the therapist (Bradway & McCoard, 1997). The therapist does not confront or interpret anything that the client does in the tray, only holding the therapeutic space so that it is seen as protected and safe. Thus, the role of the therapist is to listen, observe, and serve as a psychological container for the emotional content that becomes activated by the sandplay process. This is similar to Rogers's (1980) concept of *unconditional positive regard* that is a positive, accepting attitude toward whatever the client is at that moment. This sacred space created through the relationship and the environment is referred to as the *temenos*. When the client develops a sense of trust through the development of the therapeutic relationship, she or he can begin to use the symbols that are present in their personal and the collective unconscious.

Therapeutic Benefits of Sandplay Therapy

A question that one may ask is, "Why sandplay therapy?" Labovitz-Boik & Goodwin (2000) explored this question in their book *Sandplay Therapy*. This technique frees creativity, inner feelings, perceptions, and memories, bringing them into outer reality and providing a concrete form of their issues. This happens as their unconscious materials are brought into a three-dimensional view. It also creates bridges from the unconscious to the conscious, from the inner to the outer world, and from the nonverbal to the verbal. Thus, it can allow hidden materials to become revealed to the client. This is developed through the safety of the therapeutic relationship. The defenses of the client are allowed to diminish because the process can be nonthreatening. Because the process is mostly nonverbal, clients may view the time as playing and not involving disclosure of threatening materials. Sandplay also functions as a natural language for children and a common one for use with diverse cultures and developmental stages. Because of the variety of symbols used, the psyche of the clients with various cultural backgrounds can use images that are personal to their own experience to assist them with their healing. Finally, the process empowers clients by allowing movement from the position of victim to creator, and by affecting the course of therapy. As a creator, clients can feel as though they are in charge of the experience and begin to make changes in their lives.

Creating a sandtray is in itself a symbolic and creative act. If it happens within this free and protected space, "symbolic active fantasizing by the client stimulates the imagination, freeing neurotically fixated energy and moving it into creative channels, which in itself can be healing" (Weinrib, 1983, p. 39). Thus, engaging in the process of sandplay can be helpful in allowing clients to begin to work on issues that brought them into the therapeutic relationship. Children have a natural tendency to want to play. The sandplay process is said to facilitate healing and transformation by bringing up conflicts from the unconscious in symbolic form and by allowing a healthy reordering of psychological contents (Turner, 2005). This reordering is the "transcendent function" of ego, which is considered to be significant in Jung's theory of the self. It is defined as the ability to climb across, or transcend, the gap between the opposing positions of consciousness and the unconscious in adaptive and psychic crises (Turner, 2005). With the transcendent function, the new psychic energy or new conscious attitude is released through the external symbols used in the process of sandplay and makes change possible in client's behavior.

There are two types of unconscious material that clients may tap into while engaging in the sandplay process. The first is the personal unconscious, which is created by repression of personal events that are too painful or anxiety-provoking for conscious processing. It also includes content that has lost its intensity and were forgotten or were never full of intensity but still reached the psyche (Jung, 1960/1981). The second type of unconscious material is the collective unconscious, which is made up of instincts and archetypes. This contains the whole spiritual heritage of mankind's evolution (Turner, 2005). It appears to consist of mythological motifs or primordial images, which are inherited (Jung, 1960/1981). These forms of the unconscious are accessed through dreams, free association, and sandplay. Images and symbols are the language of the unconscious that the individual utilizes during the sandplay process. The ego of the client must be sufficiently sturdy to withstand the assaults of the unconscious and flexible enough to undergo changes. The ego strength of many children may be tenuous, and their defenses may not yet be in place (Labovitz-Boik & Goodwin, 2000). The presence of the therapist may be enough to help aid in making sturdy the client's ego as it is being reconstructed through the process of sandplay. If the process of sandplay is meant to help relax an overly rigid ego, the therapist's presence may be sufficient to help contain and hold the process for the client. It is for the therapist to determine whether the client's ego has enough strength and is able to undergo the process of change.

The ego is an active complex and is the executive organ of consciousness. The ego's function is both to recognize and assimilate the external and internal realms, and to translate the world we experience into manageable, coherent reality (Turner, 2005). Thus, we can say that the ego is the means by which individuals understand what takes place in the world around them each day. With the ego's drive to self-actualize, the constellation of the self becomes reordered to the central archetype of the self (Turner, 2005). In other words, the ego begins to become healthy and allows the changes to take place in the person and the structures of the psyche change as a result of placing the unconscious into concrete representations through the sandplay.

In sandplay, the client uses various three-dimensional representations in the form of objects with which they choose to work. Through this process, the unconscious begins to develop representations of its content through the symbols it chooses.

> Symbols that are used in sandplay are formed when psychic energy builds up and is forced down to the collective unconscious because of a crisis. The self finds an archetype that corresponds to the crisis. The symbol is based upon personal and cultural experiences. (Turner, 2005, p. 33)

The ego, through the unconscious, does the work for the client in that when it is sturdy enough, it will allow the conflict to be materialized in conscious awareness through the symbol. Symbols represent internal energy-bearing images for dispositions of humanness which, if they become visible, exert a continuing influence on the human being's development (Kalff, 1991). Through the work being done in the tray, clients develop strengths that allow them to grow and change. The symbol also bridges the ego's original misaligned position with the self and the resultant compensatory product from the unconscious providing a new perspective on how to deal with the crisis (Turner, 2005). Thus, the person's ego is better able to deal with the crisis because of the more healthy and adaptive position that result for the ego.

An archetype, which represents an underlying and universal theme, is different from a symbol which is a merely a component of the archetype. The symbols that are chosen are personal to clients and based on their own life experiences. The self is the central archetype that contains the patterns of possibility and potential for that particular person. How the particular archetype shows up is influenced by culture and the personality of the group or the individual (Turner, 2005). Archetypes are the crystallized essence, or seeds, of psychic experience. They are the essential patterns of psychic experience and should be distinguished from the images that are associated with them (Turner, 2005). The stories of mythology and the themes present are representations of archetypes that have lasted throughout time.

Children and Sandplay

Frequently, parents, schools, pediatricians, and other organizations, refer children experiencing a range of behavioral and emotional problems. Sandplay is an ideal way of working with children because it allows them to access thoughts and feelings without directly confronting these difficulties. There are several issues when working with children that differ from sandplay work with adults. The first is introducing the process of sandplay. Most of the time, this is not a difficult process. The therapist gives them the basics such as introducing the tray, talking about the sand as being wet or dry, showing the bottom of the tray as being blue, telling them they can make a picture in the sand with the toys, and discussing how they can play safely with the sand (Turner, 2005). This introduction serves two functions: to explain the purpose of the play and to establish boundaries with the clients.

Different from adults and depending on the developmental level, children may play in an interactive way in the sand. This many times involves frequent movements of objects and sometimes trying to engage the therapist. This behavior is more frequently seen in younger children usually below age 6. This is because the development of representational play cannot take place until the child's cognitive skills have reached this level. After the age of 6 or 7, the child can make a scene that holds its own action and relationship without the child physically animating it (Turner, 2005). When a child does invite the therapist to engage in the play, it is up to the therapist to use his or her clinical judgment as to how they should participate. One option is to begin by attempting to reflect verbally on what is going on in the tray. This can help to refocus the child back into the tray and remind them that it is their work. There are times when the child will insist that the therapist take part in the tray. Again, the therapist must use caution so as not to interfere in the child's process.

There are some common patterns that may be seen in a child's tray. This can be understood through the Kalff's phases of ego development. She combined her own observations of sandtrays and Neumann's (1973) phases of ego development. The first phase, called animal–vegetative, is named for the child client's use of vegetation and animals. This phase usually takes place between the ages of 6 to about 8 years but can take place at any age or developmental level. The presence of vegetation can suggest activation of the inner forces of psychological growth (Bradway & McCoard, 1997). The second phase, called 'battle or fighting phase', usually involves two opposing forces in the tray. This usually occurs between the age of 9 and 11. In this stage, children may engage the therapist as an opponent in the scene in the tray (Bradway & McCoard, 1997). They may also alternate between negative and positive feelings toward the therapist, perhaps as the result of power struggles. This coming together of opposite feelings, attitudes, and objects represents the client's recognition of these oppositions and a moving closer to wholeness. The final phase, called *adaptation to the collective,* is when the psyche takes its place outside in reality and ordinary life (Turner, 2005). This usually takes place between ages 11 and 12. In this phase, the scenes in the tray usually reflect those of ordinary life, such as towns, villages, and other outward reality. The child's ego has integrated what it has learned and comes to a temporary rest.

In sum, sandplay with children can facilitate the therapeutic process. The children typically do not need any introduction to the process. Therapists usually employ the process in combination with other techniques as they move with the client toward healing. The theoretical underpinning is based on Jung's idea that a person's psyche has an autonomous tendency to heal itself and move toward balance. The process itself is done with the use of sand, a tray, miniatures, and sometimes water. The therapist is meant to be a psychological container who employs the techniques of active listening, nonverbal communication, and silence. Sandplay is a nonverbal, nonconfrontational way of working out difficulties for the client.

MYTHOLOGY AND THE HERO'S JOURNEY

Myths are the story or language of the unconscious. The overall sand-play process is mythic because it holds the psyche's movement toward wholeness (Turner, 2005). Fantasy figures such as superheroes can be representations of important individuals in the client's life. They can also represent aspects of the "self" that are both positive and negative. The collective unconscious holds these universal myths and archetypes and allows the client to access them through the sandplay process. The use of superheroes in fantasy play lends itself particularly well to helping children with the various problems that they bring into the therapy room. This is because of the unique qualities and powers that each superhero possesses and what the particular superhero represents in our modern society. With the popularity of superheroes in the media, these mythological icons are easily recognizable and become an valuable tool for children to use within the therapeutic process. These heroes have become the equivalent to the heroes and gods of ancient mythology such as Hercules, Gilgamesh, and Zeus. The heroic myth and its symbolic representations assists in the development of the individual's awareness of her own strengths and weaknesses, in a manner that will equip her for the arduous tasks in life. (Campbell, 1956). This is done through the ego making conscious the archetypal materials that have been previously unconscious.

Joseph Campbell (1956) explored and examined myths from around the world and proposed that stories of various cultures are fundamentally the same, a concept he called the *monomyth*. Monomyth is a term originally coined by James Joyce. Campbell based this on Jung's notion that archetypes are the underlying structure of all myths. These basic elements of the myth transcend individual cultures and specific periods of time, making them universal and timeless. He saw the role of the hero as the symbol of the self and the adventure a symbol of life (Indick, 2004). The monomyth is broken down into three basic stages that are further divided into substages describing the journey of the hero. The first stage, *Departure,* signifies that destiny has summoned the hero and transferred his spiritual center of gravity from society to the unknown zone (Campbell, 1956). It is divided into the call to adventure, the refusal of the call, supernatural aid, the crossing of the first threshold, and the belly of the whale. The second stage, *Initiation,* is when the hero enters into the darkness, goes through the trials of the adventure, is aided by his supernatural helpers, and gains their reward. It involves the road of trials, the meeting with the goddess, woman as the temptress, atonement with the father, apotheosis, and the ultimate boon. In the final stage, *The Return,* Campbell articulates three possible scenarios. After attaining enlightenment, the hero could refuse the return and remain in the realm of the gods or go to another place to exist. This is because the hero may believe that the other world could not understand the newly obtained wisdom. The hero could choose to return to make humanity better and thus save the world. Finally, the hero could be brought back to the world from the new realm by someone in the realm of humanity. This return is forced because the hero is needed.

Spider-Man as Contemporary Superhero Monomyth

A contemporary example of the monomyth is the superhero Spider-Man. Originally created by Stan Lee and his partner Jack Kirby, Spider-Man first appeared in 1962 in the comic *Amazing Fantasy #15,* and the character's own series began the following year. William Indick (2004) outlines the story of Spider-Man in the context of Campbell's Heroes Journey. In Stage 1, Peter Parker is orphaned after his parents, Richard Parker and Mary Fizpatrick-Parker, are killed in a plane crash that was arranged by Albert Malik, the *Red Skull.* After their death, he is raised by Aunt May and Uncle Ben in the Forest Hills neighborhood of Queens, New York. Peter is described as a lonely weakling who is unpopular with peers and who is often bullied. At 16 years old, while on a class field trip to a Columbia University Lab, he is bitten by a genetically engineered mutant spider. As a result, he is given supernatural powers of a spider *(Supernatural Aid).* He designs a costume and adopts the identity of Spider-Man to win money as a wrestler.

The *Call to Adventure* begins for Peter when, after a wrestling match, he refuses to stop a thief that ran past him in a hallway, insisting that he was only going to look out for "number one." This *Refusal of the Call* leads to the death of his Uncle Ben by the same man that he allowed to pass him in the hallway. He comes to the realization that even with all of his superpowers, he could not have saved his uncle. Inspired by his uncle's last words, "With great power comes great responsibility," he dons his costume and seeks revenge on the man who killed his uncle, which is the moment of *Crossing the First Threshold.* The entering of the *Belly of the Whale* is when the hero, in passing the threshold, goes inward, undergoes a metamorphosis, and is born again. In the case of Peter, he must give up the idea that he is a normal man with responsibilities only to himself and don the Spider-Man costume, and he now has responsibilities to society.

In Stage 2, *Initiation,* Peter begins the *Road of Trials* by taking on the task of fighting criminals in New York City as his alter ego, Spider-Man. He encounters a wisewoman who is able to give him guidance as to what his purpose will be in life. He has a *Meeting with a Goddess,* his Aunt May, who inspires him with the phrase, "You were meant for great things." With his road of trials well on its way, Peter soon meets his *Woman as a Temptress,* Mary Jane Watson. His pursuit of Mary Jane takes him away from his road of trials and leads him into danger as his nemesis, the Green Goblin, uses her to force him into a final confrontation. During this confrontation, Peter undergoes his *Apotheosis,* the symbolic death and spiritual rebirth, in which he almost dies. He then *Atones with the Father (figure),* his Uncle Ben, by destroying his negative father figure the Green Goblin, Norman Osborn. This occurs when the Green Goblin tells Spider-Man, "I've been like a father to you." Spider-Man replies, "I have a father. His name is Ben Parker." The *Ultimate Boon* occurs in the form of an epiphany that Peter has when he realizes that the powers he has been given are meant to be in the service of others, and it seems that this may be at the cost of what he would like his life to become.

In Stage 3, *Return,* Peter enters into the *Refusal of the Return,* where he refuses to return to his superhero role of Spider-Man. A twist to his story is that he begins to lose his superpowers, a symptom of the seeming conflict between his desire to be normal and his destiny as a superhero. The *Magic Flight,* or his return to fighting crime as Spider-Man, is symbolically seen as he regains his powers and swings on his webs across the New York City. The *Rescue From Without* is described as being captured by an enemy only to be helped by him later. This occurs when Spider-Man is captured and delivered to Harry Osborn, who wanted revenge for the death of his father. Spider-Man is let go by Harry Osborn, and he is told where Mary Jane is being held by the villain, Doc Ock. Spider-Man enters into *Crossing of the Threshold* after he has returned as Spider-Man and risks his life to save the people on a runaway subway train. He ends up in a crucifixion pose that symbolically represents his role as divine and superhero. In the final battle with Doc Ock, Spider-Man is unmasked, and his true identity is revealed to Mary Jane. With his two identities revealed, he defeats the villain and is victorious in that he is accepted by the public as their hero and loved by Mary Jane. Thus, he has become the *Master of the Two Worlds*—his public life as Peter Parker and his private life as Spider-Man. In the end, the *Freedom to Live* has been achieved because Peter has the ability to live as the superhero Spider-Man, who protects the city with his superpowers that have been given to him, and as Peter Parker, the student and newspaper photographer who can have a relationship with Mary Jane Watson.

Batman as Contemporary Superhero Monomyth

Another example of the monomyth that is used later in this chapter is Batman. Originally created by Bob Kane, he first appeared in 1939 in *Detective Comics*. Batman has undergone a transformation in character over the years in the comic, television, and film genres. When first introduced in the comic books, the character was a violent avenger who carried a gun and killed the majority of his foes, but over the years he was transformed into a crime-fighting superhero who works in conjunction with the police of Gotham City.

In Stage 1, the *Departure,* Bruce Wayne receives a *Call to Adventure* at age 8 when he witnesses his parent's death at the hands of a small-time criminal named Joe Chill. As his story progresses, the reader learns that his parents were set up to be killed by Ra Al Ghul, an environmental terrorist, because Wayne Industries was polluting the planet. On the day of his parents death, the family goes to a play in which the story involves a devil dressed in a batlike costume, which scared Bruce because he had fallen down a well earlier in his life and been terrified by its inhabitants-bats. Bruce begs his parents to leave the play early, and they exit the theater through an alley, where they are confronted by Joe Chill. Bruce's *Refusal of the Call* comes when he, after going to Joe Chill's parole hearing with a gun to kill him, is beaten to it by a hit man hired by Falcone, the crime boss of Gotham City. He confronts Falcone and is told that he does not know the harshness of the world. Based on this, he gives up his wealth and drops out of society, seeking a way to fight the injustices of the world.

While on his journey, Bruce is incarcerated in a Chinese prison. There he meets his *Supernatural Aid,* Henri Duncard, who offers him a direction for his life. He offers him the chance to join an organization called the League of Shadows, which fights the injustices and corruption of the world. Bruce *Crosses the First Threshold* as he makes to trek to the compound of the League of Shadows. He learns crime-fighting techniques of martial arts, gymnastics, and disguise. Bruce's *Belly of the Whale* is when he chooses the persona of Batman because of his mentor's suggestion of becoming the embodiment of fear and turning fear into a weapon against his enemies of Gotham City.

In Stage 2, the *Initiation,* he has a *Meeting With a Goddess* when he sees his childhood friend Rachel Dawes, now the district attorney of

Gotham City. As it turns out, his meeting with a goddess is also meeting the *Woman as Temptress*. She serves as the inspiration for his entering the *Road of Trials* to fight crime against the evil of Gotham City, including Falcone and the Scarecrow, Dr. Jonathan Crane. At the same time, she serves to bring him into danger and a confrontation with his enemy, the Scarecrow. The character of Scarecrow seems to serve as the archetype of the shadow for Batman and attempts to fulfill the role of righthand man for the League of Shadows in its plan to destroy Gotham City through the poisoning the water supply with gas. He undergoes his *Apotheosis* after a confrontation in which his house is burned down by the evil League of Shadows. He is nursed back to health by his aid and confidant Alfred. His *Atonement With the Father (figure)* occurs when he confronts his former mentor and teacher Henri Ducard, who turns out to be the real Ra Al Ghul. During the battle, he not only defeats Ghul but also foils his plan to destroy the city. For Batman, the *Ultimate Boon* comes to Bruce Wayne after he has defeated Ra Al Ghul. He stands at the place where his mansion has been burnt to the ground. Standing with his friends, he is asked by Rachel Dawes what he will do now. He holds a picture of his parents and says that he will rebuild and thus continue his role of protector of Gotham as Batman.

In the final stage, the *Return,* we must look to the plots of the original comic books. In the comic's series, Knightfall, Batman becomes paralyzed after a fight with an enemy called Bain. Through the series Knight Quest, Batman asks a friend Jean Paul Valley to become the character Batman. He does so, but he is the opposite of Bruce Wayne in that he is violent and kills others. Bruce begins to heal but has his *Refusal of the Return* in which he does not assume the role of Batman. The *Rescue From Without* occurs when Bruce undergoes training with Lady Shiva, an expert in the martial arts and a killer. She gives him confidence through training but also wants him to kill so that she knows he is ready to return. Bruce tricks her into thinking he has killed, and she directs him to where Azbat is hiding. The *Magic Flight* occurs when again dons the Batman costume and defeats Azbat, his replacement. The *Crossing of the Threshold* occurs when Bruce becomes Batman and begins again to fight the crime of Gotham City. He becomes the *Master of Two Worlds* as both Bruce Wayne, the billionaire who runs Wayne Industries, and Batman, who fights crime. He has both sides to his personality—his shadow of the Batman and the light side of Bruce Wayne. He now has the *Freedom to Live* with both sides of his life.

In the following section, I will demonstrate the use of the superhero archetype, specifically, Batman and Spider-Man in the sandplay-based treatment of two children.

CASE STUDIES

Joey

Presenting Problem

Joey was a 5-year-old White boy referred to the clinic by his biological mother due to concerns about his behavior at home and in the preschool setting. A week before intake, he was asked to leave his school program because of behavior described by his teacher as "out of control." Joey's caretakers described him as an aggressive, destructive, and unsafe child whose self-directed aggression took the form of biting, choking, and hitting himself. There were also episodes during which Joey directed his aggression toward teachers, parents, and peers without apparent provocation. At home, Joey's problematic behavior included climbing on the furniture and curtains while pretending to be Spider-Man. He had also shown a disregard for his own safety by repeatedly jumping into the deep end of the local swimming pool, knowing that he could not swim. The mother was looking for individual therapy and parent counseling to understand and help her son.

Background Information

Joey was the only child of a full-term but unplanned pregnancy; his parents were never married and subsequently ended their relationship when Joey was 2 years old. Following the parental separation, Joey had limited contact with his father, whose history included depression, domestic violence, and substance abuse. The mother had a history of medical problems that required surgery. Joey's mother initially became concerned during his infancy because of frequent tantrums. By the time he was 3 years old, his mother observed strong reactions to any negative affect, characterized by head banging, screaming, and rapid shifts in mood. Although this behavior briefly appeared to subside, Joey once again began to experience difficulties when he entered school at age 4. At that time, his mother unsuccessfully attempted to implement multiple forms of discipline including time-out, removal of possessions and privileges, and early bedtime. None of these forms of discipline had much effect in reducing his negative behaviors.

Clinical Conceptualization

On the basis of information gathered through interviews with his mother, review of relevant medical and school records, family observation data,

individual play assessment, and psychological testing, Joey was displaying symptoms consistent with a diagnosis of Adjustment Disorder with
Disturbance in Mood and Conduct, later corroborated by the treating psychiatrist. Psychological testing performed through the local school system
revealed borderline intelligence, information processing delays, anxiety,
irritability, and emotional lability. This lability, along with unpredictabil-
ity, aggression, impulsively, and dangerous behavior was consistent with
a family history of mood disorder. Joey also received a psychiatric evaluation and was subsequently placed on medication to help with his
impulsivity and dangerous behavior. Treatment would focus on helping
him cope more effectively.

Treatment: Beginning Phase

The therapeutic alliance was established within a few sessions; however,
Joey required clear structure and boundaries to feel safe in the playroom.
He appeared to have considerable difficulty focusing on and remaining
with any one activity for long. This shifting from toy to toy and activity
to activity appeared to be anxiety-based; however, it subsided as Joey's
comfort level increased. He also tested the limits of safety both by throwing toys and threatening to hit the clinician—behaviors that continued
throughout the beginning phase of his treatment.

Joey played predominantly with puppets such as dinosaurs, snakes,
or dragons, which would either attack or devour the clinician or each
other. Joey also pretended to be Spider-Man, who would fight "bad
guys"—including the clinician, who were attacking him or attempting to
steal his treasures. Because of continued aggression at home, Joey under-
went a psychiatric evaluation and was prescribed medication. The medication seemed to quell the aggressive behaviors, and it was therefore
determined that in conjunction with his comfort in the playroom, Joey
could be introduced to the sandtray. This transition marked his entry into
the middle phase of treatment.

Middle Phase

After 2 months in treatment, Joey's behavior, both at school and at home,
had improved, and the frequency of his aggressive outbursts had diminished. Although Joey enjoyed playacting Spider-Man, he also created multiple sandtrays that he then flooded, engulfing the vegetation and animal
figures with water. These initial trays seemed to reflect both his internal feelings of being out of control and the perceived chaos his life. The
trays were dynamic, characterized by movement and seemingly random
aggression. This type of play continued for several weeks.

At one discernible point, Joey began to focus on human rather than animal figures, aligning them against each other in opposing armies. The battling figures, which included army men, animals, and warriors, gave way to superheroes. This theme continued for the next several months.

Final Phase

In what were to be the latter series of sessions, Joey chose to work exclusively in the sandtray. He appeared to be highly focused, almost driven. An important shift in his sandtray play was marked by the creation of more expansive themes, as opposed to the simpler scenario of opposing sides. The figure that he favored, and which most likely represented himself, was Spider-Man. Early on in his treatment, Joey had playacted the character of Spider-Man, who fought the bad guys. Through the symbolic miniaturization of the Spider-Man figure in the sandtray, however, Joey was better able to project his fantasies and conflicts, as well as work on issues involving family and peer relations and his negative self-image. By the time therapy ended, Joey was observably and reportedly less aggressive, better able to identify his feeling, and enjoying improved relationships with others.

Reflections

When Joey began treatment, he was having great difficulty adjusting to the separation of his parents and the loss of his father; his relationships with family, teachers, and peers were also troubled. He was a sad, fearful, and angry child who used aggression to cope. His initial use of the superhero Spider-Man appeared to reflect a strong need for control over his sense of powerlessness related to these events in his life. Within the family, Joey was given an inappropriate level of power—similar to that which Peter Parker received when he was bitten by the radioactive spider. Joey's entry into therapy was much like Campbell's "call to adventure." Joey valiantly responded to the call by using play therapy to develop self-awareness and the ability to control both his behavior and emotions. Whether knowingly or unknowingly, Joey, like Peter Parker, finally realized that "with great power comes great responsibility."

In the sandtray, Joey used Spider-Man in several important therapeutic ways. It can be speculated that he chose the character of Spider-Man as a means of forming a connection with his father, whom he perceived to be a powerful figure. This was particularly difficult for Joey because he longed for a relationship with this man who was apparently disinterested in him. Joey also worked on the resulting anger and sadness through Spider-Man's battles in the playroom and in the sand-tray. The character of Spider-Man was also utilized to represent the power given to him by his mother, which in turn, frightened him. As Spider-Man, Joey could symbolically fight with the figures representing people in his life, and could then reconcile with and connect to them. By working together with some of these other figures to build houses in the sandtrays, Joey could symbolically build the stability he longed for in his life. For Joey, Spider-Man was both a hero who helped him and the heroic part of himself who could rebuild family ties and mend hurt feelings.

Isaac

Presenting Problem

Isaac, a 6-year-old African American male was referred by his biological mother who had concerns about his aggressive behaviors at home and at school. Although she described Isaac as a loving child, she also indicated that he aggressed toward both her and his brother. This aggression took the form of hitting, kicking, and breaking objects, such as toys and furniture. Isaac also experienced episodes of sadness and crying spells, which he related to missing someone. Isaac's teachers described him as occasionally friendly, yet inconsistent, unfocused, inattentive, and aggressive toward peers.

Background Information

Isaac was the second child to parents who were married at the time of his birth; the full-term pregnancy was uncomplicated. His older brother had been previously diagnosed with a mood disorder and was receiving treatment at the same clinic as Isaac. Isaac was described as an "easy" baby, who, as a child at about age 3, suffered the traumatic loss of his biological father due to sudden heart failure. The traumatic nature of this event was compounded by the subsequent emotional upheaval in the family. Before the loss of his father, Isaac was reportedly well behaved at home. In the months following the loss, Isaac's behavior at home and at school deteriorated to include fighting over toys, anxiety, difficulty following directions, theft of small items, and, according to his mother, emotional intensity.

Clinical Conceptualization

Isaac, a boy with no known family history of major mental illness, violence, or neglect, suffered the sudden loss of his father. After the death, he was exhibiting symptoms of aggression, intermittent episodes of crying along with feelings of sadness, and difficulties getting along with peers. These symptoms became disruptive and problematic both at home and at school. He was diagnosed with Adjustment Disorder with Disturbance in Mood and Conduct. A psychiatric evaluation was conducted, and the psychiatrist recommended individual therapy to address the issue of loss. Following the initial parent interview, family observation, and assessment, it was decided to focus on the loss of his father.

Treatment: Beginning Phase

In the beginning of treatment, Isaac had some difficulty engaging with the therapist. Therefore, a highly nondirective approach was implemented. Much of Isaac's initial play involved the fantasy adventures of kings, warriors, Harry Potter, and vampires. In these scenarios, Isaac typically assumed the role of leader and demanded that the clinician follow his every order. During these interactions, particularly when Isaac perceived that the clinician was not being cooperative, he became sarcastic and angry, voicing concern that his orders were not being followed. As this play continued, Isaac inquired into the therapist's thoughts about religion, particularly with reference to the afterlife. Each of these inquiries allowed for opportunities to discuss similarities and differences in opinions on the topic, as well Isaacs's feelings related to the loss of his father.

During this period of treatment, and along with his fantasy play, Isaac was introduced to sandplay. Although not particularly interested in the medium at first, he later created several scenes in the safe and contained space of the sandtray to channel his aggressive feelings.

Middle Phase

As Isaac progressed through therapy, he continued to engage in fantasy play; however, he shifted its focus to include superheroes—specifically, Batman. In these sessions, Isaac would begin by enacting adventures involving search for treasures and becoming a detective to follow clues leading to the capture of "bad guys." Isaac also became more clearly interested in the sandtrays. His initial trays contained both large predatory animals, such as lions and cheetahs, as well as mythical creatures, including dragons. The various animals protected the treasures that Isaac placed in the trays. These treasures were usually typically threatened by unknown and unseen threats. Another shift in Isaac's sandtray plays took place when he began to include human figures such as kings, warriors, and various superheroes—most notably Batman. These figures would split into opposing armies, which would eventually work together to protect each other.

Final Phase

In the final stage of therapy, Isaac worked exclusively in the sandtray. It seemed that he was beginning to work on his issue of loss and many of the feelings that had become connected to this experience. This was done through use of the Batman figure along with other superheroes. In many of his trays, Isaac created scenes of isolation, in which the various characters were compartmentalized by physical manmade barriers, such as walls and buildings made of stone and sand. As he continued to work in the sandtray, these barriers were slowly broken down, and the characters began to interact with each other. Batman became the leader of the group, and led the heroes on missions to protect great treasures such as magic stones, tombstones, and ovens that made their food. Isaac was able to talk about Batman's feelings of sadness related to being alone and isolated from friends. In his final tray, Isaac created a harmonious family scene in which all of the characters helped each other—without the need for aggression.

Reflections

Isaac experienced the early-life stress of losing a father. This tragic event represented his "call to adventure," parallel to the story of Batman, who lost his parents at an early age. Both Isaac and Bruce Wayne were painfully affected by the tragedy and attempted to make sense of their respective worlds. Early on in treatment, Isaac was angry about developing a relationship with a new man (the therapist), who was clearly not his father. Through his play both with and as Batman, Isaac as the loner became a detective who symbolically searched for the "bad guys," However, Isaac's Batman soon sought the assistance of Dick Grayson, who later assumed his crimefighting identity of Robin. In taking on a companion, Isaac learned that just as Batman needed help, so too, did he need the assistance of the therapist.

In the sandtray, Isaac worked through issues in a similar way as he had done through his fantasy play. His early trays depicted warring characters, possibly related to the conflicted and painful feelings that he was experiencing in relation to the events in his life. When Isaac introduced the figure of Batman, he was unconsciously linking himself, and thus identifying, with a character whose early life was marked by tragic loss. Both he and Batman felt alone, isolated, and angry because of the tragedy. Yet the tragedy also allowed each of them to work through their painful feelings and to establish a posttrauma identity. Isaac became more capable of verbalizing the anger related to the loss of his father and the loss of an opportunity to know him. By initially containing and compartmentalizing these feelings until he was ready to experience them, Isaac gained the ego strength and defenses that allowed him to work through the loss. He came out of therapy with a better understanding of himself and his life experiences—a master of two worlds with the freedom to live. The conscious and unconscious work that Joey and Isaac did in the sandtray, and the positive effect it had on their lives, reflects the power of both the technique and the relationship between client and therapist to facilitate the healing journey.

REFERENCES

Ammann, R. (1991). *Healing and transformation in sandplay: Creative processes become visible.* La Salle, IL: Open Court.

Bettelheim, B. (1975). *The uses of enchantment: The meaning and importance of fairy tales.* New York: Vintage Books.

Bradway, K., & McCoard, B. (1997). *Sandplay: Silent workshop of the psyche.* New York: Routledge.

Campbell, J. (1956). *The hero with a thousand faces.* New York: Meridian Press.

Chethik, M. (2000). *Techniques of child therapy: Psychodynamic strategies.* New York: Guilford Press.

Cunningham, L. (2005). *What Is Sandplay Therapy?* Retrieved January 7, 2006, from http://www.sandplay.org/what_is_sandplay_therapy.htm

Davies, D. (2004). *Child development: A practitioner's guide* (2nd ed.). New York. Guilford Press.

Hegen, G. (2005). *The sandplay collection.* Retrieved January 13, 2006, from http://www.sandplay.org/symbols/index.htm#the_sandplay_collection.htm

Indick, W. (2004). Classical heroes in modern movies: Mythological patterns of the superhero. *Journal of Media Psychology, 9,* 1–13.

Jung, C. G. (1981). *The structure and dynamics of the psyche* (R. C. F. Hull, Trans.). Princeton, NJ: Princeton University Press. (Original work published 1960)

Kalff, D. M. (1991). Introduction to sandplay therapy. *Journal of Sandplay Therapy, 1,* 7–15.

Labovitz-Boik, B., & Goodwin, E. A. (2000). *Sandplay therapy: A step-by step manual for psychotherapists of diverse orientations.* New York: Norton.

Landreth, G. L. (2002). *Play therapy: The art of the relationship* (2nd ed.). New York: Brunner-Routledge.

Neumann, E. (1973). *The child.* New York: C. G. Jung Foundation.

Rogers, C. R. (1980). *A way of being.* Boston: Houghton Mifflin.

Turner, B. A. (2005). *The handbook of sandplay therapy.* Cloverdale, CA: Temenos Press.

Weinrib, E. L. (1983). *Images of the self: The sandplay therapy process.* Boston: Sigo Press.

Winnicott, D. W. (1992). *Through paediatrics to psycho-analysis: Collected papers.* New York: Brunner/Mazel.

CHAPTER FIVE

The Incredible Hulk and Emotional Literacy

Jennifer Mendoza Sayers

Created by Stan Lee and artist Jack Kirby in 1962, the Incredible Hulk is a creature whose alter ego, Dr. Robert Bruce Banner, is a victim of both scientific and emotional abuse. Scientifically, the origin of the Hulk was the result of exposure to a gamma bomb explosion following Bruce's attempt to save a reckless teenager, Rick Jones. This single act of heroism cursed the reclusive scientist to transform during moments of anger into a hulking beast often persecuted by military intrigue and villainous exploitation.

Emotionally, the Hulk persona originated from Bruce's abusive relationship with his alcoholic father, Brian Banner. As an adolescent, Bruce imagined the Hulk character to console the mistreated youth with the promise that "Hulk will smash them all." The Hulk, who thus began as a projection of Bruce's powerlessness, eventually manifested after prolonged and chronic stress as a creature who could assert his power and dominance. Within Bruce Banner, however, there remained a struggle between the two irreconcilable and split-off facets of Banner's personality—the Hulk disdains Banner's timidity and emotional suppression, whereas Banner loathes Hulk's brutish rage. With the help of Dr. Leonard Samson, Bruce Banner attempts to accept his emotions and evolve into someone who is in control of their expression.

In a clinical context, the "Incredible Hulk syndrome" refers to this splitting-off of opposing emotional tendencies in attempts to reconcile and integrate them into personality. Successful resolution of this syndrome results in adaptive emotional expression—particularly of anger—and as described in this chapter, greater "emotional literacy."

THE ROLE OF EMOTIONS

Potter-Efron and Potter-Efron (1995) identified four styles of anger that are present in the Hulk syndrome:

- Masked anger, in which individuals habitually deny or minimize the anger they feel and may substitute other emotions such as anxiety or guilt (Bruce Banner)
- Explosive anger, a pattern of extended suppression of negative emotions that eventually results in rapid, exaggerated, and often destructive release of uncontrolled rage (the Hulk)
- Chronic anger, a style that holds the emotions of anger for extended periods often resulting in physical ailments (Banner's frustration and conflicted relationships).
- Healthy anger, a style that recognizes anger as a useful signal to a problem and is expressed in a manner that can be understood by others, thus moving toward a solution including personal ownership and self-empowerment (the goal toward which Banner strives)

The legend of the Incredible Hulk illustrates that mild-mannered Bruce Banner had a problem from the beginning. Originating from the disconnection from others and the absence of healthy relationships in childhood, Bruce never learned to effectively express his emotions. Like many toxic substances or traumatic experiences, the gamma rays that Bruce Banner was exposed to merely exacerbated his already-present inability to express emotions unless provoked to the point of rage. Although academically and intellectually gifted, Bruce lacked the capacity to differentiate anger from other emotions.

Progressing from the primitive expression of raw emotion toward the adaptive use of emotion as a tool for problem solving requires practice, support, and healthy role models, all of which Bruce Banner lacked. The healthy anger style referred to, emphasizes that anger is best used as a signal of a problem rather than as a means of resolving it. Mastery of this awareness and the ability to implement it requires trial-and-error learning that begins with identifying or defining the problem. It takes considerable and ongoing practice to generate choices that eventually lead to a solution and the effective expression of emotion—particularly anger. When children (or green monsters) tantrum, they are in a stage of emotional reaction, during which they lose control of themselves and become unable to process incoming information. Whereas time-out strategies that separate the child from the environment provide the opportunity to safely exhaust the rage, the child also needs to learn how to use other means to communicate thoughts and feelings so that he or she can have needs met and find a more effective solution to the problem. The Hulk's rage and the child's tantrum both provide a false sense of power that is ultimately destructive to the self and to others.

EMOTIONAL LITERACY

Emotional literacy, the ability to identify and express different emotions quickly and accurately, sometimes referred to as emotional intelligence (Steiner & Perry, 1997), results from learning to recognize and express emotions adaptively. By recognizing and distinguishing one's own emotions and learning to differentiate those of others, feelings can be processed more accurately, and personal and interpersonal solutions can be more easily generated. When instead, emotions are "one big muddle"—avoided or limited to anger responses (or both), a key element of being human is lost (Bettleheim, 1975), and we are left to function at the level of the beasts. More than likely, the use of different words for emotions evolved into human discourse to facilitate problem solving. When someone can recognize that what is labeled as anger may actually be, for example, fear, confusion, hurt, disappointment, or all of these feelings, they can more easily generate effective solutions.

Emotional literacy grows simply through the identification and use of words that describe feelings. Regardless of a person's age, it does not matter which feeling is identified first when learning to recognize emotions. A broad spectrum of emotional labels that match corresponding feelings facilitates the process of learning to differentiate emotions and therefore build an "emotional vocabulary," which can then be employed in problem solution. For example, rather than bursting out in anger, children can be taught to identify other possible feelings they are experiencing, such as fear or confusion. In doing so, their behavioral response may be quite different. In the event that this "emotional honing process" does not occur in the course of normal development, therapeutic intervention can help someone who is an emotionally unskilled to develop emotional literacy. Below are two exercises that address development of self-awareness and empathy, the key factors of emotional literacy (Goleman, 2005).

Reframe emotions as tools (such as on a tool belt) and increase the use of feeling words in daily discourse by helping clients to describe the last time they felt angry. As the incident is described, make note of all the other possible emotions involved (e. g., disrespect, embarrassment, confusion, hurt, disappointment) and ask clients to clear their minds. As they do so, suggest that they imagine (visualize) a similar situation in which they felt an emotion other than anger and what they did in that situation to feel better. If "got mad" is the only strategy they offer, discuss the Hulk syndrome and specifically, how limiting and destructive anger can be. By exploring alternate emotional responses, the client can develop and plan to generate alternate solutions to difficult situations to situations that provoke anger.

Help the client to perceive accurately the verbal and nonverbal cues of others and use a variety of emotional tools to communicate and problem solve. The capacity to strengthen the client's ability to recognize feelings in daily discourse is accomplished by using an exercise that is a variation on a child's stained-glass window coloring game. In a group at of least two (e. g., therapist and child; siblings or adult and child), instruct one person to scribble in loops all over a white piece of paper while someone else starts a "key" page by drawing a column of small squares. One person chooses a color from a box of about 16 crayons or markers and decides what feeling word (e. g., *happy, sad, mad*) accompanies that color. After selecting a word, the client is asked to color in a space in the first page and describe a time when he or she felt that way. When each one has given an example and colored a space, the next person selects a color, a feeling word, and describes a situation reflecting the feeling chosen. Guidance to match the feeling accurately with the word may be necessary, but of course any color–feeling matches will suffice. An alternate exercise is a variation on the standard Anger Log—that is, recording the circumstances in which the client felt or expressed anger and its impact on all involved. Integration of the results of this exercise with those in the previous step provides the client with a means of recognizing and expressing feelings other than anger. This assists in relapse prevention.

Another simple method for increasing emotional literacy is to use either a sheet or poster of different facial expressions. The sheet should be located where it can easily be seen. Emotional literacy is facilitated by covering or crossing out the "angry" face (because the child already knows how to do this well) and inventing any type of game or contest to see how many other feelings can be identified, just like vocabulary is built using the week's spelling word in a sentence, feeling words are practiced in context. Even younger children can usually describe what they can do to help themselves feel better when they are scared, confused, hurt, or disappointed (Steiner, 2003) and may not be able to describe how to control their anger. Getting into a habit of using many feeling words triggers alternate solutions and limits the Hulk in us all from "smashing" things.

These exercises illustrate that people acquire new skills through direct instruction, modeling, and behavioral practice (Ginsburg & Opper, 1969). Similarly, complete emotional development includes learning to express feelings fluently to facilitate problem solving and interaction with others (Cirillo et al., 1989). The acquisition of emotional literacy results in learning to use, monitor, and express emotions successfully. These processes have specific neuropsychological correlates in brain structure and development.

NEUROSCIENCE AND EMOTION

From a physiological standpoint, the Hulk syndrome mirrors the physical development and influence of the emotional brain centers. Research in brain–behavior connections elucidates the processes involved in emotional expression and suggests that it is tied to learning processes (Kolb & Whishaw, 1996). Learning and memory pathways both connect through several central brain structures—the thalamus, hippocampus, amygdala, hypothalamus, basal ganglia, and limbic system. It would then appear that at a basic, hardwired level, learning, memory and emotions are interconnected.

Information processing theory suggests that details about the world travel from the senses to the thalamus, which then relays it directly to the upper neocortex where incoming signals are recognized, sorted, and assigned meaning. These filtered signals are then sent back down to the subcortical limbic system that triggers the appropriate visceral (emotional) response. In the course of development, and cued by social situations, we learn to reason before we react (Kolb & Whishaw, 1996).

Other components of this neural emotional network have been identified. The pathways involve the hypothalamus (meaning "lower room") positioned in the diencephalon (primitive subcortical forebrain) just below the thalamus ("inner room"). The thalamus contains pairs of nerves that influence eating, drinking, sleeping, waking, sexual behavior, and organization of the flight-or-fight and rage reactions. Developmentally, the expression and suppression of basic emotions progresses from the hypothalamus up through the basal ganglia, which serve to organize feelings consistent with behavior and thus controls their expression. From the diencephalon, through the basal ganglia, direct communication into the cortex of the temporal lobe, tasks begin to be divided, that is, the right hemisphere appears to recognize emotions, especially facial expressions, more efficiently. The highest level of organization, the cerebral cortex (or association cortex) separates humans from other animals in that humans have more cortical connections in relation to body size than any other animal (Beaumont, 1983). This affords humans relatively more insight, planning, and the sophisticated processing of conscious experience.

At a more primary level, aside from the complex information processing pathways just described, an emergency pathway processes emotional information exponentially faster by bypassing the higher cortical areas. This primitive pathway routes information directly from the thalamus to the amygdala, a small, almond-shaped structure in the limbic system, which serves as an emotional alarm. The amygdala appears to evaluate the incoming information for danger potential, rapidly and crudely assessing the perception of threat level. This instantaneously labels something as "bad" or "hurtful" without rational understanding of the "threat" (Atkinson, 1999).

Once stimulated, the amygdala triggers an adrenaline distress signal throughout the brain activating the flight-or-fight response within milliseconds. At this level, humans react very similarly to most animals—from fear to blind rage. The survival benefit to this rapid reaction has been significant over the millennia and supersedes the slower, more complex information processing track in protecting the individual and maximizing defensive efforts. However, in complex social situations, this rapid, beastlike response is not as useful. The instantaneous labeling of a perceived trigger as "bad" or "harmful" and explosive reaction before any higher level thinking occurs can be destructive to relationships as well as personal integrity. As simpler, subcortical pathways become flooded with adrenaline and overwhelm rational thinking, the beast in us dominates the rational thinker; when this happens, we fail to learn applications that could better serve our needs.

Developing from the expression of raw emotion, the use of emotion as a tool in problem solving requires the control gained from higher cortical brain structures. Raw emotions are only experienced "simply" (e. g., happy, mad, sad) if they are experienced at all. To refine raw emotion into a more complex, modulated interpretation of feelings, brain structures within the neocortex must become involved. Cognitive interpretation generated from the structures within the neocortex transform animal impulses produced by limbic structures back into the modulated control of emotional expression characteristic of human social interaction.

Neuroscientists (Kolb & Winshaw, 1996, p. 420) define emotion as an "inferred state" comprising three principle components: physiological state, overt behaviors, and the cognitive processes inferred from self-report. The Hulk syndrome is an illustration of a poor interconnection between these systems. Using the primitive emotional track, the amygdala makes its snap judgments based on the similarity of a current situation to past events that once scared us and thus contains an emotional memory. The hippocampus, once thought to be the source of emotional memories, only registers factual and contextual information and then connects to the amygdala where basic emotions are then stored (Atkinson, 1999). When the amygdala assesses the danger level of a current situation, it does so at a primitive level, not at the sophisticated level of the neocortex, which has learned to sort and analyze complex information. Thus, if any element in the current situation is crudely similar to the stored, relatively simple emotional templates—such as a voice tone, a visual contour, a smell, or tactile impression—a rapid, neurochemical response ensues. This can endear one individual to another with a warm feeling of familiarity, such as reminding someone of a loved one, or unleash an emergency alarm of emotional explosion—"Hulk will smash them all."

Stress only serves to enhance the triggering of the amygdala because of the action of stress hormones (Atkinson, 1999). By definition, victims of posttraumatic stress syndrome, regardless of the source of the trauma, frequently show hypervigilance and heightened emotional reaction as well as dissociative reactions that disconnect the original trauma from the later emotional reaction. A simple case example of this phenomenon occurred several years ago while I was routinely evaluating a 65-year-old woman for posttraumatic stress following a car accident. While drawing a stick-figure house, she became distressed and started to disassociate saying, "No, this is the train." Under the influence of the stress of the car accident, the drawing process triggered memories of her experiences as a Holocaust victim at age 10—previously long forgotten memories of the train that took her to the concentration camps. This illustrates how strong emotional memories can be separated from rational emotional responses of daily life. It is not always an angry beast that lies inside waiting to be triggered. It can also be deep sadness or fear.

The expression of anger as a reaction to a real or perceived threat is common to many species. Anger serves several positive survival purposes as a protective energetic motivator. This basic emotional reaction triggers the flight-or-fight autonomic responses and, in turn, causes an override of the higher order brain areas that control slower, more complex forethought and decision-making. Quick, unimpeded response allows a far greater behavioral reaction than would otherwise be possible (Guyton, 1971). However, this quick behavioral reaction can both provide strength and wreak havoc in social settings.

In addition to its survival role, anger is also an indicator that needs are not being met. When one person in a relationship becomes angry, it serves to establish a boundary or limit. As a primitive emotional tool, humans use anger to impress on their clansman a line across which they should not cross. Thus, anger serves to strengthen social relationships through the establishment of social contracts—from simple limit setting to complex rituals (Learner, 2005).

The social impact of this basic anger reaction is complicated. Anger frequently masks other more complex emotions, resulting in the use of a global label and singular emotional response to express many other emotions. David Banner's anthem "you wouldn't like me when I'm angry" is reflective of this process. Many people may describe themselves as angry when they are actually experiencing other feelings such as disrespect, disappointment, jealousy, embarrassment, loneliness, or guilt. The quick physiological and emotional response that protects humans in emergency situations may also contribute to a state of mislabeled confusion and nonproductive or even self-destructive behavioral reactions.

The Incredible Hulk syndrome illustrates in a simple story the destructive result of this incomplete skill development. The story's familiarity with both children and adults makes it a quick and efficient means to convey both the social and physiological error and point the way to a therapeutic solution. A variety of case studies illustrate this use of the well-known story in therapeutic settings.

CASE STUDIES

Rudy was a 12-year-old referred for counseling because of anger outbursts and poor impulse control. He came willingly and admitted that he would act out aggressively when he did not get his way or did not feel he was being heard. He gave several examples and recounted that he had participated in counseling from age 7 to help him cope with his parents' contentious divorce and with school problems. He reported that he had difficulty getting to sleep at night and had chronic conflicts with his older brother.

During the initial session, Rudy described the typical pattern of communication in his family, particularly between his father and brother. "You have to be loud to be heard," Rudy explained, after reviewing the relaxation methods he had learned in previous counseling sessions—taking a time out or reading. I asked Rudy to think about whom he regarded as a hero. He readily identified with the Hulk and quickly saw the parallel between his temper outbursts and the path of destruction left when the Hulk turned into the green monster. Rudy quickly understood that in an effort to get his point across, he actually was not being heard at all, and he was also suffering the consequences for his aggressive acting out. We discussed "mild-mannered Bruce Banner," and Rudy was given a sheet of faces titled "How do you feel?" I crossed out the picture representing "angry," and Rudy agreed to do what Bruce Banner wished he could do—express any other emotion and save anger as an option. He already knew how to get angry very well, but he also knew what to do when he felt hurt, disappointed, or afraid. I complimented Rudy in that he could readily identify alternate responses.

By allowing Rudy to hold onto his choice to get angry while helping him expand his expression of all the other emotions he knew, his expressive emotional literacy improved. In subsequent sessions, he was able to recount examples of successful interactions with his brother and father during which he felt he was being heard without having to turn into a green monster. By progressively dividing up the "big muddle" of emotions he experienced, his anxiety level dropped as well, and he felt less threatened and more competent to express himself. This reduced Rudy's need to both strike first and get back at those who hurt him.

Lynn was a 38-year-old housewife and the mother of an 8-year-old son and a 3-year-old daughter. The victim of incest at a young age, Lynn had become pleasantly passive, people-pleasing, and highly anxious. She had tried a variety of medications over the years but continued to experience weekly, and sometimes daily, anxiety attacks. She recounted that when angered, she usually let it go for fear of confrontation. Lynn added that "When I get angry I know I'm going to have physical symptoms." This in turn, triggered feelings of inadequacy and loss of control, followed by anger because she "could not get her words out." Lynn recognized that she blamed others because she was afraid to face the source of the problem. When ignoring, worrying, and blaming failed to resolve the interpersonal stressors, she exploded in anger: "I just want to scream loudly and punch someone."

After discussing assertive communication strategies, I introduced Lynn to the Incredible Hulk syndrome. I explained that both Bruce Banner and the Hulk have one strategy for dealing with stress-avoidance and violence, respectively. Neither of these strategies was effective, and both resulted in heightened anxiety. As the fear of expressing strong emotion becomes overwhelming, expression of that emotion can have an addictive purging effect (Goulston & Goldberg, 1996). I explained that the ability to experience feelings throughout the day rather than rely on denial, minimization, or blame, could lead to more effective problem solving and anxiety reduction.

Over many months with therapeutic support and guidance, Lynn learned to separate and express several emotions such as hurt, disappointment, guilt, confusion, embarrassment, and fear. As she became more emotionally literate and had more confidence in "getting words out," she became the green monster less often. Simultaneously, she was able to recognize that the anxiety, confusion, and fear she had felt as child and young teen originated with the sexual abuse that occurred over several years. Once she was able to direct the source of her anger appropriately toward the perpetrator and identify associated feelings, her anxiety level diminished. Discussion of the Hulk syndrome helped Lynn to identify the pattern of destruction she was inflicting on herself and her family. The story also helped her to more easily understand the need to express her feelings as they occurred, rather than "being mad and letting them build up into a rage." Neither medications nor behavioral interventions in the absence of this much-needed understanding were effective. Lynn became better able to process her feelings and generate more effective problem-solving strategies.

Pat and Charlie were married for 16 years and although they expressed loving devotion to each other, but they had a history of explosive incidents that significantly affected their relationship. Like many couples, both partners brought a history of parental criticism and loss to the relationship. I believed that this long-term conditioning created a pattern of hair-trigger subcortical reactions that defended them against the fear of abandonment that was triggered by conflicts in the relationship. As tension increased, culminating in violent outbursts, both Pat and Charlie were on autonomic overload, each aggressively defending themselves from attack. Their internal emotional processes were perpetuating a cycle of conflict that neither spouse wanted.

Although this couple benefited somewhat from several cognitive behavioral interventions including time-out, fair fighting, and assertive listening, they were incapable of breaking the cycle of anger–withdrawal–anger that threatened their relationship. There are few emotion-centered approaches to couples therapy. Based on the cognitive–behavioral premise that changing thinking changes behavior, few therapeutic strategies take into consideration the hardwired nature of anger triggers, assuming that the rational neocortex is dominant over the emotional limbic system. Hence the name Rational Emotive Therapy coined by Albert Ellis (1988). Similarly, pure conditioning models fail to address the complex social aspects of intimate human relationships. There are not many mature human relationships that can be consistently described by stimulus–response diagrams alone.

Pat and Charlie both had complaints about each other's neglect of the relationship. When asked to give an example, Pat stared stoically. Charlie volunteered an incident in which Pat screamed that she felt insulted and hurt that Charlie kept mementoes of past relationships in the top drawer of their dresser. Charlie came home and was shocked to find that all of his pictures and men's adult magazines had been thrown away without his knowledge. Pat recalled that Charlie suddenly turned red and screamed at her, "Are you out of your mind? Those things were valuable and meant a lot to me. How could you do that to me?!" Charlie said he felt an immediate tightening of his muscles just recalling the incident. Pat said that she remembered feeling like a fool, asking herself why she married

Charlie at all when he spoke to her that way. Charlie chimed in that he felt a whole new level of rage welling up in him when she turned her back and walked away.

By briefly describing the Incredible Hulk story to the couple, the issue of anger management was introduced in a lighthearted, and thus non-accusatory fashion. In this way, both Pat and Charlie could own their part of their extreme emotional reactivity. By recognizing the destructiveness of Bruce Banner's defensive rage reaction, they became open to refocusing on supportive strategies that first and foremost fostered a sense of mutual safety. When both Pat and Charlie learned to talk more clearly about their feelings at the moment they occurred, developing more emotional literacy and fluency, they no longer felt threatened. By preventing a feeling of threat from welling up from the limbic system, their internal alarm system remained turned off. This allowed them to shift from a defensive, nonrational fear reaction to the more extensively connected, rational, nurturing neocortex. By expanding the emotionally expressive skills of each partner, they were able to relax their defenses and explore the wider range of emotional expression. Pat and Charlie learned to respond to their respective partner with emotional expression while recognizing their own feelings. When each partner learned to identify and express a variety of feelings, both could let down their responsive guards and generate appropriately modulated responses.

Dan was a divorced father of Laura, an athletically active 13-year-old. Although he moved away from his former wife and child, being absent from Laura's life for about 2 years, he had worked diligently over the subsequent 2 years to regain a role and a relationship with his daughter. He had succeeded in establishing an amiable relationship with his ex-wife, Chris. Before his separation and divorce, Dan coached many of the sports teams Laura enjoyed. They had a close, working relationship where Laura knew how to please her father. He was her "buddy" and loved all the time he spent playing with her.

As Laura grew older and needed more complex discipline, Dan became more absent, according to Dan's wife. Chris recounted that Dan would walk away and ignore Laura when she misbehaved rather than intervene. Chris would ask Dan for help, and he would "blow up," yelling, rather than intervene rationally. Laura began to irritate her father to gain attention from him until he again exploded with anger.

Dan's explosive behavior was characterized by yelling commands. Chris, explained that she and Laura often felt as if they were not good enough and incapable of living up to Dan's expectations. She commented that his "walking away meant that you either did things his way or that he would have nothing to do with you." Dan truly wanted to rekindle his relationship with his daughter and improve the one with his ex-wife. When the Hulk syndrome was introduced to him, Dan quickly recognized that his frustration in attempting to control his daughter and communicating his feelings to his ex-wife resulted in them regarding him as a "green monster" rather than a loving mentor and co-parent. Laura typically reacted to her father's anger by either pushing him away or finding ways to irritate him. When Dan was introduced to the idea of expanding his skills rather than turning into another incarnation of himself, he became more optimistic and effective in communicating with both Laura and Chris. More important, and consistent with his need for personal control, he said that he appreciated the personal responsibility component to this strategy.

CONCLUSION

The Incredible Hulk syndrome illustrates both the errors made and the solutions generated in the course of learning to express emotions, particularly anger. Both Bruce Banner as an everyman character and the Hulk as the raging child within, simply illustrate the developmental struggle to overcome powerlessness and modulate primitive rage reactions. The solution that Bruce strives toward is gained with the acquisition of emotional literacy—learning to identify accurately and express different emotions. This learning process is mirrored in specific neuropsychological correlates in brain structure.

The Hulk syndrome also simply illustrates the dual neuropsychological tracks characteristic of human emotional expression. The basic emotional reaction, the Hulk track, triggers the flight-or-fight autonomic responses. The Dr. Banner track consists of higher order brain areas that control slower, more complex forethought and decision making. By briefly introducing the Incredible Hulk story to children, adults, or couples, the complex issue of anger management can be described in a lighthearted, nonthreatening fashion. In this way, each person can own his or her part of the extremes of emotional reaction and recognize the destructiveness of the defensive anger response. Identification with a comic book character creates less resistance to refocusing effort toward more effective communication strategies. The therapeutic use of the Hulk syndrome provides a vehicle for effective learning and a means for fostering a sense of personal control and safety.

REFERENCES

Atkinson, B. (1999, July/August). The emotional imperative psychotherapists cannot afford to ignore. *Networker*, 22–33.

Beaumont, J. G. (1983). *Introduction to neuropsychology.* New York: Guilford Press.

Bettelheim, B. (1975). *The uses of enchantment: The meaning and importance of fairy tales.* New York: Knopf.

Cirillo, L., Kaplan, B., & Wapner, S. (1989). *Emotions in ideal human development.* Hillsdale, NJ: Erlbaum.

Ellis, A. (1988). *How to stubbornly refuse to make yourself miserable about anything, yes anything!* New York: Carol.

Ginsburg, H., & Opper, S. (1969). *Piaget's theory of intellectual development.* Upper Saddle River, NJ: Prentice-Hall.

Goleman, D. (2005). *Emotional intelligence: Why it can matter more than I.Q.* New York: Bantam Books.

Goulston, M., & Goldberg, P. (1996). *Get out of your own way: Overcoming self-defeating behavior.* New York: Berkley.

Guyton, A. (1971). *Basic human physiology: Normal function and mechanisms of disease.* Philadelphia: Saunders.

Kolb, B., & Whishaw, I. (1996). *Fundamentals of human neuropsychology.* New York: Freeman.

Learner, H. (2005). *The dance of anger: A woman's guide to changing the patterns of intimate relationships.* New York: Harper Perennial.

Potter-Efron, R., & Potter-Efron, P. (1995). *Letting go of anger: The 10 most common anger styles and what to do about them.* Oakland, CA: New Harbinger.

Steiner, C. (2003). *Emotional literacy: Intelligence with a heart.* Fawnskin, CA: Personhood Press.

Steiner, C., & Perry, P. (1997). *Achieving emotional literacy: A personal program to increase your emotional intelligence.* New York: Avon Books.

Superheroes and Unique Clinical Applications

CHAPTER SIX

Holy Franchise! Batman and Trauma

Michael Brody

> People say that what we're all seeking is a meaning in life; I don't think that's what we're really seeking. I think that what we're seeking is an experience of being alive.
>
> —(Campbell, 1988)

In May of 1939, a new superhero was introduced in *Detective Comics*. Unlike his alien predecessor, Superman, he was human and vulnerable. His name was Bruce Wayne. He developed his mind for science and conditioned his body for strength. His huge inheritance provided the means to equip a crime fighter's laboratory to equal those of *CSI* and yet maintain secrecy. Searching for the perfect symbol to both frighten and disguise himself, Bruce chose the bat. He did not, however, choose his life's work—it chose him! Witnessing with his own "shocked" eyes his parents' murders, he vowed to avenge their deaths with a war on crime. Thus, Batman was born. Like most superheroes (Superman's separation from his parents; Spider-Man being stung by a radioactive spider; the Hulk's unfortunate presence in a laboratory during an explosion), Batman has his origins in psychic trauma, a mostly Freudian construct (Brody, 1995). It is the sequelae of the trauma that makes for the individuality of each superhero. The psychic trauma that these myth-like characters suffer and recover from is also part of a larger process that promotes increased strength through adversity. Batman, with no special powers, succeeds in his revenge quest through hard work and discipline, as he validates Erickson's psychosocial developmental task of Industry versus Inferiority.

Batman's creator, Bob Kane, had an immediate hit, and more than 60 years later, the success continues: the film *Batman Begins* (Nolan, 2005) became a multimillion-dollar-grossing blockbuster, and a younger generation watches *Batman the Cartoon* on television. Indeed, a new and even darker version of the caped crusader in comic book form now sells for more than $12.

As a young fan of the Caped Crusader, and later as a psychiatrist/educator, Batman became more to me than a comic book icon. He brings insight and healing to my patients, understanding to my students, and, above all, meaning and encouragement to us all. By considering how he evolved, as told by the "origin" stories in both the first comic book version, as well as the movie that revived the franchise, we can better understand the universal psychological phenomena of psychic trauma and appreciate the therapeutic impact of this true very human superhero.

Batman (Burton, 1989) begins with a solution (we watch the superhero rescue a family) and climaxes with the problem (Bruce Wayne's helpless witnessing of his parent's murder). The film tells the story backward. Pauline Kael (1989) in her review of the film praises Michael Keaton's portrayal of Bruce Wayne—Batman—as the only human being in the movie; he gives it (his role) gravity and emotional coloring. I agree when she states, "This is a man whose mission has taken over his life" (p. 84).

The very first Batman story appeared in comic book form as *The Legend of the Batman and How He Came to Be* (Kane, 1939) and more clearly illustrates the trauma and the preparation for the mission than the Keaton film. In the first comic panel, the Wayne family is confronted by a robber who advances on Mrs. Wayne. Dr. Wayne begins to protect his wife, and in the second and third panels, we see the villain murder them both. We see the back of Bruce's head. He is watching the entire scene from a direct frontal position. The next two panels are of Bruce with wide, tearful eyes viewing the horror unfolding before him.

PSYCHIC TRAUMA

Freud's (1920/1955) work on psychic trauma remains valuable in understanding Bruce's mental state at the moment he watches his parents' demise. Freud wrote about the flooding of the psychic apparatus with large amounts of stimuli and the experience of helplessness due to the ego being overwhelmed. Anna Freud (1967) focused more on the experience of helplessness on the part of the ego and felt that "suddenness and unexpectedness" (p. 223) are essential, as well as a tangible sign of the disruption of the ego. She highlights the importance of developmental concerns and how external traumas can be converted into internal ones if they connect with fulfillment of either deep-seated anxieties or wishes. She feels that a truly traumatic event is never fully resolved and may show up later in life. We do not know from the film what immediately happens to young Bruce; we can only rhetorically question, as reporter Knox does late in the movie while reviewing old newspapers about the Wayne family tragedy, "What do you think something like this does to a kid?"

Terr (1979), in her article "Children of Chowchilla," attempted to answer that very question, describing the kidnapping of 26 children in the summer of 1976 and the long-term sequelae for them and their families. The children, ranging in age from 5 to 14 years, were held for 27 hours, transferred from their school bus to two vans and then placed in a hole with a false top and buried for 16 hours with the bus driver. Although the children did not experience any of the physical responses or emotional re-actions anticipated by Anna Freud (1967), such as paralysis and numbness of feeling, they did show signs of ego misperception and hallucinations. The children also developed long term-fears, cognitive dysfunctions, and problems with repetitive, monotonous, and ineffective play.

Reporter Knox's question was also answered by Rebecca, who was brought to this therapist as a 12-year-old with learning difficulties. She and her younger sister were each adopted from South America imme-diately after birth. During the course of our treatment, which involved talking about her social and academic problems, Rebecca became more verbal and assertive. It was during our second year of therapy that Re-becca experienced a traumatic event. While going to the bathroom during a friend's confirmation party, Rebecca was accosted by a custodian and sexually attacked. After the incident, she began to have panic attacks, ac-companied by vivid disturbing flashbacks. She refused to attend school, frightened by the bathrooms. She felt "ashamed and damaged" and no longer had "faith in anything." In therapy she "confessed" her responsi-bility and guilt for what happened and "the secret" that she had flirted with the janitor on two previous occasions. Her parents stopped treat-ment when I advised them that Rebecca would make a poor witness and that a legal trial might not help their daughter emotionally at this time. Her mother did continue to keep in touch for a while, telling me of her guilt and how she knew "something bad" was going to happen that day, when Rebecca did not kiss her good-bye. Rebecca was home-schooled until the last year of high school, venturing out of the house only for her karate lessons. I last heard from her many years later when she was in her early 20s. She asked for all her medical records. She was not only suing the Temple where the attack occurred but also her parents for not "protecting her." She ended the phone conversation by stating "You remember the Batman poster in your office? He wanted revenge, I was hurt … I know I am bitter, but I need to do this." Lifton and Olson (1976) enumerated the various sequelae of the Buffalo Creek Disaster—a flood resulting from the dumping of coal in a mountain stream and a subsequent moving "wall of black water" (p. 1) that killed 125 people and rendered 5,000 homeless. The victims described a feeling beyond protest and despair. There was a lack of continuity and connectedness. Healing did not take place over time in Buffalo Creek, and people became mentally disturbed. Lifton believed that the regenerative ability of the ego is not limitless and some traumas are beyond repair. The suddenness—isolation of the community and irresponsibility of authorities—all caused a shattering of the illusion of invulnerability and resulted in rage. The same effect occurs when children experience a parental death or divorce or are sexually abused. The shield of protective innocence cracks. A severe illness in a child is made even more devastating by the helplessness he or she perceives in his or her parents. A sense of trust in the world is lost.

DEATH GUILT

Unlike the Chowchilla kidnapping, people died at Buffalo Creek, as did Bruce Wayne's parents. Bruce Wayne, like most of Lifton and Olson's (1976) subjects, is a survivor. The investigators at Buffalo Creek report on a phenomena termed *death guilt* (p. 3), a state of mind the very same researchers had witnessed while studying victims of the Holocaust and the Hiroshima bombing. Survivors exhort themselves about having lived while others died. People with death guilt feel as though they could have saved those who perished. The guilt can become even more severe if survivors feel they were spared as a result of someone else's death. This guilt infuses itself into both the dream state and waking hours of the survivor's life. As portrayed so well in the movie *The Pawnbroker* (Lumet, 1964), these people are, living a half-life devoid of pleasure and with limited vitality. This guilt is described by Mary Bergen (1958) in a case report of a 4-year-old child who "got out" before her father murdered her mother. It is also dramatically depicted in Joyce Carol Oates (1971) morbid novel *Wonderland,* where Jesse goes to school only to return home to his murdered family. Imagine the plight of "lucky" Bruce in the film, as he escapes the robber's gun because there is no time to kill him. He escapes death because the time was used to murder his parents.

When I lecture on understanding Batman as a resilient pop culture figure in an undergraduate college class, *Children and the Media*, the subject moves on quickly to a discussion of the students' own traumatic experiences. Sudden deaths of a parent and relatives, as well as "bad" car accidents, seem to top the list of traumas discussed. Several students had witnessed a drowning and some even a shooting. Only a few students have been courageous enough to speak about date rape and sexual abuse. All the students experienced sequelae, after the trauma, mostly in the form of flashbacks and anxious memories of the event. On more than one occasion, there were stories of a narrow escape, of survival, and of accompanying guilt. One undergrad spoke about swimming with her sister in a lake far from shore, when the sister developed a painful cramp in her side. The student tried to help her older and heavier sister, but she could not keep her afloat, and the sister drowned. This happened when the student was 11 years old, and she remained haunted by the memory of that moment when her sister "let go." It was only recently that she would even swim in a pool, and if young children came into the water, she would quickly leave. After class she told the author of her struggle with guilt and depression and even of her own suicide attempts. Another student described a car wreck that occurred when he was 17 and the consequent death of two close friends. He "should have suffered the same fate," but his body was shielded from harm by one of his lifeless friends. In an office meeting, the student later told me that the class on Batman not only acted as a spark for an interesting discussion but also related to his own issues. The student told of how he could not leave home for college the year after the accident or even the following year because he felt guilty that his dead friends "would never go." He also confided that he would only drive in a car alone, never with passengers.

THE SOLUTION

The original comic describes how young Wayne almost immediately integrates his familial tragedy. In a prayer-like position, with a candle to highlight the solemnity of the occasion, Bruce vows to dedicate his life to fighting crime. Perhaps Bruce's premorbid personality was intact enough to bear any blow, and hence his quick recovery. But the solution—a Batman—indicates problems, and perhaps even a pseudo-recovery, because it is both bizarre and psychologically over-determined.

Terr's (1979), Chowchilla study described compensatory fantasies that the youngsters had about their trauma. Actual fantasies of revenge were observed in 6 of the 23 children. They wanted the kidnappers starved, put in a hole, subjected to a firing squad, and finally placed in a gas chamber.

Fantasies of heroism or omnipotence were observed in five of the Chowchilla children. Several engaged in large-scale heroic and religious daydreams. One boy, the real hero of Chowchilla, Bob, who climbed out of the pit and went for help, reenacted his heroism in a dangerous manner 18 months after the kidnapping, when he shot a Japanese tourist whose car broke down near his family's property. Bob believed that the man meant to cause his parents harm. He did not wait as he had done during the kidnapping; he acted quickly. Fortunately, the tourist was not seriously injured.

Bruce Wayne's vow to fight crime is a compensatory wish. He identifies with the aggressor and, like Bob's gun assault, he acts out this wish in the movie's first scene. There is a conversion from the passive and helpless Bruce Wayne—a child—to the active and masterful Batman—an adult—who now renders robbers helpless. As seen also in the next frames of the original comic book story, young Bruce uses sublimation to harness his rage and anger. He controls his impulses by learning to become a master scientist and training to achieve the prowess of a superb athlete.

Jen, a 6-year-old girl who was referred to me as a result of a contentious divorce and custody battle, was an example of loss of innocence and subsequent rage in a child who tried in therapy to use play as a form of compensation. Jen was depressed but had enough energy to act out, hitting other children at school and than sobbing afterward that she "didn't mean it." Her play therapy was compulsive and unchanging, directed at her "bad" behavior and the need to be placed in jail. As part of her play, she would go through various crimes (stealing, murder) and place herself in jail. Once there, she would be forced to watch a continuous running video of her bad behavior. It was significant that a sex video was part of the evidence brought out in her parents divorce trial. This did make the author wonder to what exactly Jen had been exposed. To grasp how absorbed she was in her play, Jen would often include my cat, making him a very "mean" guard.

Over time, Jen calmed down in school; her parents' lives also became more balanced, and both remarried within months of a final settlement. Her jail scenarios continued, but they later incorporated Batman and Robin action figures. While playing, she would constantly refer to Robin as a "sidekick." Soon revealing to me that her brother, who was 8, often called her that, and although she did not fully understand the meaning of the term, it made her feel mad, little, and unimportant. She stated how she felt "outside" two families. This feeling was intensified when her father's new bride announced her pregnancy. Jen began speaking of the new baby as the sidekick, which baffled her parents. In her play, rather than a cooperative relationship between Batman and Robin, there was now much fighting between the superheroes. They would often be in conflict over where to go, whom to fight, and above all who was the real boss. Batman would hit and smack Robin while calling him "sidekick."

This aggressive play continued, actually resulting in the Batman action figure losing an arm. This violent play stopped when Jen's baby brother was born, because he and her older brother were now the sidekicks. She was the valuable, "only" girl.

I believe that using only generic toys (clay, crayons, blocks, baby dolls) in my playroom office to help children tell their own story can be limiting. Instead, figures depicting film or TV characters can be helpful (Brody, 2005). Jen's case illustrates how a superhero action figure can not only be identified with but can also help a child to modify his or her story to fit inner psychic needs. In the case of Jen, Robin as sidekick had great significance to her own marginalized self. These action figures can promote play and act as a catalyst for storytelling about overcoming a trauma (parental conflict and divorce) or a slight (being called a sidekick), rehearsing for an adult role, or making the unfamiliar familiar. Action figures appearing in a medical office may also create a climate of familiarity and comfort for children because they are old and trusted friends. Figures of superheroes, both TV show and film characters, demonstrate that the therapist is in tune with children's media and their world, making the therapist an adult whom the child can possibly relate to and even trust.

As part of the crime-fighter project, Bruce decided to choose a symbol to represent his mission—a signal to scare criminals. After all, Bruce may all too readily have understood Proustian involuntary memory triggers. Rado (1942) wrote of certain sensory stimuli evoking an original psychic trauma. The children of Chowchilla avoided the stale smell of basements reminiscent of the hole of their captivity and refused to eat peanut butter, the only food the kidnappers gave them, similar to the students described earlier who avoided swimming and driving with passengers.

In terms of sensory triggers and solutions to trauma, I think of *Lisa,* who began treatment while in high school. Two months before she first came to see me, she had witnessed a drive-by shooting in which the victim, another female student, was shot not 10 feet from her. Several weeks after the shooting, she was raped at gunpoint. This author saw Lisa through college as she suffered from posttraumatic stress disorder. She attended both individual and group psychotherapy sessions for her anxiety and depression. Although she still experienced flashbacks triggered by loud noises and was unable to have intimate physical contact with anyone, she did enter nursing school, which was both rigorous and demanding.

Lisa's first job was in a local children's hospital where she elected to deal with children who were abused sexually and physically. She often described her complete desensitization to the trauma and grief of the children with whom she worked. Occasionally, there would be breaks in her emotional wall, as when she saw children with rope burns from being tied up, anal tear injuries, and even bullet wounds. These situations would overwhelm her and bring her back to the fear and memory of her own traumas. Still, she persisted with her pediatric nursing, as if helping traumatized children would give her mastery over her own adolescent tragedies. Lisa was doing a great deal of good, but she paid for her compassion with much suffering. When *Batman* (Burton, 1989) was released, this therapist urged her to see it from the point of view of Batman's solution to his trauma, becoming this wonderful, yet miserable, crime fighter. Lisa understood that Batman, although helpful and good, was compulsive and unhappy, as maybe she was with her life's work, which, like Bruce's, seemed never ending and joyless. Also like him, she was on a mission to take care of traumatized children, no matter the consequences to herself. She had to do this work because "she couldn't help herself." Although psychological insight was helpful, the need to gain control and mastery over one's trauma, through tireless (repetitive) caring, was more compelling.

In the original comic, Bruce chooses the bat as a symbol soon after one flies in the window; he sees it as an omen. Posttraumatically, the Chowchilla children and their parents looked more closely for omens. The seating arrangement on the bus and fights with a parent on the day of the kidnapping all held special meaning (like Rebecca's mother not kissing her good-bye). Interpreting the most commonplace omens as signals was an effort to predict and control terrible events. It is not really odd, then, that several panels after Bruce accuses criminals of being superstitious, he is also influenced by an omen.

Bruce Wayne's belief in omens as well as his revenge solution, is evident in the case of *Sarah*, whose father brought her to see me when she was just 5 years old, saying that she was suffering from "separation fears." Sarah was born with a facial defect to a mother who initially felt only disgust and fear for the child; she worried that Sarah would be a lifelong target of humiliation and teasing. Sarah may have internalized some of her mother's fears because she refused to stay in school without her mother nearby. The administrators were growing impatient because other children began to ask their parents to stay with them. The author not only spent years working with Sarah, who would compulsively create new and "better" faces for Mr. Potato Head, but with her mother who suffered from a severe depression. Like the Chowchilla parents, Sarah's mother believed that her role in the accidental death of a treasured pet early in her pregnancy served as a "signal" that her baby would be "bad." At about 10 years old, Sarah began to play with other dolls in therapy, settling on Batman after her parents took her to see the 1989 movie with Michael Keaton. She became fascinated with the idea of revenge, because Batman's solution to his parents death was to make all criminals pay. As a teenager, Sarah began to talk of all the insults and humiliation that she experienced and her feelings of rage in their regard. She suffered from the open insensitivity of her peers. And while body image is very much self-image to most adolescents, Sarah decided to gain a sense of self from working hard on her academics and soccer, eventually winning acceptance to an Ivy League school. It is interesting that she kept a framed poster from the *Batman* movie over her bed to remind her of his "hard work and need for revenge." Sarah did go on to law school and the rewarding work of handling only disability and workman's compensation cases. She believed that "someone has to pay."

NONINTEGRATED PERSONALITY

When we first meet Bruce Wayne in the movie *Batman* (Burton, 1989), he is in a fog-like state. He is at a party distracted and constantly being helped by Alfred, his loyal butler and caretaker. Although immediately attracted to Vicki Vale, he is nonresponsive when she asks if he knows who Bruce Wayne is? Apparently, Bruce does not. His first date with Vicki starts absurdly. Vicki refers to some of the stuff in the mansion as "not you." Bruce replies, "some of it is." Bruce exudes a sense of loneliness and preoccupation. He appears to be half dead with "limited vitality." Even after sex with Vicki, we find him hanging from a bar like a bat trying to relax, probably, like many survivors, not able to feel real pleasure. The next day we find Bruce in even more of a trance, reminiscent of Kim Novak in Hitchcock's *Vertigo* (1968), another confused identity, going through a set of rituals at the site of his parent's murder. He honors the site of their deaths, rather than honoring them as people, because he is more connected to the event than to them. Still acting as if in a dream, Bruce stumbles on the Joker and his men who are assassinating a fellow mob boss. Bruce seems unaware of the flying bullets and the Joker regards his indifference with a puzzled expression.

Later in his encounter with Vicki Vale at her apartment, in a more familiar Michael Keaton style, Bruce tries to tell Vicki that he is Batman. He stutters and fails, but succeeds in tricking the Joker to shoot him in a silver plate. Bruce looks less a fool and is not really kidding, when the Joker recognizes him as "Bruce Wayne" and Bruce says "sometimes."

In *Batman Begins* (Nolan, 2005), the character emerges in full force, taking over Bruce Wayne's persona. From the very beginning of the film, the audience feels the sensation of flying. This is not the same smooth experience of flying that one has while viewing *Star Wars* (Lucas, 1977) or *Superman* (Donner, 1978), because the flight is constantly shifting, and we get a feel for the blindness of a bat. One speculates as to Bruce's need not to see, or possibly to view with another sense when others cannot.

Because he witnessed his parent's murder, Bruce may want to cover his eyes. Both Feiffer (1965) and Kael (1989) remarked on how the Batman's mask, in the comic and movie respectively, reveals only eye slits. Again, is it an attempt at blindness or, like wearing sunglasses, does it help the wearer avoid being seen by others? Perhaps this is a paranoid notion, but what is one to make of Bruce in the movie, looking through a one-way mirror and videotaping everything that occurs in the mansion? Even the Batman logo has confused and frustrated its audience. One has to be very field-independent to pick the bat out of the background. Some see teeth or even Mickey Mouse, but no bat. Is this another perceptual trick similar to the U. S. Air Force's use of a batlike design for the B-2 Stealth Bomber?

Pauline Kael (1989) was misinformed when she stated that the "picture doesn't give us any help on the question of why Bruce Wayne is creating an alternate identity" (p. 84). Bruce needs the extra identity to heal and act out his rage. He needs the menacing armored costume and various Bat Toys. This equipment allows Wayne to overcome his inhibitions and be active. He is no longer a bumbling, depressed half-person. He is no longer uncertain when he says, "I'm Batman." Batman is more pathological than a Halloween or Mardi Gras costume but less so than a Mr. Hyde or Son of Sam. Bruce appears to be in the throes of a dissociative phenomenon, but not of total identity diffusion. In fact, at this point in the movie, various aspects of his character seem to fuse, seemingly responsive to Vicki's love—apparently something Robin was only moderately successful at achieving. Bruce appears quite serious and dresses in black, moving ever closer to his Batman identity. In fact, after he recognizes the truth about his parent's murderer, Bruce Wayne no longer appears in the film; there is now only Batman.

The trauma of Bruce's parents' deaths is filmed in slow motion from a low angle, as if in the mind's eye of a child who sees the danger first. Is it no wonder that during the exciting battle that ends the film, when the Joker accuses Batman of "making me," Bruce replies, "You killed my parents, you made me first." He is one—Bruce Wayne and Batman; he is alive. But is he OK, satisfied? No! The film closes with a bright Bat Signal. Things are clearer, but nothing has been resolved. As the beautiful Vicki goes off in the Rolls Royce with champagne and Alfred, we see Batman standing alone, on guard, mission not completed, masochistically isolated and staring out at the night.

This last scene in *Batman,* filled with obsession, mission, and masked identity, reminds me of *Jody,* a 14-year-old with depression and anorexia who had been sexually abused from age 10 by her uncle. Although her parents knew of the abuse, it was kept a family secret, as the culprit, a local celebrity, brought many perks to the family in the form of free tickets, dinners, and even jobs. Jody suffered memory and sensory flash-backs of both the pain and humiliation of the sex acts, as well as rage for what had been done to her. She also confessed to being preoccupied with sexual thoughts and compulsively masturbating, which relieved tension but gave her little pleasure. Most of the time she walked around in a fog, numb to people and her surroundings. She felt emotionally dissociated not only from her trauma but also from her own body, which was deteriorating as a result of starvation. Her anorexia was a "mask" to disguise her sexuality. She needed to be removed from her desires, sexual guilt, and womanhood. She wanted to feel no connection between herself and her emaciated body, which she regarded as contaminated and the source of all her troubles. In therapy, she quickly assumed the role of the "good" pseudo-compliant patient. This "as if" (Deutsch, 1942) ingredient of most borderline patients is what makes therapy so stormy. Without an inner core of their own, patients often mirror their therapists. This action functions as resistance to any real therapeutic work, leading to endless discussions about the therapist and rarely promotes progress. After learning of my interest in Batman from a news article, she, of course, quickly became a Dark Knight fan. Instead of interpreting her compliant yet resistant transference interest, I pointed out how she, like Bruce, was immune to physical and psychic pain, as well as pleasure. There was a real therapeutic breakthrough when Jody saw the image of Batman on the big screen standing by himself, compulsively looking for the next criminal, instead of going off in the car with Vicki. This scene provoked in Jody a sadness but also positive insight. Unlike Bruce, she was in psychotherapy and could change her numbness and drive to starve herself to more depth of feeling and control.

DISCUSSION

Jules Feiffer (1965) focused on Batman's humanness—Batman bleeds, he hurts, and he needs to persevere to triumph over adversity. It was both easier and more difficult to identify with Batman than the immortal heroes with various superpowers. Feiffer even suspected the children who were involved with Batman had healthier egos. To be a fan of Superman was easier and safer. You did not have to be good in science, like Batman. For Superman to escape from a tight situation, superstrength or X-ray vision were enough. To be a fan of Superman was like rooting for the Yankees instead of the vulnerable Dodgers. Comic book critic Feiffer also credited Batman's initial popularity to Bob Kane's superior story lines, creative villains, and what he called a cinematic (how prophetic) eye in his drawings, with angle shots and long shadows (p. 27).

Caruth (1968), in her masterful explanation of Superman as a modern-day myth, began to appreciate developmental forces as the appeal of the early comic book heroes.

> The comic books, specifically the action comics, with which I am primarily concerned here are of particular appeal to the older latency and preadolescent child, who is in more of a transitional phase between primary, and secondary fantasy interests, between infantile sexuality and latency, between role playing and identity formation. (p. 8)

To appreciate Superman, primary process must predominate because of its reliance on prelogical magical thinking. It is the thinking of dreams, fantasy, and fairy tales; X-ray vision and Kryptonite. Batman's appeal relates to secondary processes that are logical and reality based. He has no superpowers and is therefore realistic and plausible. Although a very young audience struggles between primary and secondary process thinking, Batman may help toward the realistic shift. Fantasizing about flying, lifting cars, or being bulletproof does little to promote growth and inner resilience. In essence, a youngster has to become her own superhero based on her own human resources and talents.

Caruth (1968) declared comics to be an "integral part of today's literature for children" that "fulfills an important psychic function" (p. 10). Like myths and fairy tales, they provide an externalization of inner conflicts. The child can now see his inner difficulties more clearly and reflect on a variety of solutions.

Batman's myth further adds evidence to Erikson's (1968) developmental conflict between the opposing challenges of industry over inferiority. School-age youngsters, according to Erikson, must begin to turn their dreams, play, and drives into skills and success. Although Erikson's list (trust versus mistrust, autonomy versus shame, initiative versus doubt) of developmental tasks parallels Freud's psychosexual stages (oral, anal, phallic, latency), Erikson's are psychosocial and external as they relate to cultural and societal norms. It is crucial for an elementary school child to begin to feel competent, which, in our competitive American culture, is integral to one's sense of self-worth and belonging. Although Batman does not seem to have much trouble with self-esteem or a need for acceptance, as a human superhero, he does offer his readers some guidance. Batman gives instructions on how to overcome limitations and adversity by hard work and mental discipline. No superhero special powers are needed, just a Michael Jordan or Tiger Woods work ethic, as well as a firm grasp of technology, athletic skills, and strong sense of purpose.

One must also appreciate that in addition to Batman's psychological appeal as a dramatic and tragic character, he is, of course, a great source of entertainment, which through the years continues to reflect the current culture. For example, as he did earlier with comic books, in the 1960s, Batman conquered television. Camping it up, using retired Hollywood stars as villains—Cesar Romero as the Joker, for example— and Lichtenstein-like cartoon captions during fights, the Caped Crusader and a ridiculous Boy Wonder were a tonic to the violence of the real-world 1960s. Susan Sontag (1966) explained that the hallmark of camp is the spirit of extravagance. Camp is playful; it proposes a comic vision of the world that the TV show certainly promoted.

On a personal note, as a young child, I became easily hooked on the Caped Crusader (Batman), after I was punished for trying to fly out of my bedroom window wearing a cape with a big S on it. I turned to Batman with enthusiasm. Batman was more real to a 6- or 7-year-old than the Green Lantern, Submariner, or the Flash. Batman demonstrated the value of hard work, persistence, and possibility. I liked his alternate identity lifestyle as a rich playboy. I did not quite know what that was, but Bruce did have a lot of "stuff" and even a butler to clean up after him. Batman's anger and rage was also seductive to a kid being pushed around by family dynamics and societal circumstances. Clark Kent, on the other hand, seemed foolish, a do-gooder, awkward, and poor.

As I "grew up," Batman continued to appeal to me, even after reading *Seduction of the Innocent* (Wertham, 1955). Chapters including "Retooling For Illiteracy," "Design For Delinquency," and "Homicide at Home" stressed the homoerotic appeal of Batman and his young sidekick Robin. They spend their time rescuing each other and living an idyllic life in the Wayne mansion. Wertham, a psychiatrist, believed the story line was a "wish dream" of homosexuals (p. 192). He did not believe that the colorful-costumed (red and green) Robin was created to brighten up the gloomy dark Batman and to serve as a source of identification for young adolescents. Instead, he viewed Robin more as a sex partner than as a sidekick to the superhero. Wertham further described the violence and the antifeminism of the Batman character. He related numerous clinical anecdotes about homosexuals who identified with Robin. Although he had many interesting insights into the violence in children's comics, it was most unfortunate that Wertham became so obsessed with Bruce's sexuality. Like many experts of that era, he was wrong in thinking that homosexuality was both pathological and contagious. Also, Batman's problem was not one of sexual orientation but more a question of balance. There was a lack of sexual interest, all sublimated compulsively into his rage and crime fighting.

It should be noted that Wertham did not succeed in having Batman banned, but he did succeed, with the aid of the Red Scare and the

Comic Book Code, in ruining my childhood with the outlawing of such EC Comics favorites as *Weird Science* and *Tales of the Crypt*. But it is also necessary to confess that later in life, when I had my turn testifying before congressional investigators about the violence on children's television (*Playing With Death*, 2000), I invoked Dr. Wertham's name as a great protector of children.

Throughout my career, I have used popular culture as a teaching device. For most people, popular culture is real-world information. I would show video clips from the *Wonder Years* (Baldwin, 1988) and *Beverly Hills 90210* (Adams, 1990) to medical students to discuss adolescence. I used *E. T.* (Spielberg, 1982) and *Bambi* (Hand, 1942) to describe separation fears to nursery-school teachers and college counselors. I even enlisted the Cookie Monster to demonstrate Freud's concept of the oral stage as well as Erikson's ideas on mistrust to psychiatric residents. With my patients, I have formulated psychological interpretations employing scenes from films such as *The Bridge on the River Kwai* (Lean, 1957) to illustrate obsession with TV shows such as *Nip/Tuck* (Murphy, 2003) to highlight the destructiveness of narcissism.

As a therapist, I have seen superheroes appear in patients' dreams and associations. Such was the case of *Eric*, an executive and unhappily married husband who dreamt of Wonder Woman saving him from his "false" marriage. In associating to the dream, Eric revealed that as a child, his mother, a "big powerful woman," allowed him to read only one comic a month. He chose *Wonder Woman* because he admired her strength and because "she seemed very real to him." After understanding the parallel of Wonder Woman to his mother and later his controlling wife, Eric unconsciously went one step further, starting his own stealth airplane company. It was only later in therapy that Eric connected his huge financial success to Wonder Woman, who flew her own invisible plane

I have also used Batman in my teaching of medical residents. For more than 5 years, I met weekly with senior medical residents at a small general hospital and discussed the psychology of their interactions with patients. A subject that came up often was the giving of bad news. There was fear and much anxiety associated with this all too common task, and, as a result, it was usually handled poorly. Unfortunately, their supervisors were often poor role models, avoiding it when they could and shifting the burden to their younger protégés. The way information is given, especially bad news, can be traumatic. The patient's and family's emotional systems become overloaded as they become immobilized and stop receiving any information. Words such as *cancer, bypass,* and *transplantation* act as bombs or bullets. To help these residents better understand the impact of this "informational trauma," I used the origin story of Batman, describing the various sequelae that he suffered as a result of being overwhelmed by the sudden impact of what he witnessed. Once again, through the use of popular culture, to which most of the young residents easily related, I was able to describe how one's patients can experience a similar trauma if medical information is not presented in a calm, slow, and patient manner. Bad news hurts, but when presented face-to-face with time for the patient to absorb the information and possibly ask questions, the blow can be softened. As their teacher, I emphasized that human interactions like this make not only for a good doctor, but also a successful one.

CONCLUSION

Batman successfully taps into the unconscious of my patients and students because his psychology remains credible. Batman's symptoms and recovery are all consistent with the vast psychiatric trauma literature. Batman is also a true superhero for all media and times. Batman's external state reflects many of our own internal struggles. From his isolation to his metaphorical elements, which are both psychologically motivated and metaphysical, his story provides transcendence into the sublime—the mysterious! Batman is an inspiration and a true myth. Batman sheds light on all of our stories. He is a source of comfort, helps us along our inward journeys, assists in understanding and resolving our traumas, and guides us in seeking our identity and the experience of being alive.

REFERENCES

Adams, C. (Director). (1990). *Beverly Hills 90210* [Television series]. United States: Spelling Television.

Baldwin, P. (Director). (1988). *The wonder years* [Television series]. United States: New World Television.

Bergen, M. (1958). The effect of severe trauma on a four-year-old child. *The Psychoanalytic Study of the Child, 13,* 407–429.

Brody, M. (1995). Batman: Psychic trauma and its solution. *Journal of Popular Culture, 28,* 171–178.

Brody, M. (2005). Play, toys and the "Gates." *American Academy of Child and Adolescent News, 36,* 120.

Burton, T. (Director). (1989). *Batman* [Motion picture]. United States/United Kingdom: Guber-Peters.

Campbell, J. (1988). *The power of myth.* New York: Doubleday.

Caruth, E. (1968). Hercules and Superman: The modern-day mythology of the comic book. *Journal of the American Academy of Child Psychiatry, 7,* 1–12.

Deutsch, H. (1942). Some forms of emotional disturbance and their relationship to schizophrenia. *Psychoanalytic Quarterly, 11,* 301–321.

Donner, R. (Director). (1978). *Superman* [Motion picture]. United Kingdom: Alexander Salkind.

Erikson, E. H. (1968). *Identity: Youth and crisis.* New York: Norton.

Feiffer, J. (1965). *The Great Comic Book Heroes.* New York: Bonanza Books.

Freud, A. (1967). Comments on psychic trauma. In *The writings of Anna Freud.* New York: International Universities Press.

Freud, S. (1955). Beyond the pleasure principle. In J. Strachey (Ed. & Trans.), *The standard edition of the complete psychological works of Sigmund Freud* (Vol. 18, 1st ed.). London: Hogarth. (Original work published 1920)

Hand, D. (Director). (1942). Bambi [Motion picture]. United States: Walt Disney Productions.

Hitchcock, A. (Director). (1958). *Vertigo* [Motion picture]. United States: Alfred J. Hitchcock Productions

Kael, P. (1989, July 10). The city gone psycho. *The New Yorker,* 83–85.

Kane, B. (1939). The legend of Batman. *Detective Comics.* New York: National Periodical Publications.

Lean, D. (Director). (1957). *The bridge on the River Kwai* [Motion picture]. United Kingdom/United States: Columbia Pictures Corporation.

Lifton, R., & Olson, E. (1976). The human meaning of total disaster. *Psychiatry, 39,* 1–18.

Lucas, G. (Director). (1977). *Star wars* [Motion picture]. United States: Lucasfilm.

Lumet, S. (Director). (1964). *The pawnbroker* [Motion picture]. United States: Landau Company.

Martinson, L. (Director). (1966). *Batman the movie* [Motion picture]. United States: Twentieth Century Fox.

Murphy, R. (Director). (2003). *Nip/Tuck* [Television series]. United States: Hands Down Entertainment.

Nolan, C. (Director). (2005). *Batman begins* [Motion picture]. United States: Warner Bros.

Oates, J. C. (1971). *Wonderland.* New York: The Vanguard Press.

Playing with death. (2002). Hearing before the U.S. Senate Summit on Public Health and Violence in the Media (testimony of Michael Brody).

Rado, S. (1942). Pathodynamics and treatment of traumatic war neurosis. *Psychosomatic Medicine, 4,* 362–368.

Sontag, S. (1966). *Against interpretation.* New York: Farrar, Strauss & Giroux.

Spielberg, S. (Director). (1982). *E.T. the extra-terrestrial* [Motion picture]. United States: Universal Pictures.

Terr, L. (1979). The children of Chowchilla. *The Psychoanalytic Study of the Child, 34,* 547–623.

Wertham, F. (1955). *Seduction of the innocent.* London: Museum Press.

CHAPTER SEVEN

Making a Place for the Angry Hero on the Team

Harry Livesay

> I know what you mean about anger. Sometimes I just wanna fight some-
> thin' because it's the only way I know how to relate to my teammates.
> It's the only way I feel . . . validated.
> —Wolverine, from an imaginary conversation among Batman, Robin,
> Wolverine, Spawn, and the Punisher (O'Brien, 2005)

When a child, particularly a boy, is angry or aggressive, it can be difficult for adults to listen patiently and provide the necessary emotional support. Parents and teachers can often feel threatened by the boy's anger, sending the mixed message that anger is a "normal" human emotion, but that it is also something to be feared and controlled. In the pantheon of superheroes, the "angry hero," as personified by characters such as Batman, the Hulk, and Wolverine, is often the recipient of this same mixed message from society—one that both fears and needs them. Like these angry heroes, angry male children may often feel isolated from their peers and social support systems because of a "grievous injustice," such as a traumatic experience, the stigma of psychopathology, family disintegration, poverty, racial persecution, or simply being identified with the self-fulfilling label, "problem child."

In my practice as a school-based health center social worker, a common occurrence is a desperate referral from a parent, principal, coach or teacher about a boy "whose anger is out of control." In these situations, it is more often than not the case that the boy's anger is a coping mechanism he uses to contend with divorce, domestic violence, bullying, blended families, academic underachievement, negative peer pressure, and the multitude of external stressors of home and school.

Early in my clinical work with these angry boys, I had to overcome not only the great age difference between my clients and myself, but also the seemingly superhuman task of bridging the power disparities that resulted from culture and language barriers. In retrospect, the solution was simple and on my play table all along: a plastic figure of Batman, a premium from a fast-food kids meal.

I am reminded of an angry and resistant 8-year-old client who had been referred to me as a last resort by his teacher and his mother. Initially sullen and detached, his demeanor changed dramatically when he picked up this plastic figure and excitedly asked me if I had "Robin and Joker too?" Sensing an open window of common ground, I asked my young client a key question, "What do you know about Batman and the Joker?" Over an hour later, my client was still enthusiastically recounting his recollections, thoughts, feelings, and opinions of the many Batman cartoons he had seen. I wondered why Batman had succeeded when my clinical skills—empathic listening, emotional validation, unconditional positive regard, and therapeutic play had failed. As my client eagerly made clear, "Batman is *tight!* Batman is *cool!* Batman is *scary!* Batman gets his mad on and kicks some butt!" In other words, Batman is angry like me.

Employing my own great interest in superheroes and therapeutic play, I have since used my clients' interest in angry superheroes such as Batman, Wolverine, the Hulk, and others to build relationships, establish trust, and provide my angry young male clients with a safe foray into the universe of fantasy violence. In so doing, I have helped them come to terms with their anger without the frustration and shame that angry boys often encounter in home and school environments.

It is not my intention to exclude girls or to minimize the similar role that anger plays in disrupting their relationships with parents and teachers. In the universe of superheroes, the angry superheroine, from Catwoman to Aeon Flux, has also played the role of outsider alongside their male counterparts. However, in both society and in superhero culture, different standards continue to exist for the expression of anger between the genders. We see this in the historical context of parents being more accepting of anger in boys than in girls (Gibbard, 2001) and within the cultural framework of the male superhero expressing anger in harmful ways in the name of social justice (Fingeroth, 2004).

Although these gender-based role biases are seemingly weakening, allowing girls to express feelings of anger, this double standard still apparently exists in the world of superheroes. Fingeroth (2004) expressed this dichotomy by noting that "whereas Batman and Spiderman would take personal tragedy and transform it into socially useful aggression . . . a superhumanly powerful woman [Elektra, in his case] could only be powerful in the service of evil" (p. 91).

My focus on therapeutic play with male children in the context of the angry superhero is based primarily on my experiences in working with angry male children and my belief that society continues to create angry boys. This is consistent with the work of Pollack (1998), who in his book *Real Boys* noted that society pushes boys to "suppress their vulnerable and sad feelings . . . and express the one strong feeling allowed them—anger" (p. 44). Although society tolerates and encourages boys to incorporate anger into their play, it conversely requires them to stay in control of any other emotion by becoming what Pollack referred to as a "big wheel," by achieving "status, dominance and power [and acting] as though everything is alright, as though everything is under control, even though it isn't" (p. 24).

Pollack, with the support of Mary Pipher, author of *Reviving Ophelia* (1994), suggested that unwritten rules reinforced by society compel boys to cloak their emotions and to hide their fear, shame, and compassion beneath macho exteriors. Pollack's *boy code,* similar to the notion of the masked superhero, demands that boys "hide their true feelings behind a protective mask of stoicism and bravado . . . the only emotion that they can legitimately let show is anger" (Pollack & Cushman, 2001, p. 104).

In this chapter, I hope to provide parents, teachers, clinicians, and other supportive adults with some practical information that can be used in getting to know the boy behind the mask of the angry superhero by identifying the core feelings underlying the anger and, in doing so, help "unlock the mask through (emotional) connection, listening, and empathizing" (Pollack & Cushman, 2001, p. 105). As the Justice League benefits from the unique talents of Batman and the X-Men are made more powerful through Wolverine's participation, so, too, can angry male children be allowed to become valued members of the team at home and at school, through acceptance, understanding, listening, and guidance and by enhancing their self-esteem and security.

THE ANGRY SUPERHERO

The angry hero, or the hero motivated by anger, is a literary concept that dates back to antiquity. One the first and most famous angry heroes can be found in Homer's *Iliad,* in the form of Achilles, the Greek hero of the Trojan War and "a formidable warrior, possessing fierce and uncontrollable anger [who is] filled with grief and rage" (Achilles, 2003) when his friend and lover Patroclus is killed by Hector. The angry hero, or antihero—from Achilles to Dirty Harry—is a fictional character that has characteristics of a villain or an outsider. Although portrayed somewhat sympathetically, antiheroes can be awkward, antisocial, alienated, obnoxious, passive, pitiful, obtuse, or just ordinary; but they are always, in some fundamental way, flawed, unqualified, or failed heroes (Anti-hero, n. d.).

This tradition of heroes, "whose roots are in [a] grievous injustice—real or perceived or both—done to them" (Fingeroth, 2004, p. 121) is a popular genre, spanning the history of comics in the 20th century. This school of superheroes are provoked into the role vigilante or righter of wrongs because of a violent loss or change (Daredevil), childhood fury generated by some traumatic event (Batman and Punisher), or a scientific catastrophe (Wolverine, the Thing, the Hulk). Because of the recent wave of superhero films, television shows, Web sites, and video games, these angry heroes continue to fascinate, excite, and inspire boys. Of these various heroes, Batman, the Wolverine, and the Incredible Hulk have enjoyed a recent renaissance in popular culture, in the hero play of male children, and in my own clinical practice.

Since his introduction in 1939, Batman, the mysterious and menacing protector of Gotham City, has been emulated by and incorporated into the fantasy and superhero play of generation of males. Created by DC Comics artist Bob Kane, Batman is one of the more psychologically complex and intriguing of the superheroes. Batman's development into an angry hero stemmed from witnessing the murder of his parents and his subsequent oath to rid the city of the evil that took his parents' lives. Batman channeled his anger into a regimen of intellectual and physical training in the areas of chemistry, criminology, forensics, martial arts, and gymnastics, as well as theatrical skills such as disguise, escapology, and ventriloquism.

Batman's anger and subsequent desire for vengeance are the keys to his transformation into a superhero. According to DC Publisher Paul Levitz,

> Batman isn't a guy who finds himself endowed with superpowers and simply says I'll do good with them because I'm a good person. This is a man who watched his parents die and then had to decide how to respond. He's tortured by feelings of guilt and anger . . . yet he sets out to become a transformative being, someone who can change the world. (Batman Begins, n. d.)

Although the circumstances that motivated Batman to be a superhero are extreme, his continued popularity, stated actor Christian Bale, the most recent portrayer of DC's "Dark Knight," is due in large part to "our ability to relate to (his) pain of loss, outrage at injustice, and the need for an outlet through which to vent anger and turn negative emotions into positive actions" (Batman Begins, n. d.).

A differently motivated but highly admired angry hero can found in Marvel Comic's Wolverine. Introduced in 1974 by Len Wein and John Romita Sr., Wolverine rose from relative obscurity to become one of Marvel Comics' most popular characters. Wolverine is one of a number of mutants who possess both natural and artificial superpowers, including strength and a physical regenerative capacity. Wolverine also possesses animal-like senses and reflexes and has three forearm-length claws on each hand. Although his origins have been altered in subsequent story-lines, common lore has it that he was kidnapped because of ultra healing powers and made part of a project called Weapon X. The torture he endured during the experimentation, which resulted in the grafting of an unbreakable metal alloy to his skeleton, triggered a fierce, animal-like nature characterized by a ready willingness to use deadly force. His efforts to come to terms with past trauma and his angst-filled inner conflicts have made Wolverine a prototype of angry heroes for the 21st century.

Completing the angry hero trinity is a character that has been described as "the distilled essence of anger" (Fingeroth, 2004, p. 121), another Marvel Comics creation, the Incredible Hulk. Created by Stan Lee and Jack Kirby, the Hulk first appeared 1962. The result of a Nuclear Age experiment gone wrong, military scientist Dr. Bruce Banner was exposed to an enormous dose of gamma radiation that causes him to transform into the rampaging Hulk (Hulk, n. d.).

The Hulk possesses an incredible level of superhuman physical ability. His capacity for physical strength is boundless, with his strength increasing proportionally to his level of emotional stress and anger. The Hulk has a high resistance to physical damage as well as to extreme temperatures, poisons, and diseases. Similar to his Marvel counterpart Wolverine, the Hulk can regenerate damaged or destroyed areas of tissue at an amazing rate.

Although the Hulk is classified as a superhero, he and Dr. Banner share a Jekyll and Hyde–like relationship. In later versions of the origin stories, writers have portrayed the character as a symbol of inner rage and Freudian repression, with the Hulk's existence as a by-product of Bruce Banner's long-term abuse by an emotionally unstable father (Hulk, n. d.). This depiction of the Hulk's character as the wounded child justifies his rage-powered rampages as an outlet to deal with his deep emotional pain. Specifically, according to Fingeroth (2004),

It's a response frustrating to child and adult alike. It is the existential cry of humankind, the reason even the rich and accomplished suffer angst and depression. Is it biochemical? Is it spiritual? Whatever the reason, something is wrong, something we can't name or define, and something that a run in the park or a drink or a visit to a brothel or a house of worship won't cure. It just . . . hurts to be alive. That's where the primal scream of Hulkdom comes in. At the very least, one can cry out in anger and defiance: I am here! I hurt! Make it stop! (p. 126)

THE APPEAL OF THE ANGRY HERO

During the 1970s and 1980s, as comics were struggling to maintain their consumer base, characters and stories became grittier and darker. While DC Comics was destroying and condensing its multiple earths and universes, Batman returned to his Golden Age role of a morally ambiguous and sinister vigilante. Also, during this period, while Marvel introduced Wolverine, it was also producing other new angry heroes, including the Punisher and the more sinister Daredevil. Keeping in the tradition of the antihero, these characters were all deeply troubled from within. This trend is thought to have been a reflection of the cultural cynicism of the later 20th century, "when the idea of a person selflessly using his extraordinary abilities on a quest for good was no longer believable, but a person with a deep psychological impulse to destroy criminals was" (Superheroes—Deconstruction, n. d.).

In his book, *Killing Monsters: Why Children Need Fantasy, Super Heroes and Make Believe Violence,* Jones (2002) described evolution in superhero culture as the result of the "audience's growing taste for rampant passion . . . even the kids who want the simplest dramas of good and evil want their heroes to express a baseline of anger" (p. 206). Jones makes the case that the appeal of angry cultural heroes is a by-product of the growing fear and frustration that children feel in our culture. He noted, "It's natural to respond to anger with a defensive anger of our own or a fear of where it will lead. We respond more effectively, when we first ask, why are kids so angry?" (p. 206). Fingeroth (2004) referred to a nationwide survey of violent youth by Dr. Helen Smith, who concluded that "a tremendous number of young people compare school to prison" (Smith, 2000). Fingeroth concurred with Smith's conclusion and lamented that many of today's youth feel angrily imprisoned by uncontrollable circumstances, seemingly unreasonable adult expectations, and violence in the world.

Jones's book also provides—in the story of former DC Comics editor and school teacher Ruben Diaz—a remarkable example of how children look to role models in popular culture in coming to terms with these feelings of anger, fear, and hopelessness. Diaz, who grew up in a South Bronx public housing project, describes himself as the stereotypic inner-city bully. According to Jones's account of Diaz's story, he grew up in the 1980s with no father and a working mother who couldn't be around much. Afraid at school and on the street, he spent his teen years in his apartment watching TV, listening to rap music, and reading comic hooks. He saw little in a negligent government, a decimated educational establishment, or a crime-obsessed news media to make him think that society had much use for a non-White, low-income teenager. He found his most meaningful models in gangster rappers and superheroes. In their different ways, both demonstrated how individual anger could be channeled into the power to confront corruption and change the world. And both, Diaz realized, "were created by commercial storytellers in not—quite—respectable fields who were willing to say what kids were really thinking and fantasizing" (Jones, 2005, p. 209).

As in the case of Ruben Diaz, we see that young males are naturally drawn to angry representations in our culture for direction and validation of their own feelings of anger. For me, this explains the continuing fascination my young male clients have for Batman, Wolverine, the Hulk, and their angry brothers in the pantheon of cultural icons because they provide them with fantasies of being a larger and more powerful self than they actually are. Along these lines, Jones argued that

> being something; superheroes, monsters, army men ... can nourish those fantasies. They provide symbols of power—powerful feelings they can "become"—that their usual experiences cannot .... especially at around age four or five, as children become more conscious of themselves as individual, trademarked superheroes can be the perfect surrogate selves. (p. 70)

For boys dealing with anger and the inevitable social challenges that accompany it, the angry superhero provides "the final common pathway for a boy's strong feelings" (Pollack, 1998, p. 44) via his own imagination by letting him *be* what he sees in these angry heroes—he can be glamorous, invincible, powerful, and express the poignant need for acceptance.

ANGER, AGGRESSION, AND BOYS

Children's anger presents challenges to parents and teachers who look on it as baffling, exhausting, and upsetting. According to Jones (2002), "There is no emotion that we feel so uncomfortable with in our society as anger, no other emotion than we dread more in our children. But anger can be creative too. It can be an energizing force. It can kick us back into action after a defeat, push us through obstacles, [and] knock our fears out of our minds" (p. 69). In their early years, many children receive the message that anger is "bad" or something to be stifled, suppressed, or ignored. Parents and teachers must remember that just as there are many things in our adult lives that make us angry—being cut off in traffic, losing something important, the demands on our time and attention, or being frustrated by the stressors of daily life—there are likewise many things in children's lives that make them angry, and their reactions are normal. Children respond with anger when they feel helpless or powerless. The feelings of helplessness are often accompanied by embarrassment or shame, loneliness, isolation, anxiety, or hurt.

Children often respond with anger to these types emotions because they feel helpless in comprehending the situation and helpless or powerless to change it. In this way, their anger is a response to feelings of frustration as well. Consider the example of a boy who demonstrates oppositional or defiant behavior as a way to way to deal with feelings of dependency, fear, or loss. A child who feels hurt by a loss may become angry as a way to avoid feeling sad and powerless. This culturally determined male ideal has been referred to as the "sturdy oak" response (David & Brannon, 1976), the expectation that boys do not openly share their emotional pain and instead conceal it beneath a façade of strength and imperturbability.

In Pollack's view (1998), anger then becomes the primary conduit for boys to channel their feelings of hurt, fear, and sadness. He suggested that

> it is through anger that boys express their (feelings) of vulnerability and powerlessness. The more tender feelings seem too shameful to show and boys turn to anger as the easiest feeling to express.... Understandably it is very challenging for most men to express or experience emotions other than anger since, as boys they are encouraged to use anger to express the full range of their emotional experience. (p. 44)

Parents and teachers should remember also that anger is not the same thing as aggression. Anger is a feeling and is generally a temporary emotional state caused by an underlying emotion, frustration, unmet need, fear, or a combination of these. Aggression is a class of behaviors, historically associated with predatory conduct, domination, defense, and competition (Moyer, 1968). Some parents and teachers can confuse the two and make an effort to punish anger because they do not like aggression. In fact, research on neurological and behavioral differences between the sexes indicates that all aggression by boys is not necessarily something to be feared. In fact, for some boys, aggression may be an important mechanism for male–male communication (Gurian & Stevens, 2005). According to these authors, boys who aggress against each other often demonstrate joyful behavior with the intimacy of such physical contact. In the context of this notion of *aggression nurturance*, Gurian and Stevens indicated that boys nurture themselves and others through aggressive gestures and activities. Given the hormonal and neural makeup of males, "it's often the case for boys (and men) that aggressive gestures (which we've called 'karate kicks') are as nurturing as words, as bonding as hugs" (p. 93).

This is not to say that all aggression in boys should be accepted as nonharmful behavior, as Jones noted when he said "aggression also taps into real anger, even when it starts out playfully. Play fighting can turn into real fighting. A kid may not know how much damage he can do or might use roughhousing as a pretext to hurt someone" (Jones, 2005, p. 69). Aggression, when it results in harm to others or damage to property, requires immediate attention from parents and teachers and should necessitate immediate consultation with medical and mental health professionals. On the other hand, children who are referred for help in controlling their anger may often demonstrate aggressive or destructive behavior as a way to compel an adult in their life to get involved and provide the needed attention.

SUPERHERO PLAY

In an essay on the nature of children and their play, television celebrity and child advocate Fred Rogers shared the belief that "a large part of children's making and building play comes from the desire to feel in control of the outside world and the inner self" (Rogers & Sharapan, 1994, p. 14). This desire to feel in control is a key element in the creation of a positive individual identity in children and in ensuring their healthy emotional development. Superhero play, according to Jones (2002), helps to foster these feelings of being in control. As Jones noted,

> They provide symbols of power—powerful beings they can become— that their usual experiences cannot. . . . There is a special power inherent in cartoon characters and action figures; they are individualized and yet universal, human yet superhuman, unique visual symbols that can be held clearly in the mind's eye and are instantly recognized by everyone. (p. 70)

Similarly, famed cartoonist and essayist Jules Feiffer (1965) explains in his pioneering work, *The Great Comic Book Heroes,* that our cultural fascination with superheroes can be traced to our societal realization of the complex and scary realities of living in 20th-century America:

> The advent of the superhero was a bizarre comeuppance for the American dream. Horatio Alger could no longer make it on his own. He needed "Shazam!" Here was fantasy with a cynically realistic base: once the odds were appraised honestly it was apparent you had to be "super" to get on in this world. (p. 18)

Author Danny Fingeroth (2004), concurred with this philosophy of our cultural need for superheroes, advising "that even in their 'real' heroes, people need to see powers and abilities far beyond those that the rest of us—even the best of us—are capable of displaying" (p. 33). Thus, superheroes in addition to offering opportunities for expression and creativity also encourage and empower children in fostering a sense of control.

For children of the post–September 11 era, superhero play can also provide a way for them to reveal needs, fears, and difficulties, as well as means to overcome psychic pain. In this context, Jones (2002) cited his experience in working with a 5-year-old survivor of sexual abuse, who in dealing with this trauma would create fantasies of great power, while professing, "I'm so fast I can run faster than a car so he can't catch me! I'm so strong I'll hit him with those flowers and because I'm strong the flowers with knock him out!" (p. 67). Through the use of superhero play, this child begins the process of healing by becoming his own rescuer and transforming fear and rage into more positive and hopeful feelings. In a sense, he provides a means of infusing power into his life story and for the first time, perceiving himself as a winner.

By becoming their own version of Batman, Superman, or Spider-Man to defeat a Joker, Lex Luthor, or Green Goblin, children create new endings not only to routine daily problems in home and at school but, as we have seen, to the most complex ordeals as well. Superhero play can help to foster a sense of control—significantly, at time in children's lives when they feel quite vulnerable and powerless.

Superhero play can also promote socialization and emotional bonding in children by tapping into themes of central importance to their lives. According to her observations of children's storytelling efforts using superheroes and Greek gods in an urban primary school, Dyson (1996) suggested that the appeal of superheroes in children's play is due to the universal themes in their stories. Comparing the exploits of superheroes and Greek gods in classroom learning efforts, she asserted that their stories "offer consistent characters whose qualities and exploits become familiar as they appear and reappear in story after story. Good guys and bad guys, great quarrels and grand rescues, marriages, births, and deaths—all are powerful playground fare" (p. 493).

In my own experience with angry boys, the universality of the basic themes of good versus evil and 'saving the day', transcend race, age, socioeconomic level, and culture as a result of the child's intuitive understanding that it's fun to be a superhero! I find that children and adolescents who are resistant to direct exploration of their thoughts, experiences, and feelings, respond positively and excitedly to superhero play. The reason for this is that this storytelling helps children to experience their thoughts and feelings more completely. In relating the adventures of a favorite hero and villain, children can safely experience the excitement and hazards of superhero life and provide adults with a tool to "learn what is uppermost in the child's mind at that moment" (Rogers & Sharapan, 1994, p. 15). As supportive adults, we can also use superhero play to promote attachment; teach empathy, acceptance, and forgiveness; and assist angry children in making sense of the perplexing and contradictory world in which they live and gaining understanding of themselves and their place in this world.

THE ANGRY HERO ON THE TEAM

Another aspect of our captivation with superheroes is their "family appeal," or what author Fingeroth (2004) defined as a team appeal of "individuals banded together with the purpose of combining their powers and abilities, usually against a threat that is too great for any one of them to handle on their own" (p. 103). Superhero teams and families (the X-Men, Fantastic Four, Justice League, and The Incredibles) permeate our popular culture and "both reflect and inspire the families that we ourselves wish we could belong to and/or wish we could escape" (p. 101). In the world of superheroes, many teams have been created over the years to share adventures, role model egalitarian behavior, and provide a playground "where characters could attract new fans while entertaining established admirers" (Daniels, 1995, p. 127).

Popular superhero teams have included DC Comic's Golden Age lineup of heroes in the Justice Society of America, a family of teen sidekicks of adult heroes who banded together to form the Teen Titans, and a team of varied alloyed robots known as the Metal Men. Marvel Comics, too, has made the superhero family a cornerstone of its publications during the last 40 years with the Avengers, the Fantastic Four (who share the distinction of being superheroes who are actually related to each other), and, in more recent years, the widely popular X-Men.

The gold standard for superhero teams is DC's Justice League of America (JLA), created in 1960 by DC editor Julius Schwartz. The JLA, whose membership has included a core group of heroes including Superman, Batman, Wonder Woman, Flash, and the Green Lantern, was initially shown as "cheerfully cooperative and often so crowded together they had little room for temperament or even personalities" (Daniels, 1995, p. 126). With the move to more realism in comics in the 1970s and 1980s, the dysfunctional aspects of the JLA family came to light. Wonder Woman briefly lost her powers and team membership status. Superman took greater interest in social issues and in his daytime job as a television reporter. Batman, the avenging Dark Knight, returned to the Batcave, shunning the camaraderie of the JLA headquarters.

Batman and the Justice League

In its recent incarnation on television and in comic books, the Justice League, formerly the Justice League of America, is a leaner, meaner organization whose membership is by invitation only. In the new and improved Justice League, Batman, although still a core group member, struggles to fit into the organization. The angry and often abrasive Dark Knight is unable to bond with his fellow team members or to form what Morris and Morris (2005) identified as a complete friendship with other heroes.

> It's not just his high standards. It's not just his failure on the part of other people. A good measure of the responsibility seems to lie on his doorstep. Such a friendship requires a large personal investment. This is almost impossible for Batman after the promise he made to his dead parents. He has given so much of his time and effort to his crime-fighting quest that he doesn't have much time left for friends. (p. 115)

Much like the angry child whose time and energy is directed toward coping with a family trauma or living with the challenges of a behavioral disorder or learning disability, Batman simply may not have the emotional resources or understanding to invest in membership with the group. For Batman to function and succeed as a member of the League, he must first find friendship with himself. Morris and Morris (2005) state:

> If there is any sort of perfect friendship available for Bruce (Wayne) or Batman, perhaps it is here, in the solitude of the relation of himself to himself. Bruce Wayne is committed to good, which means that he commits himself to Batman. In his case, we find not one soul in two bodies, but one soul, two personae, two identities, two presentations to the world. Because of this all-consuming nature of his mission, it seems like this may be all that is possible for him at the level of true friendship. (p. 116)

Like the angry child, Batman often does not feel a bond with his fellow superheroes because of his past traumas and inner turmoil. Batman must also cope with dual systems of limits, boundaries, and expectations as a member of the Justice League that he finds frustrating and confining outside of his "home environment" in the Batcave, where he feels in control.

Despite this emotional detachment from his fellow members, the key to Batman's successful role as a member of the Justice League is in his own unique contributions. Although he has no superpowers of his own, his peers understand that he has a highly scientific and analytic mind, often generating logical solutions to seemingly insoluble problems that lead the Justice League to success. His fellow heroes understand that he works better alone and in the shadows, but when he commits his skills and talents to his team, Batman is a fierce and ardent crusader against crime—all members of the team benefit by simply letting him be who he is, rather than trying to change him.

Although it would be encouraging to conclude this account of Batman's relationship with the Justice League on a positive note, unfortunately in the world of superheroes, everything and anything can change. Currently, all is not well in the DC Universe with the current *Infinite Crisis* storyline that is reshaping the world of Batman and the Justice League. The JL has disbanded, in large part because of Batman's discovery of a past betrayal by his fellow Leaguers. This betrayal resulted in Batman's mistrust of the team and in his creation of a surveillance satellite that is tearing apart the DC world as we know it. How these events will affect Batman and his participation in the revamped Justice League remains to be seen.

Wolverine and the X-Men

Because of their enduring and currently resurging popularity with new fans, Marvel Comics' X-Men rivals the Justice League for its instantly recognizable logo and roster of multicultural, multipowered meta-humans. Created in 1963 by comics pioneers Stan Lee and Jack Kirby, the X-Men has produced multiple comic book series, several popular cartoon shows, video games, and a successful series of films.

Founded by the paraplegic telepath, Dr. Francis Xavier, the X-Men, under the cover of Professor Xavier's School for Gifted Youngsters, the original roster of X-Men included Cyclops, Marvel Girl, Angel, Beast, and Iceman. Like the Justice League, X-Men has been reformed and reconfigured many times during the last 40 years. Setting it apart from other superhero family teams has been an undercurrent of social and political conflict that draws the mutant heroes together in battling the problems and prejudices of the so-called society of normal human beings.

The X-Men have boldly gone where no other superhero team has gone before by openly equating and presenting antimutant prejudice with racism, homophobia, and anti-Semitism. Thus, the members of the X-Men come together as a family of outsiders because their own families and communities are afraid of them. Wolverine first appeared as a member of the X-Men in 1975. Victimized by the evils of so-called normal human society, Wolverine developed neither an affinity for his fellow mutants nor an ability to play well with them. Initially his character was presented as a misanthropic loner, whose resentment of authority underscored his continued conflict with X-Men leader Cyclops. His feral rages and use of lethal force set him apart from his more rational and controlled teammates.

Yet Wolverine is still viewed as a sympathetic character because of the inner pain and hurt that is the essence of his ostensibly uncontrollable fury. According to Fingeroth (2004), the rationale for his continued acceptance by the X-Men and his appeal to audiences is the realization that

> Wolverine is fighting for every persecuted mutant. And if mutants are seen as the handy metaphor for any and every persecuted subgroup a person could belong to in reality or in fantasy, then Wolverine is the father, or big brother standing outside our house as the marauders advance—who protects us from evil. The anger has been channeled and has transcended from mere petulance and become the salvation for all that is good and well intentioned in us. (pp. 136–137)

In more recent years, through Hugh Jackman's successful characterization of the character in three films, Wolverine's evolution into a more misunderstood and less ferocious antihero is in large part due to the X-Men team's acceptance, understanding and compassion for him that fuels his own moral growth. According to Evans (2005),

> it is not easy for a person possessed by the inner demons that appear to drive him. Wolverine has suffered a great deal as a victim of a disturbing medical experiment that wiped out most of his memory. Wolverine initially seems uninterested in helping [Professor] Xavier and his group. His own personal agenda is all that counts. He seems motivated by inner rage than by any desire to do or be good. However, as he becomes a part of the [X-Men] community he seems to care about them and their cause. (p. 169)

Clearly, what we can learn from the X-Men's example of acceptance and understanding of Wolverine is that anger often times come from pain, both physical and emotional. Additionally, beneath the anger and the pain is a person who very much wants to belong if we are willing to look past our own fears and difficulty accepting the anger in someone else.

The Hulk

The Hulk, the most unlikely of team players because of his "over-gendered and under socialized, half-naked and half-witted raging" (Jones, 2002, p. 15), would never feel at home in a place so systematic and disciplined as the Justice League or one as politically and socially conscious as the world of the X-Men. For the Hulk's particular talents, a team—the Defenders— was created to showcase this hero's role as an outcast, a team created as a place for those heroes that "not only didn't get along but actually hated each other" (Defenders, n. d.).

The Defenders first appeared as a team in 1971, when its founding members, the Hulk, the Submariner (Marvel's King of the Seven Seas) and Dr. Strange (Marvel's Sorcerer Supreme of the Earth) gathered to battle an alien wizard. Despite their intense dislike of each other, the three decided to remain a team. The enduring popularity of the team is credited to the creativity of Marvel writers Erik Larsen, Kurt Busiek, and Al Gordon. However, according to Marvel Comics pioneer Stan Lee, the Defenders' beginning ranks as the most democratic of all superhero teams origins, with the idea of this team of misfit heroes suggested by the Marvel fans themselves.

Described as the antithesis to Marvel's supergroup, the Defenders have no charter or bylaws, no permanent headquarters, no mission, and very little regard for each other. The Defenders' ranks soon grew adding among other notable Marvel loner and oddball heroes, Nighthawk, the Gargoyle, Silver Surfer, and Daredevil. Due to the group's unofficial nature, any individual who assisted them could be considered a member, but only a select few fit the two major criteria of true membership—they consider themselves Defenders and they are accepted by the continuing core group (Defenders, n. d.).

The Hulk's sometimes-uneasy alliance with this group continued, off and on, until the Defenders disbanded in 1986. Like many other hero teams, however, the Defenders have been reborn and reconfigured many times, all the while carrying on the team tradition of being at each other's throats. The Defenders was recently resurrected in 2005 in a comic miniseries featuring Doctor Strange attempting to reunite the Hulk, Submariner, and Silver Surfer in a story line focusing mostly on humor with the heroes spending as much battling danger as arguing and criticizing one another.

Although a group of very angry individuals with superhuman powers promotes feelings of uneasiness within adults, the angry child can readily identify with the freedom and acceptance of being part of a team in which it's not only acceptable to get angry, but doing so is greeted with support and encouragement. The Defenders offer Hulk a place where his anger is not a destructive force but a natural, healthy, appropriate, and life-enhancing emotion (Paul, 1995). What the Defenders lack in anger management skills, they more than make up for with their apparent non-judgmental acceptance of fellow outsiders into their ranks. Perhaps the Defenders, in understanding and accepting anger as part of who they are, comprehend something that Justice League and the X-Men do not: that teams, like families, friendships, and people, are basically flawed in some way. And although team members can argue, fight, and raise hell with each other, it doesn't mean they cannot be a team.

As caregivers, counselors, and educators, do we practice such acceptance with our angry boys? If our angry boys are capable of this insight about each other, it makes one wonder who the real outsiders are.

CASE STUDIES

Joshua

Five-year-old Joshua was referred to my office by his mother for challenges with anger management. Joshua, who lived with his mother and her male partner, had a history of aggressive and what his mother identified as "acting-out" behavior at home and school, particularly when dealing with adult authority figures, which included his mother, his mother's partner, and his teachers at school. He was particularly resistant to their attempts to set limits and boundaries around play, time spent watching television, playing video games and spending money. Additionally, Joshua's teachers were reporting problems with impulse control and interpersonal conflicts with peers, especially during group learning activities, when Joshua, refused to follow the rules.

During our initial individual counseling session, I asked Joshua what television shows he liked and what games he liked to play. Joshua advised of his great interest in the Cartoon Network and the network's Toonami programs featuring Japanese animae-style cartoons such as *Dragon Ball Z* and hero-themed shows such as *Batman* and the *Justice League*. In a subsequent session, I asked Joshua if he would like to play with some Justice League action figures from my toy chest. The figures included the "core" heroes from the television show—Batman, Superman, Wonder Woman, Green Lantern, Flash, Martian Manhunter, and Hawkgirl—as well some other DC characters who do not appear on the cartoon show, including some of Batman's foes—Supergirl, Batgirl, Cyborg, Robin, the Joker, Catwoman, and the Penguin.

I asked Joshua to use as many characters as he wanted to tell me a story about the Justice League. Joshua showed an early preference for the character of Batman, who was usually the focal point of his story about the Justice League, combating the Joker and the Penguin. During play, Joshua would include other heroes such as Robin, Flash, and Hawkgirl in minor roles, with these characters usually being rescued by Batman.

When I attempted to include other hero figures as rescuers in our play, Joshua would become more aggressive, pushing the other heroes out of the way. He showed a particular aversion to the inclusion of Green Lantern into the story, reacting with anger and saying, "We don't want him here!" and striking the Green Lantern figure with the Batman figure.

Because of his hostile reaction, I attempted to explore in his story what Green Lantern had done to receive such an unwelcome response from Batman. Joshua related that Green Lantern was, "always being mean" to Batman. Joshua recalled an episode of the cartoon show when Batman and Green Lantern had argued about "being in charge" and Green Lantern not wanting to do what "Batman wanted."

After some additional clarification of the events in his story, including how Batman and Green Lantern resolved their fight, I asked Joshua if this had ever happened to someone he knew. Joshua then related his own experiences of getting into fights at school with peers, particularly with a male peer, Andre, who was, "real bossy with me." Joshua also shared feelings of frustration related to his perception that, "Andre is always talking mess with me." I then asked Joshua if he could tell me what Batman does when Green Lantern gets bossy with him. Joshua advised, "Batman gets real quiet and gets by himself in the rocket." Clarifying Joshua's understanding of Batman's response, we both agreed that Batman had never hit or yelled at Green Lantern, and we determined that Batman was giving himself a *time out*, similar to what Joshua's mother did when he would exhibit defiant or oppositional behavior at home. We agreed that like Batman, Joshua also would not hit or yell when Andre (Green Lantern) exhibited domineering behavior. Following Batman's example, Joshua could notify another team member, his teacher, and seek help in dealing with Green Lantern. We also agreed, that with his teacher's permission, Joshua could give himself a time out.

In subsequent sessions, we explored other ways Batman could deal with Green Lantern's bossy behavior, and Joshua recalled from his memories of the cartoon show, that Batman had been successful in getting the other heroes to go along *with him* when, "he knew stuff they didn't know." In our storytelling efforts, Joshua (Batman) would share his knowledge and experience with the other heroes on battling The Joker and The Penguin and how to defeat them. We then explored ways that Joshua could do this in the classroom as well. We agreed that like Batman, Joshua could share his interests and experiences, (*the stuff he knew*), with the classmates in his learning group. In addition to the action figures, we also incorporated a Justice League storybook with a central theme of *success* being the result of teamwork and cooperation.

Through Joshua's interest and knowledge about Batman and the Justice League, I was able to establish trust and learn about his feelings of anger, frustration and sadness related to the negative-attention seeking behavior of his school peer. Additionally, through storytelling and therapeutic play with the Justice League action figures and related readings, we were able to identify and alternative skills and behaviors that Joshua could implement at school and at home to achieve more positive outcomes.

Gregorio

Seven-year-old Gregorio was referred for counseling by his mother who disclosed a recent history of disruptive behavior and sibling rivalry toward his younger brother. His mother also shared a history of impulsivity and attention control problems, particularly in school. Upon initial assessment, Gregorio disclosed feelings of fear and sadness related to recent nightmares of unknown persons in the family home.

During individual counseling sessions, Gregorio was given the choice between several sets of action figures with which to engage in therapeutic play/storytelling. Indicating a preference for the X-Men figures, Gregorio was asked to tell a story about them. Gregorio's initial storytelling focused around his memories of the plots and action scenes from the movie. Through exploration and clarification, Gregorio expressed personal identification with, and later took the role of the Wolverine, a loner. Gregorio insightfully compared the relationship with his own family to that of Wolverine's and the X-Men 'family' noting, "He's in the [family] group but he gets mad with them." Continued exploration revealed ongoing tension and conflict with his younger sibling, whom he represented by Cyclops, a character he believed received more positive attention from parent figures of Dr. Xavier and Jane Gray. Additionally, Gregorio disclosed feelings of fear of the Toad, whom he called "the frog dude" and who resembled the unknown person(s) in his nightmare. Through continued interactive storytelling, Gregorio began to confront his fears of "the frog dude." As Wolverine, he could defeat the Toad, with help from parent figures, Dr. Xavier and Jane Gray, as well as Cyclops, who represented his brother.

Using Wolverine and the X-men in therapeutic play helped Gregorio by reinforcing feelings of safety and comfort within the family, while assisting him to improve relations with his younger sibling and mother. Eventually, Gregorio reported no further nightmares while his mother reported improved relations between him and his siblings. Additionally, through cognitive reframing of Gregorio's X-men story, I was able to assist him in adapting and expanding his X-men stories to encompass his role on the "team" at school, incorporating his teacher and peers as other characters such as Storm and Nightcrawler.

CONCLUSION

Superhero play can be a powerful instrument for angry male children to recognize, express, and work through painful experiences, thoughts, and feelings. By tapping into superhero fantasies and imagery, parents, teachers, and counselors can help to unlock thoughts, beliefs, memories, and feelings that are the source of these children's anger to foster hope and understanding, helping the angry boy rejoin the team. By so doing, our littlest angry heroes can once again connect with those around them with renewed and constructive, rather than destructive, power.

Understanding a child's identification with an angry superhero and their shared experience of a felt injustice, can be of great use to the adults who live, love, or work with an angry child. Understanding this affinity for heroes such as Batman, Wolverine, Hulk, and other angry champions can facilitate our efforts as supportive adults in helping angry boys to verbalize their needs, feelings, challenges, and difficulties within the context of the superhero adventure. This is especially the case with children and adolescents who have experienced trauma, abuse, and betrayal at the hands of both adults and peers.

Bridging this age and cultural gap can begin with simple exploratory questions such as, "What television shows do you watch?" "What movies do you like?" "What video games do you play?" and then taking on the role of "audience" as the child shares stories of, knowledge of, and enthusiasm for his or her favorite superheroes. Upon determination of an angry child's favorite superhero, that child can then be encouraged to delve deeply into his or her and that superhero's world through the familiar play activities of art, storytelling, action-figure play, comic books, game cards, puzzles, Colorforms, and board games to further facilitate this process, therapists are encouraged to do the following:

- **Keep up with the current superheroes:** Talk to your children, watch their favorite shows with them, go to a comic book store, browse the video and PC game section of media stores or rental shops, watch Cartoon Network and the WB Network and visit their Web sites. Find out which heroes are "hot," especially the heroes you remember that have been rediscovered by your children.
- **Have some superhero *cues* in your home, classroom, or office:** These can include action figures, posters, toys, games, age-appropriate comic books and activity and storybooks. Let your angry hero know that your mutual space is a "hero haven."
- **Join in the superhero play:** Explore your angry hero's interests, favorite characters, storylines, shows, and movies and share yours as well. It is also acceptable to test understanding your angry heroes on the difference between what's real and what's pretend.
- **Set limits and boundaries for superhero play:** Direct adventurous and risk-taking behaviors for use with action figures, drawing,

clay, paint, coloring, collage, and storytelling. Don't sidestep or prohibit violence or aggression in superhero play but do ask why violence or fighting was or is necessary. Explore, discuss, explain, reframe, and teach.

- **Encourage expression of all feelings, thoughts, frustrations, beliefs, opinions:** Make superhero play a place to drop the mask and share secrets as well as secret identities. Share your thoughts, feelings, and beliefs in nonjudgmental and validating ways by asking questions such as, "What happened to [Batman, Wolverine, Hulk] was very interesting. Do you think that could happen in real life? To someone you know? To you?"
- **Stress the importance of teamwork:** Share experiences of what it means to be a member of the team and why it is important to allow others to be on the team as well (Booth-Church, 2003). The reemergence of superheroes in the mediums of cartoons, movies, and computer games has provided teachers, counselors, parents and other supportive adults with a way to help angry boys conquer fear and make sense of a confusing world and foster the skills and knowledge with which to feel in control.

In recounting his own challenges with a troubled home and school environment, Gurian (Gurian & Stevens, 2005) recounted:

> At home, my family struggled near poverty. My parents fought. Their discipline … was physical and brutal. Their marriage struggled, and I began running away from home at nine years old. In school, I was called "incorrigible," summoned many times to the principal's office, a discipline problem. By fifth grade I had seen a psychiatrist and been put on Ritalin. When I was a boy, I liked Superman, Batman and Spiderman. My school friends and I traded our comics on the playground, in our back yards, our homes. In the fourth grade, I discovered the Fantastic Four. The special power of one of the Four mesmerized me; he could stretch his arms and legs elastically. Even when his enemies tried to kill him, he would not be torn apart, he could not be broken.… I know now that I wanted to be a superhero, unbreakable and bold. (pp. 1–2)

Gurian's experience is still common in the lives of the incorrigible, out-of-control, impossible, and angry boys of today; who find in superheroes fulfillment of "a powerful human need to be valued, accepted, included and understood" (Fingeroth, 2004, p. 60). If we want our angry boys to grow, learn, and be in control of their actions, we can start by allowing them, in the fantasy world of superhero play, to leap tall buildings, get the bad guys, defend the earth, and make the world safe for democracy and, in doing so, become more powerful and emotionally healthier beings in the real world.

REFERENCES

Achilles. (2003). *Columbia Electronic Encyclopedia* (6th ed.). Retrieved February 12, 2006, from http://www.cc.columbia.edu/cu/cup/

Anti-hero (n.d.). Retrieved March 25, 2006, from http://en.wikipedia.org/wiki/Anti-hero

Batman Begins: The Origins of the Dark Knight. (n.d.) Retrieved February 5, 2006, from http://movies.monstersandcritics.com/features/article_8259.php/Batman_Begins_The_Origins_Of_The_Dark_Knight

Booth-Church, E. (2003, February/March). When good kids play the bad guy [Children's module]. *Scholastic Parent and Child, 10,* 45–46.

Daniels, L. (1995). *DC Comics: 60 years of the world's greatest heroes.* New York: Bulfinch Press.

David, D., & Brannon, R. (Eds.). (1976). *The forty-nine percent majority: The male sex role.* Reading, MA: Addison-Wesley.

Defenders. (n.d.). Marvel Directory. Retrieved March 27, 2006, from http://www.marveldirectory.com/teams/defenders.htm

Dyson, A. H. (1996, Fall). Cultural constellations and childhood identities: On Greek gods, carton heroes and the lives of school children. *Harvard Educational Review, 66,* 471–495.

Evans, C. S. (2005). Why should superheroes be good? Spider-Man, the X-Men, and Kierkegaard's double danger. In T. Morris & M. Morris (Eds.), *Superheroes and philosophy: Truth justice and the Socratic way* (pp. 147–160). New York: Open Court Press.

Hulk. (n.d.). Retrieved March 20, 2006 from http://en.wikipedia.org/wiki/Hulk

Feiffer, J. (1965). *The great American comic book heroes.* New York: Bonanza Books.

Fingeroth, D. (2004). *Superman on the couch: What superheroes really tell us about ourselves and our society.* New York: Continuum.

Gibbard, W. B. (2001, Winter). Anger management in children. *Kids Doc, 8, 2,* 1–4.

Gurian, M. & Stevens, C. (2005). *The minds of boys: Saving our sons from falling behind in school and life.* New York: Jossey-Bass.

Jones, G. (2002). *Killing monsters: Why children need fantasy, superheroes and make-believe violence.* New York: Basic Books.

Morris, T., & Morris, M. (Eds.). (2005). *Superheroes and philosophy: Truth, justice and the Socratic way.* New York: Open Court.

Moyer, K. E. (1968). Kinds of aggression and their physiological basis. *Communications in Behavioral Biology, 2A,* 65–87.

O'Brien, P. (2005). Superhero vigilantes: An imaginary conversation between Batman, Robin, Wolverine, Spawn and Punisher. Retrieved March 11, 2006, from http://crossoveruniverse.com/forum6.htm

Paul, H. (1995). *When kids are mad, not bad.* New York: Berkeley.

Pipher, M. (1994). *Reviving Ophelia: Saving the selves of adolescent girls.* New York: Ballantine Books.

Pollack, W. (1998). *Real boys: Rescuing our sons from the myths of boyhood.* New York: Henry Holt.

Pollack, W., & Cushman, K. (2001). *Real boys workbook: The definitive guide to understanding and interacting with boys of all ages.* Henry Holt.

Rogers, F., & Sharapan, H. (1994). How children use play. *Education Digest, 59,* 14.

Smith, H. (2000). *The sacred heart: Understanding and identifying kids who kill.* In G. Jones (Ed.), *Why children need fantasy, superheroes and make-believe violence.* New York: Basic Books.

Superheros—Deconstruction of the superhero. (n.d.). Retrieved March 13, 2006, from http://en.wikipedia.org/wiki/Superheroes–Deconstruction_of_the_superhero

A Super Milieu: Using Superheroes in the Residential Treatment of Adolescents With Sexual Behavior Problems

Karen Robertie, Ryan Weidenbenner,
Leya Barrett, and Robert Poole

The Onarga Academy is a residential facility specializing in the treatment of youth who have demonstrated sexually abusive behavior. Program I, Field of Dreams, works with clients who are between 12 and 16 years old and their families. The population is highly heterogeneous in nature, with a wide variety of mental health issues, family backgrounds, behavioral and emotional problems, abuse histories, and legal issues. Common diagnoses include oppositional defiant disorder, conduct disorder, attention-deficit/hyperactivity disorder, bipolar disorder, adjustment disorder, depressive disorder, posttraumatic stress disorder (PTSD), and many others. Deficits in cognitive, emotional, and social development are often the norm rather than the exception. Many clients have also had significant personal histories of abuse, neglect, abandonment, and loss. Many clients need to work through myriad difficult family issues; still others need to learn how to mourn the loss of a family system that they have never known. These clients also represent a highly heterogeneous group from across the state, defined primarily in terms of their problem behaviors and the subsequent response by legal and social systems. These problem behaviors are often self-reinforcing and difficult to extinguish (Kahn, 1990). Many clients have been placed in residential treatment as a last resort after failing to make progress in outpatient therapy, other residential treatment centers, or both. As a group, they tend to have low self-efficacy, low frustration tolerance, and often little internal motivation to change.

The client population, as a whole, is not antisocial in personal orientation, although a certain percentage of these clients certainly are (Isaac & Lane, 1990). Within the context of their sexual development and behavior. if not other aspects of their lives, these clients share the following core issues: (a) seeking out of short-term "feel goods" (immediate gratification) despite a pattern of increasing long-term "feel bads" (personal consequences); (b) thought processes predominated by self-serving cognitive distortions and problematic attitudes designed to continue abusive behavior despite all costs; (c) seeking to gain covert power and control over others while demonstrating little power and control over themselves, their feelings, and their behavior; (d) singular motivation to maintain problem behaviors and avoid consequences; (e) avoidance of self-examination; and, above all (f) resistance to personal change and identities that are intricately linked to issues of control, revenge, anger, and power (Lane, 1991). In summary, the client population often begins treatment with schema that are criminal in nature. Within the colorful context of the comic book/superhero metaphor, they begin treatment with belief and value systems more aligned with the villainous Legion of Doom than with the Justice League of America.

TRADITIONAL RESIDENTIAL TREATMENT

The treatment process for youth who demonstrate sexually abusive behavior involves the introduction of new schema—beliefs, values, and behavioral patterns that are more heroic in nature (i.e., prosocial, empathic, sharing, communicative, honest, and promoting of healthy sexuality). Cognitive–behavioral methods are generally considered the best practice when working with this population because these methods have proven consistent, effective, and efficient in practice (Stickrod et al., 1984). There are many ways to teach the same sound cognitive–behavioral concepts that are the foundation of accepted treatment practices, such as the sexual offense history, the cycles of problem behaviors, and relapse prevention plans (Bays & Freeman-Longo, 1989).

Residential treatment centers make use of the treatment culture and peer milieu by capitalizing on the principles of social learning and reality theories. Because this client population often has difficulty with social and emotional connection, our program also employs experiential methods including techniques drawn from narrative and expressive therapies. Those working with the program have long prided themselves on the ability to individualize treatment to individual clients' needs, but there is also a need to develop and implement interventions on a programmatic rather than individual level. The Field of Dreams program thus attempts to use as many interventions as possible to optimize the chances of treatment success. (Kendall, 1991). From a social learning perspective (Bandura, 1986), treatment success requires the following:

- The client must focus attention on the new cognitive schema or behavioral patterns (or both).
- The client must learn and understand the new cognitive schema or behavioral pattern.
- The client must perceive the new cognitive schema or behavioral pattern as having consequences that are desirable and attainable.
- The new cognitive schema or behavioral pattern must not conflict too strongly with the client's existing self-image.
- The client must perceive himself or herself as capable of successfully adapting the new cognitive schema or behavioral pattern.
- The new cognitive schema or behavioral pattern must be practiced and reinforced.
- This is particularly powerful when the new cognitive schema or behavioral pattern has consequences that are naturally occurring.
- The acquisition of new cognitive schema or behavioral patterns is greatly facilitated by the practice of effective role modeling or vicarious learning (or both).
- Effective role modeling and vicarious learning are methods best employed by "valued others"—individuals that the client holds in great esteem.

INCORPORATING THE SUPERHERO
AND SUPERVILLAIN

For the purpose of effective role modeling or vicarious learning, valued others can include actual members of the client's support network as well as other admired individuals, celebrated or personal, living or dead, real or fictional (Bays et al., 1990). The use of comic books and superheroes as a treatment metaphor therefore has many advantages in terms of a client learning and adapting new cognitive schema or behavioral patterns. Comic book heroes are highly salient in popular culture. Even people who are not comic book fans are aware of popular media superheroes such as Spider-Man, Superman, Batman, and the X-Men. The personal histories, mythologies, and personalities of these superheroes resonate with and are familiar to teenagers. Clients readily identify with superheroes and discuss their adventures with the same sense of seriousness and shared experience as a fantasy football league discusses the weekly exploits of their favorite athletes. With a bit of selective editing and imagination on the part of the therapist, the cognitive schema and behavioral patterns introduced to clients by superheroes can be practical, prosocial, and immediately reinforcing. It can be a few short learning steps to move from a mind-set of "do unto others before they do unto you" to "with great power comes great responsibility."

Heroes and villains are not defined solely by their amazing powers, colorful costumes, or impressive code names, but by their actions and the choices that they make. Superheroes seem to enjoy a certain edge over their villainous opponents not so much in terms of overt superpowers and resources but in terms of more covert advantages. First, there is the immutable concept of karma. The universe tends to provide positive consequences for positive behaviors and negative consequences for negative behavior. This Golden Rule is the underlying principle behind most world religions and philosophies because it arguably is "good." Whereas the superhero is making his own luck, the supervillain is usually spreading the seeds of his eventual destruction—it is just a matter of time. Second, there is teamwork. Villainy is essentially a solitary undertaking, driven by a singular self-centered agenda. The superhero can always depend on his friends and teammates to watch his back when he is in trouble, providing strength during those rare moments of weakness. Superman can always count on his any of his many superfriends to come to his aid when presented with the inevitable kryptonite-laden trap; however, the likes of Lex Luthor, Green Goblin, and the Joker find no solace or protection in their mindless companions. Third, there is motivation. Superheroes are motivated by primarily benevolent goals such as upholding the common good, seeking justice, and helping others as best they can. Supervillains, however, are primarily motivated by their own selfish desires, their self-destructive patterns of behavior and quite often by their own megalomaniacal fixations, obsessions, and psychoses. Because of this, supervillains first turn on society, then on each other, and finally on themselves. How successful might the Riddler have been at grand larceny if he did not feel compelled to send puzzle clues forecasting his crimes to test his wits against those of the Batman? Why don't any of Spider-Man's many supervillain enemies commit crimes outside of New York City to avoid the wall crawler's inevitable involvement? Why hasn't any of Flash's Rogues Gallery decided to shift his antipathy toward some other hero—any other hero—who is not capable of attaining the speed of light? The answer is, because this would involve self-examination, self-evaluation, and personal change—concepts beyond the ken of the so-called criminal mind. Fourth, there is also the feasibility and desirability of the hero's and villain's respective goals. The heroic motivation is often driven by the need for atonement, powerlessness, or revenge. This is a form of benevolent wish fulfillment with built-in checks and balances. Although the superhero is motivated by a desire for return to the status quo, the supervillain is never satisfied—he or she always wants more, be it more power, more control, more revenge, or more evil. Some of the most notorious of the supervillains, including the Joker, General Zodd, and Doctor Doom are never satisfied and are always stirring up more trouble as soon as they are vanquished and should otherwise retreat. Superheroes are the redeemers; they are not the ones in need of saving. In this regard, they are quite unidimensional.

Something interesting happens to a supervillain when he steps outside of his established role as a villain. From the point when a supervillain ceases to be a protagonist and therefore acts as an antagonist, or hero, of his own story, he immediately becomes more human, more identifiable, better defined, more easy to relate to, and, hence, a more effective treatment ally. This character is no longer restrained by the limitations of his former villainous motivation and therefore becomes capable of learning, growing, and developing; superheroes in contrast, are static.

There are many such stories of redemption within the history of comics. The mighty Avengers have had several members who started their careers as supervillains such as the Black Widow, Hawkeye, Quicksilver, the Scarlet Witch, and the Swordsman. At one point, three out of four members of the Avengers roster were reformed villains working under the tutelage of none other than Captain America. The Suicide Squad took many supervillains—such as the Bronze Tiger, Dead Shot, Captain Boomerang, Count Vertigo, and Poison Ivy—out of their usual dark roles and transformed them into an elite American espionage force acting on behalf of the government. The Thunderbolts went even further; taking previously established villains such as Baron Zemo, the Beetle, the Fixer, Goliath, Moonstone, and Screaming Mimi and establishing new superhero identities for themselves such as Citizen V, Mach One, Techno, Atlas, Meteorite, and Songbird, respectively. Most of these transformed evildoers felt more comfortable and stronger in the role of hero than they ever felt in the role of villain. Imagine that.

As this discussion highlights, both superheroes and supervillains can be used in the service of psychotherapy with residential clients by encouraging them to replace maladaptive and destructive schema with a more heroic (functional, prosocial, effective, and empathic) self-identity. New cognitive schema and behavioral patterns are facilitated by the use of superhero-related interventions based on role modeling and vicarious learning (Bandura, 1997). The following are a collection of treatment interventions developed for our program's treatment toolbox.

CORNERSTONE SUPERHEROES

The "Nexus Cornerstones" are the core ideals and values that undergird treatment at the Onarga Academy, and are based on the premise that clients can make healthy changes by learning to live their lives based on responsibility, courage, care and concern, and honesty. Each of these Cornerstones, exemplified in the lives of superheroes, then lays the foundation for the Center Stone of growth. Peter Parker, aka Spider-Man, learns the lesson of the first Cornerstone, *responsibility*, the hard way as he watches his beloved Uncle Ben die at the hands of a criminal whom Peter failed to thwart. Transformed from a self-centered teen into a great hero, Uncle Ben's message of "with great power comes great responsibility" follows him on all of this Spider adventures. These adventures have been inspirational for many of our clients who slowly come to accept personal responsibility for their behavior and thoughts. The second Cornerstone, *courage*, is represented by the man without fear, Daredevil. Blind, although his other senses are now enhanced, Matt Murdock is no stranger to victimhood. His credo, "one can only be brave by admitting your fears and facing them," has been helpful for clients who enter treatment with a large number of fears, both real and imagined and who struggle to address their sexually offensive behavior.

The third Cornerstone, *care and concern*, is represented by the Man of Steel, Superman. Sent to Earth from the doomed planet of Krypton, Clark Kent is raised on the values of truth, justice, and the American way. Although criminals regard Superman as weak, his compassion is his greatest asset. Our clients often enter treatment with a wide variety of cognitive distortions that impair their ability to reach out for and accept help. "How can someone actually care for me when I have committed unspeakable acts?" they wonder. Care and concern are particularly difficult lessons for them to learn if they have been abused. The fourth and final Cornerstone, *honesty*, is represented by Batman—a very human superhero. The millionaire playboy Bruce Wayne is simply a façade for the vigilante Dark Knight who lives outside the law. If one lives outside of the law, honesty is imperative; otherwise, you either are or are perceived to be a criminal.

With the four Nexus Cornerstones introduced and equally represented by the various superheroes, the Center Stone of growth is revealed. Our goal throughout treatment is to assist our clients in learning to make healthy choices in all aspects of their lives. We strive to teach them how to make healthy choices about sexuality, family dynamics, teenage peer pressure, and their identity. We ask them to be responsible, honest, and courageous and to demonstrate care and concern—in essence, we want them to grow. For our Center Stone, growth, we find the one person who represents our clients in the truest sense—the reluctant superhero, the Rocketeer, a relatively ordinary individual who tries to do the right thing at the right time during an extraordinary adventure. Our clients symbolize the ordinary guy, trying to do the right thing, making healthier choices, during their extraordinary adventure called treatment. The story of the Rocketeer takes place in the 1930s, just before the United States entered World War II. Cliff Secord, despite being poor, stumbles onto an experimental jet pack developed by eccentric millionaire and aircraft designer Howard Hughes. He tries out the dangerous jet pack and, with the good sense to wear a helmet, takes off on adventures against the Nazis as the Rocketeer. Armed only with a two guns, he grows and matures as both a superhero and person.

So what does it take for our clients to be superheroes?

- Having enough courage to do the right thing when running away seems much easier.
- Having enough care and concern to fight for others when you could be looking out for only yourself.
- Having enough honesty to uphold the rules when you could be living outside them.
- Having enough responsibility to handle great power.
- Having the capacity to keep learning from mistakes, growing stronger and better.

Role-Play Group

Another treatment modality that utilizes the superhero genre as the catalyst for change is the role-play group. The group leader, a therapist, selects a small group of clients and assigns each an individually created superhero identity with powers that are representative of the client. Each client can be responsible for creating a representation of their superhero, via drawing, sculpting, or whatever creative media are available.

For example, if a client is intelligent, witty, or strong, his or her superhero may be super smart, funny, or strong, respectively. A physically impaired client may either use that impairment as a strength or have a compensatory skill. Each superhero is also given an assigned amount of karma, based on the concept that "you get what you give and you give what you get." The clients' level of karma is raised or lowered by the leader, based on their performance in the role-play—supportive behavior garners karma, whereas selfishness results in its loss. The group leader then assigns a scenario and nemesis for the group which usually involves a problematic situation that is related to a real-life problem. For example, if clients are having difficulty getting along with each other, they must work together in the role-play scenario to defeat a nemesis. Clients are encouraged to strategize and problem solve until they begin to figure out what works and what does not. The group activity culminates when the group leader decides that the goal has been accomplished; this may be a win, lose, or draw situation. This then sets the stage for the next role-play session, which is again tailored to fit the current treatment focus for the clients.

As an example of the power of this technique, the following letter was written by a group of five clients, dubbed the Freedom Force, whose motto was "fighting for a second chance."

> The Freedom Force would like to reassure all of you that we are here to protect all of you from harm and that we don't want to hurt any of you. Even though we look scary, we are actually very nice people, and we would like to get along and be friends with all of you. So, please, when you see us, don't run away from us or scream because we look different, or be afraid of us. Please let us do our job and don't try to fight the villains who attack the city even if one or all of us are hurt because we don't want you to suffer the same consequences as us. We fight then because we have powers and strengths that could overcome the people who are trying to attack the city. We use our powers to overcome evil mutants, villains, gangs, thieves and insane super human beings.
>
> Thank you,
>
> Dragon, Ampere, Crucible, Private Eye, Meteor

Superhero Month

Superhero Month began as a way to structure the time in between summer school and the beginning of the regular school year. The initial week of activities was expanded to 4 weeks when we considered the wealth of information and interventions that were available. Because of the heat and humidity of the central Illinois summer, we scheduled indoor activities centered around superhero-related movies, TV shows, videos, books, and songs. Each morning, we viewed a video, after which the clients completed a worksheet, highlighting the treatment messages in the movie—the heroic themes. In the course of the discussions, clients were encouraged to incorporate the Nexus Cornerstone values linked to the particular superhero. For example, *Daredevil* led to a discussion of courage and fear,

The Incredibles led to addressing the parallels between superheroes and clients, and *The Rocketeer* demonstrated the relationship between superheroes and everyday people. In an effort to highlight some of the more unique superpowers in the world of superheroes, we also watched the movie *Mystery Men*, old Batman and Spider-Man television episodes, and cartoons such as *The Tick, Teen Titans,* and *The Justice League.* Finally, an in an effort to leave no medium unexploited, we also included a "superhero story hour," during which we read books such as *Atomic Ace He's Just My Dad,* by Jeff Weigel and *Super Dog: Heart of a Hero* by Caralyn Buehner.

The role-playing, movies, and stories were very exciting and therapeutically productive and culminated in the *big even*t-each client designing his own superheroes. After being asked, "If you could be a superhero, what would your superpowers be?" The group leaders created a matrix with which each client could pick five powers (and two limitations mirroring their own struggles) totaling 50 points. The next step was for clients to draw their superhero, which we facilitated by providing comic and coloring books as well as *The Marvel Encyclopedia,* and the step-by-step *Draw the Marvel Comics Superheroes* by Klutz Press. By encouraging clients to combine different elements from existing superheroes into their own hybrid drawings and to use *Model Magic* by Crayola for three-dimensional figures, we opened avenues of creativity and allowed for creative problem solving. Once a client designed his superhero, he was encouraged to create a biography by addressing the following questions:

- What is his secret identity?
- What are his powers?
- Where did he get his powers?
- Why does he fight crime?
- Who is his supervillain nemesis?
- Where do they battle?
- How does the battle end?
- How are you like your superhero?
- How are you unlike your superhero?
- How are you like your supervillain?
- How are you unlike your supervillain?
- Is there someone in your life who is like your supervillain nemesis?

From the clients' answers to these questions, it became obvious that superhero choice and biography mirrored their own identities and struggles. Finally, and because of the proliferation of superheroes and superhero paraphernalia during this special month, winners of a subsequent social skills game were awarded superhero certificates, and scavenger hunt participants were given superhero pencils, notebooks, and miniatures—it was amazing how far superhero clip art could go as therapeutic incentive.

Interestingly, enthusiasm for the project spread to many of the program staff (child-care workers, case managers, therapists) who were encouraged to participate and create their own superhero alter egos.

The Results of Superhero Month

As the previous discussion suggests, Superhero Month was wildly popular and therapeutically helpful. The following are a few illustrated examples.

Hurricane

Hurricane's (Figure 8.1) dominant power is his "wave blast"—the ability to control water and hurricanes. He wraps water around his wrists when he is fighting evildoers, and water potentiates his strength. Hurricane resembles his creator, both physically and emotionally, and like his creator, reacts with anger and aggression when forced to discuss his abusive past. Hurricane's creator dreams of growing up to be a fireman, saving people by using water, and having a hope-filled future.

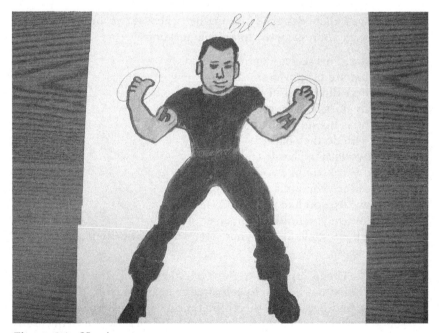

Figure 8.1 Hurricane.

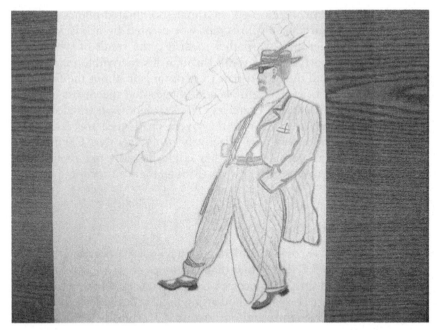

Figure 8.2   Deuce.

Deuce

Deuce (Figure 8.2) is a loner and former criminal, whose parents' death was partly his fault—it is extremely difficult for him to discuss this. Deuce, a smart, lucky, and suave character, much like his creator, is also cool under pressure and a snappy dresser. Both are intellectualizers, who distance themselves from their feelings and who began their adventures as tragic loners who nevertheless long for contact. Like his creator, Deuce struggles to reconcile his victimization of his half-sister.

Other Superheroes

Lightning Bolt was the powerful, intelligent, and invisible super-alter-ego creation of an extremely anxiety-ridden client whose inner tension seemed to crackle around him like lightning. *Ghoul* was the ghostly creation of a boy who experienced unspeakable sexual and emotional abuse since early childhood and who did not perceive himself as being human. Although this client made remarkable strides in coping with PTSD, he struggled to feel a part of the milieu. *Sonic Siren's* titanium claw and sound-barrier-shattering voice helped him (and his creator) to cope with feelings of powerlessness that were expressed in sexually aggressive behavior. Both

Sonic and his creator were raised on a male-dominated planet and had difficulty around girls. *The Marksman* was created by a boy who lost his father to murder and his mother to drugs, the result of which was a dedication to protecting the weak through his incredible marksmanship. Both Sonic and the Marksman were optimistic about the future. It is clear from these brief descriptions and images that the clients invested much of themselves into the exercises. The lessons they learned were integrated throughout treatment as they were challenged to make good choices, interact positively, and effectively problem solve. Clients were continually urged to consider how they could be more like their superhero creations and to continue to work through their traumas and deviant behavior.

Everyday Superheroes

Once the clients have come to understand that superheroes are defined by their choices and behaviors, rather than costumes, it is easier to recognize superheroes in real life. Their heroics are sometimes celebrated but often unsung. They seem to rise above and attain higher ideals. They are heroes who take longer to recognize without costumes. Despite the glory of comic book superheroes, our clients often identify with everyday superheroes because it could be them.

Everyday superheroes are conducive to groups that teach morals and values. For example, a group can highlight courage. Pat Tillman, an NFL player, was honored as a man of character. He forfeited his $1.2 million contract to serve in the U.S. Army. He chose to serve his country and died for it. To highlight this sacrifice, the group discussed what courage meant and examined 40 "courage" quotes. Next, to put $1.2 million in "teenage terms," the clients were given "tokens." These "tokens" represented cars, electronics, and vacations up to $1.2 million. Then, once the "tokens" were accepted, they were asked to forfeit it, serve their country, and sacrifice their lives. Suddenly, clients understood courage and the value of the human spirit of everyday superheroes.

Another example highlighted Lance Armstrong's battle against cancer. The clients learned who Lance Armstrong was as a cyclist. They then discussed his cancer and return to racing. The clients mapped out the race course and followed Lance's progress, which culminated in his victory. The group also donated to the Lance Armstrong Foundation.

"What If?" Stories

One of the core messages that we instill in our clients is that treatment progress is the result of a seemingly endless series of choices—sometimes positive, sometimes negative. Healthy change is as much about regression as it is about progression. Although our clients understand that superheroes use their powers for good, we also challenge them to consider questions such as, "what if they had made the choice to use their powers for evil instead of good, or for personal gain and glory?" and "what if superheroes made some of the same mistakes and used the same erroneous cognitions that you [the client] currently use?"' Many of our clients made poor choices or failed to learn from their mistakes. As one of our clients was fond of saying, "The only difference between a superhero and a supervillain are the choices they make." We extended this line of reasoning to create the "what if?" technique, a simple story-based procedure in which the client is asked to imagine what would have happened if a beloved superhero made a poor choice. This in turn, provided the foundation for discussing parallels in the client's life and both positive and negative ways of solving problems. Storytelling becomes psychotherapy!

A Spider-Man "What If?" Story

What if one day Spider-Man fails to stop a robber who later that day kills his beloved Uncle Ben? After learning of the murder, Peter Parker reasons that "it's really too bad, but I didn't have anything to do with this—the robber did it and life goes on." Tired of the chump change he is earning as a wrestler, Parker decides to use his amazing spider senses, strength, and agility to become a burglar—after all, no one is being hurt, and he can hide behind his disguise. As the money begins rolling in, Parker buys a flashy sports car, becomes popular (except with Mary Jane Watson), and lies to his Aunt May about his criminal lifestyle. One night, while robbing a safe, Parker is shot and later tracked by the police back to his house, where he sees his Aunt May crying as she is being interrogated by detectives. Worried that the police would find the jewels he has stolen, Parker laments, "no, this is not fair, I am special, I had a hard life, what am I going to do?" In pain, alone, and frightened, Parker realizes that the hammer has finally come down on him—he is on his own. "So what," he says, "I don't need anyone, my life is going just fine, it's not my fault anyway."

A Wolverine "What If?" Story

What if instead of serving with the X-Men, Wolverine decides to forget his past to escape painful memories and nightmares. He decides to live alone so that he does not have to discuss painful experiences and as a result creates a vicious cycle of pushing people away, becoming even more animalistic, frightened, angry, and isolated. By exploring how Wolverine's faulty cognitive style leads him deeper and deeper into pain and isolation, clients are able to identify with him as they tell their own similar stories. Externalizing treatment issues is much less threatening for them than is direct discussion or confrontation, allowing for easier acknowledgment of negative attitudes, thoughts, or behaviors and thus opening the door for more in-depth discussions. Clients are provided with an opportunity to share the consequences of their own faulty cognitions with other members of the group, who can offer adaptive alternatives.

Each of these what-if exercises is accompanied by a worksheet, which begins with the superhero's true story. A different 'what if?' story follows, in which the superhero follows the other, destructive voice in his head In the story of Daredevil, for example; instead of bringing justice to his neighborhood through his superhuman senses, he cowers in pain after waking to discover that he is blind. Even after he recovers, Matt Murdock continues to withdraw inside himself because his blindness is too overwhelming to face. This story demonstrates the distortion inherent in the victim stance, and how clients often use it by stating "I can't" or "It's too hard." In the story of Daredevil they can see how disempowering the distortion of victim stance can be and the devastating effects it can have in one's life.

Teachable Stories

The use of comic books as teachable stories, has also been highly effective in educating and assisting clients about a variety of social issues. Many superheroes and their friends have faced personal dilemmas and struggles that can serve as a catalyst for discussion and reflection. Spider-Man was sexually abused by an older male who was showing him "special attention" as a youngster. Iron Man had personal struggles with alcoholism. Omega Man often deals with gang violence and drug abuse. Northstar is one of few openly homosexual superheroes. Mia Dearden of Green Arrow Comics disclosed her HIV diagnosis, a result of her previous prostitution. Green Arrow's sidekick, Speedy, had a heroin addiction, and Green Arrow also addressed such issues as drug abuse, racism, overpopulation, and pollution.

These social issues are not glorified or used to create a sense of martyrdom among the superheroes. They are typically addressed in a straightforward manner, much as they would be in a real-life situation. Our clients can relate to these superheroes as they face their own personal issues. Clients often feel isolated in terms of having to confront their problems, but such superheroes can serve as role models and potential motivation, suggests that clients, too, can defeat or deal with their problems. Each superhero's social issue can also be addressed in a manner designed to suit treatment programming. For example, Spider-Man's abuse issues are easily related and discussed in groups that assist clients in addressing personal abuse issues, such as our Healing Group. Mia Dearden's HIV status can be used to assist in the education of clients in sex education groups. Iron Man's alcoholism could be addressed in chemical dependency education groups.

Sandtray

Sandtray is widely used and popular with our clients who particularly enjoy the calming tactile sensations of the sand, the clearly defined limits of the tray, and the rich metaphors that the miniatures provide. Although superhero miniatures make up just a small fraction of available sandtray figures, they have found their way into countless sandtrays. Sometimes the superheroes represent the clients themselves, sometimes they are allies that help the clients overcome obstacles, and sometimes they are simply used to illustrate a battle between good and evil. No matter how the client chooses to use the superheroes, they are depicting internal processes or current issues that they are attempting to make sense of and resolve. The use of superheroes in a sandtray can also reveal the client's view of power dynamics. This may be displayed through the number of superheroes and villains present in the tray or in the specific heroes that are selected by the client. Placement of the items in relation to other miniatures in the tray may also be significant. In whatever ways a client chooses to use superheroes in their sandtray, new and exciting metaphors always emerge. These metaphors can then be brought into their everyday treatment sessions, activities, and assignments to help them develop additional insight into their issues. Our clients enjoy their sandtrays a great deal and often ask to keep pictures of them. Clients will often make this transition themselves and bring up their sandtrays outside of sessions.

Bill, the oldest of five children, had been physically and sexually abused in his family of origin where he was often made responsible for his siblings—he was subsequently placed in several foster homes. Soon after learning that his parents' legal rights to him were being terminated, he was referred for treatment for sexually abusive behaviors. In the sandtray, he created a series of scenes he called "War of the World." The first tray depicted six vehicles, all specifically selected to represent each member of his immediate family They are close together to reflect their loyalty and emotional closeness. Bill explained that the superheroes and the armored knight are people who are on his family's side, helping them stay together. The tall slender figure in the corner represented the judge who was attempting to terminate parental rights. The soldiers are protecting the judge and enforcing his orders. Bill placed several boulders around the family to represent obstacles blocking the family from moving effectively in their vehicles. His youngest sister is the tank in the back, and she actually has a boulder on top of her vehicle. He added that because parental rights to her had already been terminated, she was slowing down and starting to be more permanently separated from the rest of the family.

Bill's next tray had many of the same elements but was dramatically different in many ways. All of the items were closing in on the figure in the corner, which still represented the judge. However, the judge who was previously powerful was now considerably smaller and less threatening. Although Bill again included boulders as in the previous tray, they were no longer blocking the family's view or path. In Bill's description, he explained that the family was uniting and even though they may have been physically separated, they were still emotionally close to one another. He clarified that each snake also represented a specific family member. He identified himself as the long, black snake, covering the full length of his family. Interestingly enough, the week before, Bill disclosed that he had sexually molested all four of his siblings. It is likely that this tray is reflecting the new disclosure. Our clients often use snakes to represent sexual abuse or secrets. Bill allowed himself to reveal these issues both in his sandtray and in his discussion of the tray. Another interesting factor in this tray is the three-headed dragon. Currently in the art therapy group, Bill was creating his own superhero—a dragon named Shum. He included the three-headed dragon to represent his superhero. He placed the snake around the neck, stating that snakes were his friends and protect him. He described the superheroes as representing extended family members who were providing additional help, strength, and assistance. The family members were coming to his aid during a time of need to help fight against the judge. Bill was working through his anger, fear, insecurity, uncertainness, and pain. As can be seen, this tray was dramatically different from his previous one. There appeared to be significantly more power, aggression, and activity. When Bill spoke about these issues outside of his sandtrays, he sounded hopeful and optimistic; however, his trays belied pessimism, doubt, and lingering fear. He used superheroes as a metaphor for control and to reflect elements of his conscience (see Figure 8.3).

Draw Your Own Comic Strips

Clients have also been able to address treatment issues by drawing their own comic strips. Clients have used blank comic strips to illustrate traumatic experiences, current treatment issues, family circumstances, everyday challenges and solutions, dreams and nightmares, future hopes, and their life's events. Comic strips also allow clients to recreate their story

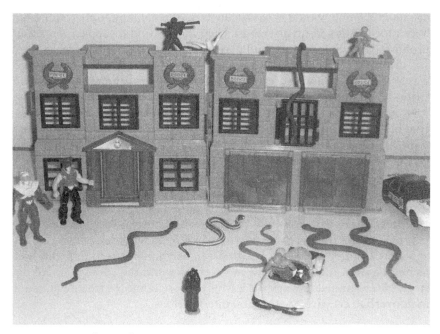

Figure 8.3   Bill's sandtray.

the way they wish it to be, which is particularly useful for changing what happens in a nightmare or a traumatic experience. When clients change their view of a past traumatic event, they are able to regain a sense of power over the circumstances and how it affects them. This intervention can be used in either a directive or nondirective fashion. The therapist may decide to give the client a particular topic to illustrate, or he may decide to let the client develop the concept on his own. This allows the therapist to tailor the activity based on therapeutic purposes, time constraints, client needs, artistic talent, or other factors.

One client created a comic strip that depicted the abuse he experienced as a child. Although he was only asked to draw his autobiography, he decided to illustrate the abusive aspects of his childhood. This particular client, whom we refer to as Steven, had experienced extensive trauma and abuse at the hands of his family. He was typically quiet, withdrawn, emotionally distant, and sad. He struggled to form attachments, and it was extremely difficult for him to talk about his past experiences. He found it challenging to verbalize any thoughts and feelings. Steven possessed amazing resiliency, despite all of the hardships he had faced. He advanced through treatment with courage and honesty that baffled us all as we watched him strive for a healthy life with or without his family of origin. His family would occasionally visit and call him, only to raise his hopes for continued involvement. Then they would disappear, breaking promises, avoiding contact, and placing him in unsafe situations

Although Steven struggled to verbalize his thoughts and feelings, he was a talented artist who created some very powerful and revealing comic strips. He told the story of his physical and sexual abuse history involving four perpetrators. The comic reflected several aspects of his abuse, including the size differential between him and the abusers and his attempts to be hypervigilant against unexpected attacks. Even on his birthday, he was not safe from the threat of violence. The comic depicts how he was groomed, coerced, and forced, to go along with the abuse and to keep it a secret. He even illustrated his pain, fear, sadness, powerlessness, and disorientation as a result of the abuse Figure 8.4.

Steven's comics allowed us to address his abuse history in a new way. It provided the treatment team with a whole new understanding of his experiences and provided access to previously unexpressed thoughts and feelings. Steven found his voice in his comics and the courage to tell his story. He continued to work successfully through myriad treatment issues in nonverbal, creative, therapeutic interventions.

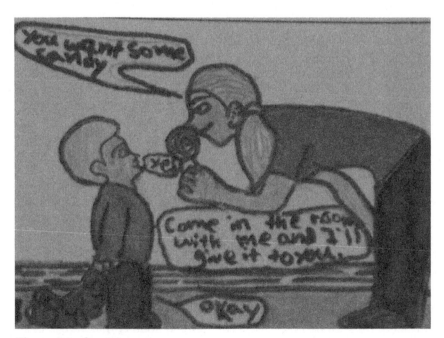

Figure 8.4   Steven's comic.

INTEGRATING SUPERHEROES INTO THE RESIDENTIAL TREATMENT CULTURE

Superheroes and their messages can be found throughout the treatment culture of our program. From posters to sandtray figures, the courage and strength that superheroes inspire is all around us and ready to be harnessed by our clients. In addition to the various techniques mentioned in the previous pages, there are endless ways to incorporate superheroes into a treatment culture. Simply adding superhero merchandise, quotes, and stories to the atmosphere of a program can introduce concepts to clients in a new way. A program culture that includes the concepts of superheroes gives the clients additional concepts and metaphors to draw from when expressing themselves. Clients may then refer to and draw on the material express their thoughts, feelings, and struggles in richer, fuller detail.

Posters

One way to reference superheroes is through posters. A particular poster used in our program displays the Incredibles and illustrates that "Evil is no match for the family dynamic." Because many of our clients come to treatment for sexually abusive behaviors, they experience extensive relationship difficulties and highly dysfunctional family ties. This particular poster reflects a basic superhero tenet: that disagreements and differences of opinions occur, but superheroes (and a family) join forces to overcome formidable obstacles. The poster, as well as others like it, suggest that together with their family, clients can face and resolve the issues that brought them into treatment.

Comic Books

Another, more obvious way of introducing clients to superheroes is through comic books. Our program expert on comics, who has a sizeable collection, developed a comic book lending system for clients who have attained a specific privilege level. They are able to check out comic books from his library for use during their recreational time. Not only does it help them develop a healthy new way to spend their free time, it also promotes the culture and knowledge of superheroes. Requiring clients to attain a specific privilege status to use the comic library supports the idea that the library is special and motivates clients to gain access.

A Spider-Man comic was produced in cooperation with the National Committee for Prevention of Child Abuse. Titled *Spider-Man and Power Pack,* it addresses the issue of sexual abuse. A young boy is with his babysitter while his parents are at a party. The babysitter starts to touch the boy in sexually inappropriate ways, and Spider-Man overhears the boy's protests. Spiderman responds to the boy's call for help, and the babysitter runs away after threatening to hurt the boy if he tells. With Spider-Man's assistance, the boy shares what happened with his parents, and then Spider-Man shares a similar story. He shares with the boy how he was sexually abused as a child and struggled with feeling responsible for the abuse as a result. Important and common aspects involved in child sexual abuse are illustrated in the comic. Reading and discussing this comic in Healing Group allowed clients to externalize their issues of abuse.

There are a variety of resources that help clients express the fruits of their imagination. *The SuperHero Comic Book Maker* by Kreative Komix is a computer program that creates single-page graphics, full multipage comics, and animated cartoons. It includes backgrounds, characters, props, text, sound, and animation. It has easy-to-follow instructions and is recommended for clients of all ages. Another creative resource is the *Make-Your-Own Comic Book* kit from Curiosity Kits. It includes blank comic book pages, generic comic book scenes, tracing sheets, colored pencils, and illustrated instructions. The pages are ready to be brought to life with creative ideas. Klutz has also published *Draw the Marvel Comics Super Heroes*. This book details how to draw a Superhero. It includes fun facts and helpful hints on how to improve your drawings. Clients love to use these resources and expand their artistic abilities.

Movies

We like to be multimedia and multimodal in our approach to treatment. Toward that end, we have often used superhero movies to illustrate a concept or demonstrate a point. This can be as simple as viewing the final battle from *The Fantastic Four* to illustrate the need to work together as a team. This can be as complex as using multiple clips from the second Harry Potter movie to illustrate the Phoenix mythology to draw the parallels between treatment progress and being born from one's own ashes.

Using movies, or sections of a movie, can often serve as an easy introduction to the group's topic as well as a vehicle for an important treatment message. We define the term *treatment message* to include messages that promote the four cornerstones (courage, care and concern, responsibility, and honesty) along with growth. Inherent in the superheroes' stories are themes of battling evil, fighting for what is right, and the triumph of good. The following is a partial list of movies (and television series), and some of the additional treatment messages that they illustrate, and like superheroes, they are everywhere!

- *Daredevil* (Johnson, 2003): persistence despite obstacles/handicaps.
- *Superman* (Donner, 1978; Furie, 1987; Lester, 1980, 1983; Singer, 2006): the true meanings of strength and heroic.
- *The Incredibles* (Bird, 2004): family dynamics and teamwork.
- *Spider-Man* (Raimi, 2002, 2004): loss issues, alternative family situations.
- *Mystery Men* (McCarey, 1935): even misfits can be superheroes.
- *X-Men* (Ratner, 2006; Singer, 2000, 2003): the concept of family of choice.
- *Harry Potter* (Columbus, 2001, 2002, Cuaron, 2004; Newell, 2005): the unlikely hero, alternative family setting, family of choice.
- *Star Wars* (Kershner, 1980; Lucas, 1977, 1999, 2002; 2005; Marquand, 1983;): you do not have to grow up to become your father.
- *Sky High* (Mitchell, 2005): the pressure to live up to parents' expectations.
- *Batman* (Burton, 1989, 1992; Nolan, 2005; Schumacher, 1995): trauma, loss, heroism.
- *The Hulk* (Lee, 2003): anger management, accepting all parts of your personality, body image.

CLOTHING

Clothing is an enjoyable accessory to help promote the use of superheroes and their message. The program has designed shirts using the moral from Spider-Man, "with great power comes great responsibility." Only those clients who have begun to demonstrate an internalization of treatment concepts receive a shirt. These clients have achieved specific treatment objectives and have made a commitment to live a lifestyle free of sexually abusive behaviors. The shirt acts as an external, tangible reminder of the lifestyle they are learning to embrace. Issues involving the legitimate and appropriate use of power as well as being responsible for one's actions are paramount themes throughout treatment that addresses sexually abusive behavior. As a result, the slogan helps clients to be even more mindful of the morals supported by their superheroes and the changes they are attempting to make themselves. The shirt also sets them apart as leaders and role models on the program. Clients view the shirts as an honor and privilege. Like the comic book library, residents are motivated to improve their status to receive a shirt and be included in this privileged group. Clients could also create their own T-shirts through the use of readily available computer software. They will appreciate your efforts, value their new apparel, and show it off. Our clients have worn their superhero apparel until it is stained, torn, outgrown, and beyond.

Superhero Merchandise

Making superhero merchandise available to clients is also helpful in generating excitement and reinforcing the therapeutic messages present in the stories and characters. A variety of superhero items can be used as prizes for contests and games. Party favors from card stores are a great source of inexpensive and fun items that depict popular superhero characters. Easily found merchandise typically includes stickers, notebooks, pens, folders, games, posters, sports bottles, and action figures. Clients are eager to earn these prizes and show off their winnings. The culture of superheroes is infectious and easily gains momentum with staff and the families of our clients. Just one example of this was the donation to the program from a client's family of a superhero chess set. They wanted to show their appreciation to the program as well as provide an item that would add to a client's experience while in treatment. The chess set is widely used, and new clients are told about the graduate and his family who donated it.

Handouts

Handouts and worksheets are frequently used during group sessions with our clients. Initially our group handouts were like any other, with ordinary fonts, no graphics, and boring text. The treatment team started to use graphics, word art, clip art, and fun fonts to add life to the group materials. This simple change to the handouts generated energy about the group topic and was fun for both the clients and staff. Clients collected the handouts and even became interested in who possess the coveted *original copy*.

With just a little imagination, you can introduce superheroes to clients in easy and inexpensive ways. To help our clients become more familiar with superheroes, one of the therapists created a series of handouts filled with superhero fun facts and quizzes. Others announced upcoming movie releases, treatment activities, and special off-grounds outings. One specific worksheet summarized information about the members of the Fantastic Four and announced an outing to see the movie. Allowing clients to learn about superheroes in fun and exciting ways helps them forget they are learning useful and treatment related concepts.

Music

Music can also be an enjoyable and exciting way to reinforce treatment issues with clients. The use of music can allow clients to connect with concepts, feelings, and attitudes that otherwise may remain one dimensional. Music helps bring their understanding of an issue to another level and makes for a richer experience. There are countless songs that relate to superheroes and suit the purposes of treatment-related activities and assignments. *Hero* by Superchic[k] is a particularly powerful and relevant song that tells the story of four adolescents who struggles to live courageous lives. After listening to the song and reading the lyrics, our clients completed a worksheet on which they identified the people in their lives who are heroes and ways they could be heroic through their everyday choices. In their worksheets, clients made significant disclosures involving previously undisclosed sexually abusive behavior.

CONCLUSION

This chapter has related just a few of the ways superheroes are introduced to our clients as they enter into and continue through residential treatment. Initially a client's understanding of superheroes may be fairly superficial. The biographies of the superheroes will begin to personally resonate with clients as their self-understanding grows. The early life experiences of the hero may act as a mirror for clients to view their own unpleasant life events. The hero's journey, transformation, and ultimate victory offer clients hope. Often clients question their ability to succeed in treatment. They are wondering if they can make the personal changes necessary to live a healthy life. They are unsure if they can bear the pain of facing the issues that led to treatment. The superhero's story gives them a road map and a picture of the destination to which they are striving. The superhero's story helps them believe that the very obstacles of their past can become their greatest assets and strengths. They find their own story in the histories and biographies of the superheroes they love to read about. Through the superhero's struggle and ultimate success, our clients find their own strength and ability to persevere. Superheroes allow our clients to distance themselves from their own pain while acknowledging and experiencing it in a fuller, more meaningful way. When clients can simultaneously distance from and experience their issues, they have the opportunity to sort through their thoughts, questions, and reactions. Clients can begin truly to resolve their issues in a safe yet genuine way. This is particularly true for our clients as they begin to address their history of abuse and neglect, many for the first time, when they enter treatment.

POSTSCRIPT

There is something heroic in the work being done with these clients. We treat clients who have been labeled "untreatable" by other facilities. We believe in changes that have not happened yet. We fight the good fight daily, against seemingly impossible odds. We seek to prevent children from being victims, thereby preventing a chain reaction of abuse and victimization. We create hope where there is none. We maintain our senses of imagination, enthusiasm, and wonder against a daily deluge of cynicism, apathy, and banality. Ideally, we work to put ourselves out of business one day.

There have been several benefits to working together to write this chapter. The first benefit was discovering that we were up to this challenging task. The second benefit was conceptualizing and creating the "Treatment Team." This took a bit of creativity and effort, but we were merely describing what was already there. The Treatment Team already comprised heroes; we just needed the capes, costumes, and credentials. We have always known that we are heroes to the clients. We were surprised to learn that we are heroes to each other as well. The third benefit was the ability to share what we have been doing with others.

REFERENCES

Bandura, A. (1986). *Social Foundations of Thought and Action*. Englewood Cliffs, NJ: Prentice Hall.

Bandura, A. (1997). Self-efficacy: The exercise of control. New York: Freeman.

Bays, L., & Freeman-Longo, R. (1989). *Why did I do it again? Understanding my cycle of problem behaviors*. Orwell, VT: Safer Society Press.

Bays, L., Freeman-Longo, R., & Hildebran, D. (1990) *How can I stop? Breaking my deviant cycle*. Orwell, VT: Safer Society Press.

Bird, B. (Director). (2004). *The Incredibles* [Motion picture] . United States: Walt Disney Pictures.

Burton, T. (Director). (1989). *Batman* [Motion picture]. United States/United Kingdom: Guber-Peters.

Burton, T. (Director). (1992). *Batman returns* [Motion picture]. United States: PolyGram Filmed Entertainment.

Columbus, C. (Director). (2001). *Harry Potter and the sorcerer's stone* [Motion picture]. United States: 1492 Pictures.

Columbus, C. (Director). (2002). *Harry Potter and the chamber of secrets*. [Motion picture]. United States: 1492 Pictures.

Cuaron, A. (Director). (2004). *Harry Potter and the prisoner of Azkaban*. [Motion picture]. United States: Warner Bros. Pictures.

Donner, R. (Director). (1978). *Superman* [Motion picture]. United Kingdom: Alexander Salkind.

Furie, S. (Director). (1987). *Superman IV: The quest for peace* [Motion picture]. United States: Red Sun Productions Pty., Ltd.

Isaac, C., & Lane, S. (1990). *The sexual abuse cycle in the treatment of adolescent sexual abusers* [Videotape or audiocassette and reference materials]. Orwell, VT: Safer Society Press.

Johnson, M. (Director). (2003). *Daredevil* [Motion picture]. United States: Marvel Enterprises.

Johnston, J. (Director). (1991). *The Rockefeer.* [Motion picture]. United States: Walt-Disney-Vig..

Kahn, T. J. (1990). *Pathways, A guided workbook for youth beginning treatment.* Orwell, VT: Safer Society Press.

Kendall, P. C. (1991). *Child and adolescent therapy, cognitive behavioral procedures.* New York: Guilford Press.

Kershner, I. (Director). (1980). *Star wars: Episode V—The empire strikes back* [Motion picture]. United States: Lucasfilm, Ltd.

Lane, S. (1991). The sexual abuse cycle. In G. D. Ryan & S. Lane (Eds.), *Juvenile sexual offending: Causes, consequences and correction.* Lexington, MA: D. C. Heath.

Lee, A. (Director). (2003). *The Hulk* [Motion picture]. United States: Universal Pictures.

Lester, R. (Director). (1980). *Superman II* [Motion picture]. United States: Alexander Salkind.

Lester, R. (Director). (1983). *Superman III* [Motion picture]. United States: Cantharus Productions, N.V.

Lucas, G. (Director). (1977). *Star wars* [Motion picture]. United States: Twentieth Century Fox.

Lucas, G. (Director). (1999). *Star wars: Episode I—The phantom menace* [Motion picture]. United States: Lucasfilm, Ltd.

Lucas, G. (Director). (2002). *Star wars: Episode II—Attack of the clones* [Motion picture]. United States: Lucasfilms, Ltd.

Lucas, G. (Director). (2005). *Star wars: Episode III—Revenge of the Sith* [Motion picture]. United States: Lucasfilm, Ltd.

Marquand, R. (Director). (1983). *Star wars: Episode VI—Return of the Jedi* [Motion picture]. United States: Lucasfilm, Ltd.

McCarey, R. (Director). (1935). *Mystery man* [Motion picture]. United States: Monogram Pictures Corporation.

Mitchell, M. (Director). (2005). *Sky high* [Motion picture]. United States: Max Stronghold Productions.

Newell, M. (Director). (2005). *Harry Potter and the goblet of fire.* [Motion picture]. United States: Warners Bros. Pictures.

Nolan, C. (Director). (2005). *Batman begins* [Motion picture]. United States: Warner Bros. Pictures.

Raimi, S. (Director). (2002). *Spider-Man* [Motion picture]. United States: Columbia Pictures Corporation.

Raimi, S. (Director). (2004). *Spider-Man—2*. [Motion picture]. United States: Columbia Pictures Corporation.

Ratner, B. (Director). (2006). *X-Men: The last stand*. [Motion picture]. United States: Twentieth Century Fox.

Schumacher, J (Director). (1995). *Batman forever*. [Motion picture]. United States: PolyGram Filmed Entertainment.

Singer, B. (Director). (2000). *X-Men*. [Motion picture]. United States: Twentieth Century Fox.

Singer, B. (Director). (2003). *X-2* [Motion picture]. United States: Twentieth Century Fox.

Stickrod, A., Hamer, J., & Janes, B. (1984) *Informational guide on the juvenile sexual offender*. Eugene, OR: Adolescent Sex Offender Treatment Network.

Story, T. (Director). (2005). *The 1* [Motion picture]. United States: Twentieth Century Fox.

CHAPTER NINE

Superheroes Are Super Friends: Developing Social Skills and Emotional Reciprocity With Autism Spectrum Clients

Patty Scanlon

What I like about Superman is that he can *fly!* I like to pretend I can fly, too! And I like that when I look at the sky, sometimes maybe Superman might be up there. And even though I can't fly, I can be nice to people, which is the other thing Superman does—so he helps me remember to do that, too. I don't know why *he* does it, but *I* do it because it makes me happy to think about him. I think [the sky's] really *pretty*, especially if you imagine you can see Superman *flying* up there. And the sky is always, always there, so I think Superman is, too, 'cause he can always, always fly.

—(Grayson, 2006)

The magic of superheroes is recognizable, pervasive, and all-powerful. Most children, adolescents, and adults have likely identified with a super-hero at some time in their lives. This is illustrated by our incorporation of various identifiable phrases into our everyday language. When one utters, "Look, up in the sky!" all eyes turn upward, and Superman can be seen flying through the air on his way to another heroic rescue. "Live long and prosper" is a familiar phrase from the long-lived *Star Trek* (Butler et al., 1966) television series and movies. "Trekkies" need not even speak but can merely indicate Spock's famous hand signal to send the message to another. Buzz Lightyear's refrain, "To infinity . . . and beyond!" is another easily recognizable expression since the movie *Toy Story* (Lasseter, 1995) introduced Buzz, Woody, and their friends into our culture. With the popularity of *Finding Nemo* (Stanton & Unkrich, 2003), Dory's encouraging mantra, "Swim, swim, swim, just keep swimming!" reminds each of us to stay focused and persist even when we feel the chips are down.

Another example of the way superheroes have permeated our culture is through their appearance on children's clothing, household items, sporting goods, and vitamins. A new movie is barely released before the star superhero begins to appear on the chests of children everywhere. Wearing clothing with the image of their new superfriend, children can pretend to take on the superhero's positive characteristics. Likewise, children's bedrooms are transformed through wallpaper, furniture, linens, and assorted accessories bearing the likeness of their new star performing powerful feats. Children quickly find comfort slumbering with their strong, brave buddies. Children need only open their bedroom door to enter a magical world where suddenly superpowers are all their own! Asking Santa (perhaps our oldest superhero) for a PowerPuff Girls bicycle means pedaling at warp speed might be just around the neighborhood street corner. Certainly, taking a flavor-filled superhero vitamin helps children to think that their body will be absorbing magical superhero superpowerful nutrients— imagine the newfound strength Johnny or Kathy might experience upon swallowing such a magical pill! To infinity and beyond, indeed!

Yet another miraculous superhero power is these characters' ability to convey meaning through metaphor. Marketing itself is a lesson in superhero culture. Vitamins, supplements, and healthy foods are made all the more attractive through their simple association with a popular superhero. The meaning within the message is that we, too, can become superheroes if we only buy that product. In *Vitamin C and Bioflavonoids: The Batman and Robin of Eye Health,* Gina White (2005) used the popular metaphor to explain how bioflavonoid is the sidekick to vitamin C. Her metaphor conjures up the image and accurate job description of Robin as the ever-loyal and hardworking sidekick to Batman and sharpens her meaning through the use of the superhero metaphor. Maleskey and McCommons (1999) described superhero vitamin E, and the Almond Board of California (2006) went further by calling vitamin E a cellular superhero of sorts on GetYourE.org. Some marketing is even more direct. We are persuaded to buy Bravo Brands' Slammers Ultimate Milk Shakes because of their association with various superheroes on their label. Their marketing material states, "All your favorite MARVEL Super Heroes™ are here in four

delicious flavors, . . . This is milk with a built in fan club . . . Vitamin forti-
fication matches Super Hero's unique powers" (Bravobrands, 2006). The
message is clear: associate your product with a superhero and you have
a built-in fan club. One might wonder, "Does *my* superhero drink this
milk?" Spider-Man's namesake milkshake is "Chocolate Web." Imagine
scaling the side of a building after drinking this powerful stuff! Yes, it is
the magical, universal appeal of the superhero that lends itself to instant
recognition and powerful understanding.

THE APPEAL OF SUPERHEROES

It is this universal attraction of the superhero with which children everywhere readily identify. Children wear their Spider-Man T-shirts, sleep on
their Buzz Lightyear pillows, and take the latest superhero vitamin, all in
an effort to achieve power. Living in an adult world, children feel less than
powerful, less than super, less a hero. Leon feels lonely in a new school
because his father's job transfer moved his family to an unfamiliar town.
Tammy is teased because her mother cannot afford to buy her the latest
clothes. Children everyday attempt to meet standards set by adults. The
mighty image of the superhero helps them to see that even from the most
unfortunate of circumstances, success and glory can be achieved.

Children in therapy often feel disempowered. By the time they reach
therapy, they already may feel they are a "problem" at home and school.
Knowing they need outside help may intensify this feeling. Children need
heroes while they are mastering difficult circumstances. It is not surprising,
then, that superheroes come to play therapy along with their real-life
admirers. Children come into the therapy office eager to show off their
newest T-shirt bearing the image of the latest popular culture superhero.
Still other children draw or paint their favorite superhero in the playroom.
Toting along a comforting stuffed Spider-Man, a prized Yu-Gi-Oh card
collection, or the hottest Star Wars figure, children introduce an important
element of their world into the therapy hour.

In whatever form they appeared, I noticed the strong identification
and admiration so many of my young clients had for their superheroes.
It was unmistakable. Seeing this theme repeatedly, I began to ask myself,
are these just manifestations of Winnicott's (1971, p. 2) "transitional object," or something more? These superheroes did not simply come to help
ease the child's transition from mom into therapy, just to be left behind
and retrieved at the end of the hour. These superheroes were with children throughout their session, often participating at some level in their
therapy. The entire Yu-Gi-Oh collection was present for therapy! With all
due respect to Winnicott, it was not just a teddy bear or stuffed animal to

which these children were clinging. Indeed, it reflected something more. It was power, the need for rescue, sometimes obsession. Spider-Man came to play therapy over and over again. Children began to teach me more about their superheroes and what special meaning they held for them. I soon realized these superheroes were becoming my very own cotherapist(s). Incorporating children's favorite superhero into their play therapy seemed natural. Sad Sarah smiled with Dora's encouragement. Shy Sam transformed into Sociable Sam with Superman's friendly assistance. Yes, superheroes provide comfort and rescue when needed. Superheroes can teach essential skills. Superheroes are best friends. All that's required is imagination.

In addition to loaning children some superpower, I also noticed that for some, superheroes were an object of fixation, an obsession. Whenever asked to draw a picture, some children would always repeat the picture they had drawn previously. Spontaneity appeared lacking in these particular children. Some were perfectionistic, obsessing over every detail in their Pokemon drawing. Others would talk endlessly about the latest movie they had seen and be able to narrate that movie seemingly verbatim. Still others would take pride in showing the latest additions to their Yu-Gi-Oh card collection and appeared unable to shift focus from it to another task. For some children, superheroes even assisted me in my assessment of their difficulties and challenges. This group of children presented with features of autism spectrum disorders (ASD).

AUTISM SPECTRUM DISORDERS

Historical Overview

Kanner (1943) first defined a category of individuals who ignored people, did not relate, had delayed or absent language (including echolalia), excellent rote memory, and obsessiveness. Around the same time in Vienna, pediatrician Hans Asperger identified a cluster of individuals he classified as "little professors" (O'Neil, 1999). Asperger noted that his patients had average to above average intelligence and could not understand social cues. However, because it was World War II Germany, it would not be until 1981 that Asperger's work would receive wider attention. London psychiatrist Lorna Wing translated Asperger's work and first used the term Asperger's syndrome in a 1981 paper on the subject, and it began to receive international recognition (Attwood, 1998). Kanner's autism, also known as "classic autism," was first defined as a diagnostic category in the *Diagnostic and Statistical Manual*, third edition (DSM–III; American

Psychiatric Association, 1980). It was not until 1994 that Asperger's disorder was defined in DSM–IV (American Psychiatric Association, 1994).

Controversy has surrounded the causes of autism, beginning as early as Kanner's writings. Kanner noted that the parents of the autistic children he observed were less than "warm-hearted" (Wolfberg, 1999). Bruno Bettelheim (1967) coined the term *refrigerator mothers* who were emotionally detached from their infants and thus drove them to withdraw into an autistic state (Wolfberg, 1999). Bernard Rimland (1964) was instrumental in dispelling this myth by proposing organic states in autism. Current controversies remain and include environmental toxins and mercury in vaccines. Perhaps the disorder is controversial because it is increasing in prevalence.

Prevalence

According to the Centers for Disease Control (CDC) (2005), the prevalence of ASD is between 1 in 500 and 1 in 166 children. Estimating 4 million live births in the United States each year, the CDC report assumes approximately 24000 children will be diagnosed with an ASD. Assuming this prevalence rate was constant over the previous 2 decades, the CDC also estimates that there are up to 500,000 individuals between the ages of 0 and 21 with an ASD. An April 2003 report by the California Department of Developmental Services indicates that new cases of diagnosed full syndrome autism in California doubled in the 4-year period between 1999 and 2002 (California Department of Developmental Services, 2003). The report notes that full syndrome autism occurs at a much smaller rate than other disorders in the autism spectrum, such as Asperger's disorder or pervasive developmental disorder—not otherwise specified (PDD-NOS), which were not included in this report. The report cautions that it "very likely underestimate[s]" (p. 6) actual prevalence rates for the California population. The Centers for Disease Control (2005) reports that autism is the fastest growing developmental disability with 10% to 17% annual growth. This makes ASDs more common than childhood cancer and Down syndrome. According to the CDC, this rise in autism has been attributed to both an increased understanding of the disorder leading to an increase in diagnosis and a substantial growth in its prevalence.

It is undeniable that the rate of diagnosis of children with ASDs is rising. Therefore, it is critical for mental health professionals to broaden their knowledge and treatment skill base. Good treatment dictates a thorough understanding of the breadth and depth of the ASDs.

Definition

The Autism Society of America (2003, 2006) defines autism as "a complex disability that typically appears during the first three years of life and is the result of a neurological disorder that affects the normal functioning of the brain, impacting development in the areas of social interaction and communication skills." Treatment and educational supports for children with autistic characteristics must use diagnostic criteria according to the DSM–IV. However, the descriptive categories of the DSM–IV merely scratch the surface in explicating the complexities of behavior in individuals with ASDs. In this context, much has been written about the limitations of a *categorical,* as opposed to a *dimensional* approach to diagnosis (Hollander et al., 1998; Widiger & Samuel, 2005). The argument is that a categorical approach is unduly limiting, and the diagnosis of autism is no exception.

> "No two people with autism are the same; its precise form or expression is different in every case. Moreover, there may be a most intricate (and potentially creative) interaction between the autistic traits and the other qualities of the individual. So, while a single glance may suffice for clinical diagnosis, if we hope to understand the autistic individual, nothing less than a total biography will do. (Sacks, 1995, p. 250)

The more common currently used term, autism spectrum disorders (Rutter & Schopler, 1992), as it is used here, refers to the diagnostic category in the DSM–IV known as the pervasive developmental disorders (PDD). This category includes autistic disorder, Rett's disorder, childhood disintegrative disorder, Asperger's disorder, and PDD-NOS. Although Rett's disorder and childhood disintegrative disorder are classified as such, they are relatively rare and follow a distinctly different course of onset than their more common neighbors on the autism spectrum. For the purposes of this discussion, only the more common PDD are addressed here. To qualify for a diagnosis of one of PDD, a child must have a delay or abnormal functioning in at least two of the following: social interaction, language as used in social communication, or symbolic or imaginative play. Autistic disorder is differentiated from Asperger's disorder by language development and cognitive skills. In autistic disorder, language does not develop normally or may be completely absent. Approximately three-fourths of those diagnosed with autistic disorder also have some degree of mental retardation, usually in the moderate range. In Asperger's disorder, there is no significant delay in language and cognitive development is normal. Otherwise, the criteria for Asperger's disorder are the same as for autistic disorder. Further, according to the DSM–IV, autistic characteristics must be present by age 3, whereas Asperger's characteristics may not be recognized until later. If full criteria are not met for either of these diagnoses but there is subthreshold impairment or late age of onset, then the classification PDD–NOS is used. The existence of this category alludes to the fact that the DSM–IV does not fully capture the range of individuals with autism characteristics.

Impairments in ASD

Individuals classified on the autism spectrum often have sensory idiosyncrasies (Rapin, 1998). One child may appear to have tactile sensory aberrations such as a higher than normal pain tolerance, hypersensitivity or hyposensitivity to being touched or hugged, or difficulty with aspects of clothing such as tags on shirts, seams in socks, or long-sleeved shirts. Auditory peculiarities include being over-or-undersensitive to certain noises. Visual and olfactory disturbances may include over-focusing on light or particular smells. Gustatory sensitivities can include limiting oneself to a particular color of food or dislike of certain textures of foods.

Emotions and mood may also be idiosyncratic in children on the autism spectrum. A child may be extremely fearful of seemingly innocuous things, such as fear of walking in the dewy grass because of small spider webs seen glistening in the sun. Others may appear to have no fear in the presence of real danger. Anxious children may twist and twirl strands of hair until it begins falling out. Others may thumb-suck well into latency age. Mood in some ASD children is depressed, and there may be unusual emotional responses such as extreme giggling or no emotional response when one is expected. A child who requires strict adherence to a 32-step bedtime ritual may "melt down" if a step is missed, resulting in a 1-hour tantrum. Others have tantrums because of difficulties with transitions. One boy regularly would not leave the waiting area to come to play therapy until he had finished turning all the pages in the children's book he was holding. These children appear to have features of obsessive–compulsive disorder. Indeed, children may be misdiagnosed with this disorder. According to Volkmar (in O'Neil, 1999), the crucial difference in diagnosis is that their obsessive behavior significantly impairs their social functioning. Some children appear flat in affect when talking about sad events, only to suddenly burst into loud crying 5 minutes later. It is as if a switch is turned on and off in the individual.

Cognitive abilities also vary widely in these children. Hyperlexic children may be able to read as early as 2 or 3 years of age (Bligh, 1995). Others may possess an extraordinary ability to memorize movies or songs seen or heard only once. Receptive or expressive language skills can be impaired. Children may range from being mute to echolalic to engaging in monologue speech. One child repeated "aloha" upon crossing a threshold because going through any door must mean "hello" or "good-bye." He had heard this new word and had taken a liking to using it. Intelligence measures in some children may reveal large discrepancies between their verbal and performance IQs. Many children on the autism spectrum have coexisting learning disorders. An example of this might be the hyperlexic child who falls in the below average range in performance measures of intelligence, such that she may qualify for an Individualized Education Plan at school. Other idiosyncrasies of language include the inability to understand jokes or idiomatic phrases. The phrase such as "step on a crack, break your mother's back" can be taken quite literally. Certainly, this might create heightened anxiety.

Socially, children on the autism spectrum may range from completely withdrawn and isolative to friendship seeking with only one or two persons. These friends may be younger or older than the child, or may even be adults. Peer relationships may be adversely affected because some children do not understand how to enter a play situation. They lack an understanding of the rules governing social situations. It is said that children with ASDs feel as if they are living in a foreign land or culture (Ortiz, 2004). Given that upward of 80% of our communication is nonverbal, it is no wonder these children have difficulty understanding social cues. Says a young man with autism, "I know that people communicate with each other through their eyes, but I cannot understand what they say" (Beyer & Gammeltoft, 2000, p. 27).

PLAY IN AUTISM SPECTRUM DISORDERS

Play behavior in children with ASDs is notably lacking in spontaneity and may consist of taking apart rather than playing with toys. These children may engage in only solitary or parallel play. Additionally, when these children engage in game play, they may quickly end the game if they see they are losing. If they continue the game to completion and lose, the child may have a meltdown.

Through play, children learn the numerous rules governing social and cultural behavior, which in turn facilitates their healthy cognitive development (Beyer & Gammeltoft, 2000; Piaget, 1962; Vygotsky, 1978). In their book, *Autism and Play,* Beyer and Gammeltoft explained how play is the bridge between the physical and the social worlds for children. They cited an example of the infant looking to its caregiver for meaning about the physical world. When a toy is moved away from the mouth of an infant, she looks not to the toy or to the hand moving it, but directly into the eyes of the person to understand and make meaning of their intentions. In so doing, the infant may wonder, "Do we know each other?

Are you smiling? Is it fun?" (p. 27). The child with autism spectrum characteristics, however, is not able to make meaning out of the many nonverbal cues available to him. Therefore, the child may focus solely on the toy itself and busy himself by watching it move. Because of this, the child remains focused on the physical world.

> That the essence of the autistic spectrum may be best captured by a restricted range of interests and a seemingly obsessive insistence on sameness may speak to the detrimental impact of social isolation. When children with autism seem to engage in pretend play, a closer examination of the behaviors involved may reveal them to be highly repetitive. In sharp contrast to the rich, thematic variations evident in the play of typically developing children, the play of children with autism seems almost obsessive in its literal repetition of identical acts. Analogous with the literal quality and the apparently meaningless repetition of speech in echolalia, the play of children with autism might be described more aptly as "echoplaylia." (Schuler & Wolfberg, 2000, p. 253)

Echoplaylia

Echoplaylia is an accurate description of how children on the autism spectrum play. Often, these children mimic various cartoons they have watched or movies they have recently seen. These characters sometimes become the object of fixation. One 6-year-old boy was insistent that I participate in his play of the latest Star Wars movie. This child directed me repeatedly to steer the starship at my command in a precise manner, while he commandeered his own starship in parallel play with me. Unfortunately, I had not seen the movie, nor could I understand his speech very well. Moreover, the "whisper in the ear" technique (the nondirective clinician steps out of the play briefly to ask the child how to respond at that moment) did not work with this child. Even if it had, I would have had to use it far too often. He expected me to know precisely what to do and when and how to do it. I was to make the appropriate "shooting" sound with my mouth at the appropriate time and at the appropriate volume. We were reenacting seemingly every aspect of a movie that I had not seen. I was an actor without a script, a movie without a director. I may not have grasped his play, but in those moments, I certainly grasped the depth of his struggle for communication and understanding in the countertransference I experienced with him. How must it be for him to attempt to convey his meaning using our language?! He needed *his* very own coach to "regularly whisper in his ear." Imagining his frustration in coping with everyday life became crystal clear to me during those play therapy sessions.

Theory of Mind

Around age 4 or 5, children normally begin to develop a "theory of mind" (Twachtman-Cullen, 2000; Wolfberg, 1999). They begin to understand that others have thoughts, feelings, and beliefs that differ from their own. Together with the development of this theory of mind, children are able to *distinguish* their own thoughts and feelings from those of others (Mundy & Stella, 2000). Experimental studies testing for theory of mind illustrate this concept:

> In the prototypical "false belief paradigm," a child is asked to watch an agent ("Sally") hide an object in one of two hiding places (Place 1 versus Place 2). Sally then leaves the room, and another agent ("Anne") moves the object from Place 1 to Place 2. When Sally returns, the child must answer the question, "Where will Sally look for the object?" To answer this question correctly the child must disregard his or her own knowledge of where the object really is (Place 2) and *think about where Sally thinks* the object is. (Mundy & Stella, 2000, p. 59)

Simon Baron-Cohen (1995) termed this ability to read the mental states of others as *mind-reading*. Conversely, Baron-Cohen used the term *mindblindness* to describe the impairment in theory of mind that persons with autism appear to have.

TREATMENT

Given the multitude of viewpoints regarding the etiology and parameters of the various autism spectrum disorders, it is not surprising that there exists a correspondingly wide variety of treatment options from which to choose. Whereas most approaches are based on learning theory and incorporate behavioral techniques, others focus on the development of communication skills. Still other treatments address the emotional component in ASDs. Described here are some of the more widely accepted forms of treatment for ASD children.

Of the behavioral approaches to treatment, applied behavior analysis (ABA) is perhaps the most popular (Ozonoff, Dawson, & McPartland, 2002; Prizant, Wetherby, & Rydell, 2000). Also known as Lovaas therapy after its founder, Dr. Ivaar Lovaas, ABA is a well-documented approach to teaching autistic children (Prizant, Wetherby, & Rydell, 2000). It is an intensive behavioral approach to teach and develop needed skills in children with ASD. Based on the behavioral theory of B. F. Skinner, ABA uses discrete trials of behavioral intervention and is conducted individually in one-on-one sessions with a trained behavioral therapist.

Treatment approaches aimed at improving communication in ASD children include Treatment and Education of Autistic and Related Communication-handicapped Children (TEACCH), Picture Exchange Communication System (PECS), and Social Stories. *TEACCH* is a highly structured, individualized curriculum using visual learning to improve communication, social skills, and coping skills (Ozonoff et al., 2002; Yarnell, 2000). In the *PECS*, the child is instructed to communicate by exchanging a picture for something desired. Based on speech therapy, PECS seeks to assist the ASD child to understand the function of communication and to attach meaning to words (Bondy & Frost, 2001). The concept of Social Stories originally was developed by Carol Gray (1995) to assist a child with ASD in understanding the rules of games and social situations. Social Stories address the theory of mind deficit in children on the autism spectrum. Each story consists of descriptive sentences that address the who, what, where, and why of the story; perspective sentences that focus on the ASD child's and others' thinking and feeling states; and directive sentences that suggest appropriate behavior (Gray, 2000). They are widely used and applicable to many types of situations because they can be easily tailored to the child and his specific needs.

Greenspan and Wieder (1998, 2000) advocated the use of the developmental, individualized relationship-based (DIR) approach to helping the child with an ASD develop his or her emotional world. Based on Greenspan and Wieder's (1998) original concept of Floor Time, they advocated that affect is the glue to all the other pieces of a child's development and that traditional behavioral approaches disregard this critical emotional component. For these researchers and clinicians, normal development in children with an ASD is sometimes just "ready to take off" and the key to helping the child is to engage him within the context of a relationship to help him move up the developmental ladder. Floor Time/DIR is an intensive approach in which caregivers and their child interact through play. Caregivers enter the child's play activity and follow the child's lead in whatever she is doing, creating mutual, shared engagement. Eventually the caregiver engages the child in more complex interactions which expand the child's "communication circles" and develop the child's emotional world with real-life interactions so affective learning can occur.

In summary, each approach described in this section has its strengths and weaknesses, its proponents and critics. As is true for all children, what works with one child may not with another. Combining therapeutic approaches is likely to yield the greatest results. Perhaps Levy (1988) summarized it best by suggesting that regardless of the treatment option chosen, the child with ASD must experience success, and it is wise to allow the child to have control over some aspect of the situation. Play therapy does just that.

Beyer and Gammeltoft described the rationale for play therapy thus: "The fact that children with autism do not play in a varied and spontaneous way should not mean that play activities cannot be a source of personal development" (p. 17).

Child-Centered Play Therapy

Why might a clinician choose to employ a child-centered (or nondirective) approach to play therapy, given that children with ASD play in an echolalic manner (Schuler & Wolfberg, 2000)? Is it counterintuitive to "let the child lead the way" if the child repetitively plays out movie scripts or cartoons with seemingly little imagination or movement? In this context, Beyer & Gammeltoft (2000) noted that

> Many children with autism seem to be at a very early developmental stage in their play. They need to be approached at their own level. You need to create a framework and set the stage for play in a way that makes it both possible and attractive. This requires special attention to aspects such as visualization, imitation, mirroring, taking turns and being concrete and specific. (p. 41)

From the outset, child-centered play therapy acknowledges and values the child's specific developmental level and needs. The child leads the way and is thus in control of the therapeutic process (Landreth, 1991). Further, because the child-centered play therapist is nondirective and accepting, she is uniquely positioned to appreciate the wide variety of play and interactional styles of children on the autism spectrum. By relating to the child in a reflective mirroring manner, the play therapist gains and conveys a thorough understanding of the child's strengths and challenges, specific interests or fixations, and unique ways of relating (or not relating) to the world. This understanding of the child's private language has been noted elsewhere to be of importance in helping the ASD child (Mittledorf et al., 2001). The clinician can then apply this knowledge to the child's treatment so that he will more willingly accept and comprehend. "My attitude of respect for, acceptance of, and faith in Brad allowed him 'to be.' In this safe, supporting, and emotionally nurturing relationship, Brad gained a sense of self.... He learned an increased sense of 'I am'" (Mittledorf et al., 2001, p. 268).

Two interesting cases of nondirective play therapy with autistic children have provided qualitative evidence of its value. The first was Richard Bromfield's (1996) use of psychodynamic play therapy with a higher functioning autistic child. Bromfield used puppets to communicate with a 6-year-old boy over the course of a 3-year therapy. The boy improved in his use of direct communication and in his acceptance and appropriate expression of his feelings. The second case involved the use of monthly psychoanalytic play therapy with a 5-year-old girl. Therapist Monica Lanyado (1996) facilitated a girl's ability to communicate her feelings symbolically with patience and careful observation. Through Lanyado's use of play therapy, the girl's communication with others increased while she made steady strides toward normal development . Each of these cases illustrates the need for play therapists to be very patient in their treatment of children with an ASD.

Virginia Axline's (1969) principles of nondirective play therapy allow the therapist to respect and support the child's unique perspective on the world. Four of Axline's principles are especially critical in the treatment of ASD children (p. 73):

- The therapist must develop a warm, friendly relationship with the child, in which good rapport is established as soon as possible.
- The therapist accepts the child exactly as he is.
- The therapist establishes a feeling of permissiveness in the relationship so that the child feels free to express his feelings completely.
- The therapist is alert to recognize the *feelings* the child is expressing and reflects those feelings back to him in such a manner that he gains insight into his behavior.

These principles provide a framework for the clinician to touch the inner world of the child with an ASD. Applied rigorously in therapy with these children, they will likely experience a relationship like no other. This is true for most children in play therapy, but it is especially relevant in play therapy with a child who has an ASD. These clients requires the patience and understanding of an accepting play therapist to invest in the relationship. By applying these core principles of child-centered play therapy, the children with ASDs are helped to realize feelings and inner states of which they may previously have been unaware. This provides a window into the realm of social and emotional life of the child with an ASD.

Further evidence suggests that the active mirroring and reflecting practiced in child-centered play therapy may help to develop empathy in children with ASDs. In an April 2003 study, neuroscientists at the University of California—Los Angeles researched the brain mechanism involved in empathy (Davis, 2003). They asked, "Why does a person reflexively wince at another's injury? Why is laughter contagious?" They used functional magnetic resonance imaging to observe subjects assigned to either mirror or observe others' facial expressions of random feelings. They found that when subjects mirrored the feelings, compared with those who only observed them, there was far greater activity in the primary motor cortex, the area of the brain governing emotion and empathy. They concluded that understanding the brain mechanism governing empathy could inform treatment of brain injury and autism. When applied to therapy with children with ASDs, labeling and mirroring feelings may help them to develop or increase their capacity for empathy.

Prescriptive Play Therapy

Charles Schaefer (2003) defined prescriptive play therapy as

> incorporat[ing] the theories and techniques of many psychotherapists into a broad framework that facilitates the development of client-specific treatment strategies. The goal of the play therapist is to construct an individualized treatment plan that matches the client's needs and situation and thus is likely to maximize therapeutic gain. (p. 306)

A prescriptive approach to play therapy is fitting for a child with an ASD for many reasons. First, these children range from those of lower intellect to those of very high intellect. It is practical to tailor treatment to the child's own manner of relating out of respect and value for that child. A child of higher intellect may prefer to engage in a game of strategy such as chess, rather than spend time in the playroom. Second, the child may need more structure from therapy than the nondirective approaches to play therapy provide. He may even be overstimulated in a play therapy room. It is the therapist's responsibility to provide a safe place in therapy, which for the child with an ASD may well be a directive, structured approach. Third, parents who seek our help often do so after much time and effort attempting to help their child through other means. Although other approaches may benefit the child, it is our responsibility to provide the most efficient treatment possible where there is one available. Fourth, and most relevant to our discussion here, children with an ASD often have obsessions. These obsessions are often about a popular cartoon character or movie superhero. What better way to engage a child than using his or her own favorite friend to meet treatment goals? As Wolfberg (1999) stated, "fascinations can be vehicles for socially interactive and imaginative play" (p. 52). In summary,

> A prescriptive approach to play therapy challenges the clinician to weave together a variety of interventions in formulating one comprehensive treatment program that is tailor-made for a particular child. ... The most important issues relate to the child's needs and ability to use and benefit from the approach or technique. (Schaefer, 2003, pp. xi–xiii)

Therapeutic Factor	Beneficial Outcome
Overcoming resistance	Working alliance
Communication	Understanding
Competence	Self-esteem
Role play	Practice/acquire new behaviors, empathy

Schaefer (1993) delineated 14 therapeutic factors of play in his book *The Therapeutic Powers of Play*. Outlined now are some of the factors and their outcomes relevant to the case illustration that follows:

As we will see in the case of Jason that follows, play therapy can help clients to develop socially and emotionally. A strong therapeutic alliance was formed and understanding was conveyed through the use of Jason's own preferred character of Superman. Jason was able to practice friendship through role-play while gaining competency through the safety of play therapy. To protect confidentiality, the case of Jason is a composite of several in which superheroes were used in play therapy with children on the autism spectrum.

CASE STUDY

Reason for Referral and Presenting Problem

Jason was referred for play therapy by his pediatrician at the request of his mother. He had been having trouble getting along with his peers at school, had low frustration tolerance, and was increasingly aggressive. He was also enuretic and encopretic.

Psychosocial, Developmental, and Medical History

Jason was a 5-year, 7-month-old boy, the younger of two siblings of professional parents in an intact family; his brother was 4 years older than he was. At intake, his parents described Jason as perceptive, helpful, and intelligent with a very good memory. They also described him as being difficult to motivate, angry, competitive, oppositional, and impatient.

The parents reported two things about Jason that they found unusual. Ever since they could remember, Jason had resisted baths, often screaming while bathing. The parents were also concerned about Jason's eating habits. He had always been a picky eater but recently had begun refusing anything but French fries. The time he took to eat an order of fries was inordinately long because he chewed them very slowly.

Family history was positive for depression and anxiety. Developmental history revealed pregnancy and birth to be unremarkable. Developmental milestones were all within normal range or early. Jason walked at 9.5 months and had begun to read at about 4 years old. His mother reported that Jason did not sleep through the night consistently until about 13 months of age. Medical history was positive for chronic ear infections beginning at 6 months until tubes were placed at 15 months.

Jason's play history revealed that he favored trains and trucks, sometimes liking to take them apart. Jason reportedly did not like losing games, so his parents avoided playing them. He mostly played alone or with his brother. No peer relationships were noted.

Case Conceptualization and Treatment Plan

Jason's presenting problems of aggression and poor peer interaction, along with his play behaviors of taking apart toys and difficulty losing, led me to consider an ASD. I also wondered about sensory integration issues because of his odd strong reaction to water and his odd eating habits. His parents and I set initial goals for treatment to reduce Jason's aggression and improve his social skills.

Jason's Treatment

Jason was looking at the children's books on the bookcase in the waiting room when I greeted him. "Hi Jason, I'm Patty," I said as I knelt down to greet him. He turned and ran by me into the counseling room as his mother laughed and I proceeded after him. Jason was quickly occupied with the various "fidget gadgets" in the counseling room, seemingly absorbed with everything. My initial impression was that it did not matter to him whether I was there or not. "You're finding some things to look at," I said. Jason did not respond. I decided to wait while Jason explored, not wanting to intrude in his space and hoping he would feel more comfortable that way. I quietly wondered to myself how long it might take him to make contact.

After a few more minutes of exploring and not responding, Jason picked up the small expandable ball, making it larger and then collapsing it. At this, he turned to me, made eye contact, and said, "You know the sun is in the middle of the Earth and the planets rotate around?" Somewhat surprised at Jason's comment, I replied, "It sounds like you know all about that." Jason nodded. He then proceeded to tell me all the correct names of the planets, while rhythmically expanding and collapsing the ball. "You're proud that you know all of them," I reflected. "Yep," Jason said, smiling sheepishly. "I'd like to find out what else you know, Jason, would that be okay?" "Sure, Miss Patty." Again, I was surprised at the interaction of this little boy who seemingly did not know I was in the room just moments before.

Jason proceeded to respond easily to my requests, singing his ABCs loudly (I remembered his mother indicating at intake that Jason loved to sing loudly in the church choir); counting as high as he could (again I was surprised when Jason counted 1 to 50 at his young age, without missing a number); and labeling various feelings. I learned how Jason missed his cat that had died 2 years earlier and about his love of trains, especially Thomas the Train. Jason seemed to have a love of knowledge and loved to talk about what he knew. In play therapy, however, Jason would act very differently.

Jason's first few sessions in the play therapy room were very quiet and long. Entering the room that first session, he stood motionless, appearing frozen just inside the door. Moving only his eyes around the room, he seemed to wonder what to do or why he was there. He tentatively moved toward the vehicles. He again seemed to disregard my presence in the room or any reflections I made as he got down on the floor to explore the trucks and the train. Soon he was intently focused on the wheels of the trucks and the other vehicles in the play therapy room. This play continued for several sessions. In these moments, he would lie on his stomach on the floor, face turned to the side with his cheek on the floor, intently watching the movement of the wheels on whatever vehicle he was investigating at that moment. It seemed no contact could be made with him at these times. I had no way of knowing if any of my tracking comments made any difference to him or even if he heard me. I continued to practice child-centered play therapy with Jason for several more weeks.

During the seventh therapy session, Jason's play changed. He noticed a red cape for the first time. Jason put it around his shoulders, quietly asking if I would tie it for him. When I had done so, he looked into the mirror at his reflection and announced, "Superman." Excited at the prospect of this interesting change in Jason's play, I reflected back, "You're Superman." At this, Jason began to role-play Superman for the remainder of the session.

The following week, I met with Jason's parents. They reported his behavior at school with peers remained the same, but there were fewer tantrums at home. When I inquired about any favorite characters of Jason's, his father exclaimed, "Oh, Superman, my gosh, he's *addicted* to Superman!" His parents went on to explain that Jason would watch the Superman movies repeatedly with his older brother. I scheduled Jason for the following week, wondering how I might enlist Superman's help.

Superman in the Playroom

Jason returned to play therapy that next week and immediately put on the red cape; I tied it for him. Again, he looked into the mirror and announced, "Superman" and began to reenact the movie he so loved. I reflected how powerful he was, being able to leap tall buildings or outrun trains. Why, he could do almost anything as long as he had the special red cape!

The following session I suggested to Jason that we try something new. Immediately I sensed his hesitation. Putting the red cape on him, I encouraged, "You could probably do almost anything wearing this cape." I asked him if any of his friends at school (knowing he did not have any) liked Superman as much as he did. He shrugged his shoulders. I replied, "I doubt that anyone knows as much about Superman as you do, Jason." He still looked skeptical. I suggested we take some time together and just talk about Superman so I could learn more about him. He seemed eager to try this. With that, we sat down at the table, and I "interviewed" Jason about Superman. I wanted to know where he came from, why he was here and what his special qualities were. Jason was an *encyclopedia* about Superman. We eventually moved to a discussion about Superman's personal qualities. We talked about "mild-mannered reporter" Clark Kent—how he was kind of different from other people and didn't quite fit in. That session talking about Superman was powerful for helping to strengthen our alliance. My understanding of Jason was communicated through the metaphor of Superman, so appropriate for him. I wondered to myself whether Jason felt like he was on a strange planet sometimes, not able to understand nonverbal communication. I wondered whether Jason's aggression was the "cape" he felt he needed to wear to defend against his own vulnerabilities in the face of his peers. Did Jason feel he could be annihilated with a small gesture or word, just as kryptonite could annihilate Superman?

The next few sessions with Jason were spent in role-play. I asked Superman Jason what character he wanted me to play as we reenacted Superman in play therapy. At times, Jason was rigid about how this play proceeded. Within this play, I commented on Clark Kent/Superman's social skills. "How polite of you to open the door for me, Clark!" "Clark, you're so nice!" Even when playing Lex Luthor, I would turn aside and comment to another "character" about how kind Superman was to fight for "Truth, Justice, and the American Way!" At times, Jason would snub my comments, rolling his eyes. Over time, however, he made fewer rejecting comments and seemed more able to hear and internalize the positive.

Eventually, I proposed we switch roles. "I'd like some practice being Superman," I said, pretending to be jealous. Jason complied. In one memorable session, Jason played villain Lex Luthor. As Superman, I apparently was being too forceful in battling my enemy. Jason suddenly stopped his play and said, "No, stop! Superman wouldn't *do* that, he's *nicer* than that! He'd let Lex win a little!" Hearing this, I wondered to myself whether this was just Jason not wanting to lose, or was this a "new and improved" Jason, who was learning to be less aggressive? As we continued to role-play, I commented on how hard it was to fight for justice and how easy it was just to be a nice guy. When we ended the session that day, I observed, "Superman is a Superfriend!" Jason smiled. The coming sessions would focus on this analogy.

Outside of treatment, Jason's parents reported a continued decrease in aggression and fewer negative reports from school. Jason was improving in his peer relationships and appeared to be developing more empathy. In therapy, Jason seemed more confident, and his Superman play was less rigid. I regularly used the term Superfriend throughout his therapy. I would ask Jason whether he had met any new Superfriends, or how was he being a Superfriend to others. We would quiz each other on how to be a Superfriend. At the end of one session, Jason asked if he could hold my hand on the way to the waiting room saying, "That's another way to be a Superfriend!"

In the last three sessions, we used small figures to set up problem-solving scenarios which we then played out. My Superman-turned-Superfriend figurine was ever-present as the role model who was always socially appropriate and kind. By emphasizing these characteristics in Jason's favorite superhero, he continued to internalize these behaviors. In one session, I suggested we pretend that Jason was Superman as we played out a peer scenario. Once again, Superman Jason responded appropriately, demonstrating his newfound social skills.

At the end of therapy, I took a Polaroid of Jason in the red cape and of my Superman-turned-Superfriend figurine to take with him. I wanted him to have a concrete reminder of his hard work and be able to look at the pictures to remind him of how he had become a Superfriend.

CONCLUSION

Superheroes have empowered children of all ages for decades. Most of us likely have fond childhood memories involving a superhero. They are universal and everlasting. Their magic speaks to our very core. For working mothers, certainly the Wonder Woman metaphor rings true. Who among us hasn't wished for superpowers to face some life obstacle? As a young girl, I vividly remember attempting to fly off the edge of the bathtub with the shower curtain draped around my shoulders! Alas, I could not fly, and I was soon discovered, along with the torn shower curtain.

Play therapists have the opportunity to embrace the various super-hero metaphors and integrate them into their work with troubled children. As we have seen in this chapter, superheroes can be uniquely applicable to play therapy with children on the autism spectrum. So many of these children have fixations related to superheroes. It is a small step to adopt them into treatment.

I continue to marvel at the wisdom of children. Deep inside, children know what they need and how to get there. They bring to therapy exactly the tools we as clinicians can use to help them. Superman, Spider-Man, Pokemon, Yu-Gi-Oh—they all come to therapy with their troubled pals. We need only to observe and facilitate the process. For Jason, the Super-man metaphor touched him deeply. By revealing this to me in his therapy, he became a Superfriend!

REFERENCES

Almond Board of California. (2006, February). Get your E. Retrieved February 12, 2006, from http://www.getyoure.org/

American Psychiatric Association. (1980). *Diagnostic and statistical manual of mental disorders* (3rd ed.). Washington, DC.

American Psychiatric Association. (1994). *Diagnostic and statistical manual of mental disorders* (4th ed., text revision). Washington, DC.

Attwood, T. (1998). *Asperger's syndrome: A guide for parents and professionals.* Philadelphia: Jessica Kingsley.

Autism Society of America. (2003). *Facts and statistics.* Retrieved February 11, 2006, from http://www.autism-society.org/site/PageServer?pagename= FactsStats

Autism Society of America. (2006). *Defining autism.* Retrieved February 11, 2006, from http://www.autism-society.org/site/PageServer?pagename= WhatisAutism

Axline, V. (1969). *Play therapy.* New York: Ballantine.

Baron-Cohen, S. (1995). *Mindblindness: An essay on autism and theory of mind.* Cambridge, MA: MIT Press.

Bettelheim, B. (1967). *The empty fortress: Infantile autism and the birth of the self.* New York: Free Press.

Beyer, J., & Gammeltoft, L. (2000). *Autism and play.* Philadelphia: Jessica Kingsley.

Bligh, S. (1995, Fall). What's in a name? *American Hyperlexia Association Newsletter.* Retrieved July 11, 2003, from http://www.hyperlexia.org/aha_labels.html

Bondy, A., & Frost, L. (2001). The picture exchange communication system. *Behavior Modification, 25,* 725–744.

Bravobrands.com. (2006, February). *Slammers® Ultimate Milk Shakes*. Retrieved February 12, 2006, from http://www.bravobrands.com/prdct_marvel.html

Bromfield, R. (1996). Psychoanalytic play therapy with a high-functioning autistic child. In G. Landreth, L. Homeyer, G. Glover, & D. Sweeney, D. (Eds.), *Play therapy interventions with children's problems*. Northvale, NJ: Jason Aronson.

Butler, R., Chomsky, M., Daniels, M., & Wallerstein, H. (Directors). (1966). *Star trek* [Television series]. United States: Desilu Production.

California Department of Developmental Services. (2003, April). *Autistic spectrum disorders: Changes in the California caseload. An update: 1999 through 2002*. Retrieved July 1, 2003, from http://www.dds.ca.gov/Autism/Autism_main.cfm

Centers for Disease Control and Prevention. (2005, February). *How common are autism spectrum disorders (ASDs)?* Retrieved February 11, 2006, from http://www.cdc.gov/ncbddd/autism/asd_common.htm

Davis, J. (2003). *Mimicking emotions creates empathy*. Retrieved April 8, 2003, from http://my.webmd.com/content/Article/63/72025.htm

Gray, C. (1995). Teaching children with autism to "read" social situations. In K. Quill (Ed.), *Teaching children with Autism: Strategies to enhance communication and socialization*. Albany, NY: Delmar.

Gray, C. (2000). *The new social story book*. Arlington, TX: Future Horizons.

Grayson, D. (2006, January). Superman is weak! In *Superman Secret Files and Origins 2005* (pp. 3–24). New York: DC Comics.

Greenspan, S., & Wieder, S. (1998). *The child with special needs: Encouraging intellectual and emotional growth*. Reading, MA: Addison Wesley Longman.

Greenspan, S., & Wieder, S. (2000). A developmental approach to difficulties in relating and communicating in Autism spectrum disorders and related syndromes. In A. M. Wetherby & B. M. Prizant (Eds.), *Autism spectrum disorders: A transactional developmental perspective* (Volume 9, Communication and Language Intervention Series). Baltimore: Brookes.

Hollander, E., Cartwright, C., Wong, C., DeCaria, C., DelGiudice-Asch, G., Buchsbaum, M., & Aronowitz, B. (1998). A dimensional approach to the Autism spectrum. *CNS Spectrum 3*, 22–39.

Kanner, L. (1943). Autistic disturbances of affective content. *Nervous Child, 2*, 217–250.

Landreth, G. (1991). *Play therapy: The art of the relationship*. Bristol, PA: Accelerated Development.

Lanyado, M. (1996). Treating autism with psychoanalytic play therapy. In G. Landreth, L. Homeyer, G. Glover, & D. Sweeney (Eds.), *Play therapy interventions with children's problems*. Northvale, NJ: Jason Aronson.

Lasseter, J. (Director). (1995). *Toy story* [Motion picture]. United States: Walt Disney Pictures.

Levy, S. (1988). *Identifying high functioning children with autism*. Indianapolis: Indiana Resource Center for Autism.

Maleskey, G., & McCommons, J. (1999). *Parkinson's disease*. Nature's medicines.

Retrieved February 12, 2006, from http://www.mothernature.com/Library/
Bookshelf/Books/23/121.cfm

Mittledorf, W., Hendricks, S., & Landreth, G. (2001). Play therapy with autistic
children. In G. Landreth (Ed.), *Innovations in play therapy: Issues, process,
and Special Populations* (pp. 257–269). Philadelphia: Taylor & Francis.

Mundy, P., & Stella, J. (2000). Joint attention, social orienting, and nonverbal
communication in autism. In A. M. Wetherby & B. M. Prizant (Eds.), *Autism
spectrum disorders: A transactional developmental perspective* (Vol. 9, Communication and Language Intervention Series). Baltimore: Brookes.

O'Neil, J. (1999, April 6). A syndrome with a mix of skills and deficits. *New York
Times Science*, p. 1.

Ortiz, J. (2004, March 10). *Asperger's syndrome and autism spectrum disorders in
children and adolescents*. Workshop sponsored by Health Ed, Indianapolis,
IN.

Ozonoff, S., Dawson, G., & McPartland, J. (2002). *A parent's guide to Asperger
syndrome and high-functioning autism*. New York: Guilford Press.

Piaget, J. (1962). *Play, dreams, and imitation in childhood*. New York: Norton.

Prizant, B., Wetherby, A., & Rydell, P. (2000). Communication intervention issues for children with autism spectrum disorders. In A. M. Wetherby & B.
M. Prizant (Eds.), *Autism spectrum disorders: A transactional developmental perspective* (Vol. 9, Communication and Language Intervention Series).
Baltimore: Brookes.

Rapin, I. (1998). Progress in the neurobiology of autism. *CNS Spectrum, 3*, 50–57.

Rimland, B. (1964). *Infantile autism: The syndrome and its implications for a
neural theory of behavior*. New York: Appleton-Century-Crofts.

Rutter, M., & Schopler, E. (1992). Classification of pervasive developmental disorders: some concepts and practical considerations. *Journal of Autism and
Developmental Disorders, 22*, 459–482.

Sacks, O. (1995). *An anthropologist on Mars: Seven paradoxical tales*. New York:
Plenum.

Schaefer, C. (1993). *The therapeutic powers of play*. Northvale, NJ: Aronson.

Schaefer, C. (2003). Prescriptive play therapy. In C. Schaefer (Ed.), *Foundations
of play therapy*. Hoboken, NJ: Wiley.

Schuler, A., & Wolfberg, P. (2000). Promoting peer play and socialization: The art
of scaffolding. In A. M. Wetherby & B. M. Prizant (Eds.), *Autism spectrum
disorders: A transactional developmental perspective* (Vol. 9, Communication and Language Intervention Series). Baltimore: Brookes.

Stanton, A., & Unkrich, L. (2003). *Finding Nemo* [Motion picture]. United States:
Pixar Animation Studios.

Twachtman-Cullen, D. (2000). More able children with autism spectrum disorders: Sociocommunicative challenges and guidelines for enhancing abilities.
In A. M. Wetherby & B. M. Prizant (Eds.), *Autism spectrum disorders: A
transactional developmental perspective* (Vol. 9, Communication and Language Intervention Series). Baltimore: Brookes.

Vygotsky, L. (1978). *Mind in society: The development of higher psychological
processes*. Cambridge, MA: Harvard University Press.

White, G. (2005, October). *Vitamin C and bioflavonoids: The Batman and Robin of eye health.* Retrieved February 5, 2006, from http://www.allaboutvision.com/nutrition/vitamin_c.htm

Widiger, T. A., & Samuel, D. B. (2005). Diagnostic categories or dimensions? A question for the *Diagnostic and Statistical Manual of Mental Disorders—Fifth Edition. Journal of Abnormal Psychology, 114,* 494–504.

Winnicott, D. W. (1971). *Playing and reality.* New York: Routledge.

Wolfberg, P. (1999). *Play and imagination in children with autism.* New York: Teachers College Press.

Yarnell, P. (2000, November–December). Current interventions in autism—a brief analysis. *Advocate.* Retrieved February 21, 2006, from http://www.unc.edu/~cory/autism-info/autitrea.html

CHAPTER TEN

Superheroes in Play Therapy With an Attachment Disordered Child

Carmela Wenger

My clinical population is diverse. I work with toddlers, preschoolers, school-age children, adolescents, and adults. Among the children I treat, presenting problems include triangulation in the midst of acrimonious divorce, adjustment to an adoptive placement, coping with a life-threatening or terminal illness, attempting to adapt to the mental illness of a parent, recovering from physical and sexual abuse, and witnessing severe and occasionally lethal family violence. Irrespective of the presenting problem, these clients, particularly the young ones, have experienced significant threats to the security of their attachments.

Invariably, the nature of these children's circumstances has brought them in direct contact with the Child Welfare System. In my own experience, the greatest challenge has been dealing with its various factions and representatives including judges and magistrates, child advocates, attorneys, and parents. As I have attempted to understand and contend with the very powerful and contentious forces that seem intent on defeating each other, I have come to recognize that it is the children who are so often forgotten. In the course of this work, I have experienced emotional challenges similar to those of my young clients and have often imagined a superhero coming to my rescue.

Themes of good and evil are played out as professionals with strongly held convictions about whether children should be returned to their birth parents, demonize, and devalue each other. These "heroes" take up all of the energy, delegating the true victims—the children, to the role of helpless bystander. This is parallel to the unfolding relationship that I attempt to develop with the children, who are often retraumatized by the legal and child welfare systems.

In a sense, these children and I embark on a hero's journey. In this context, I have to differentiate from the overall system in order to focus on my client. I must avoid the therapeutic trap of overidentifying with my client and crusading against, rather than collaborating with, the system, the birth parents, the foster parents, and the child advocacy attorney. My client's task is to find her own inner hero to heal—my role is to be an ally on that journey.

When a child is referred to me, the first crucial intervention I make is to offer a corrective experience. From the developmental–neuroscientific perspective, corrective experiences create new circuitry in the brain, which in turn, contributes to behavior change. In the safety of the therapeutic space, the child, not the child welfare system or the agenda of its agents is the focus of my attention. The client is neither used to meet my needs nor is he evaluated for a third party. My only goal is to understand this child's view of the world, his coping strategies, and his defenses. I define my role clearly as a therapist rather than as an evaluator. As the American Professional Society on the Abuse of Children recommends, I maintain a strong boundary between the role of evaluator and the role of therapist (Deaton & Carsel, 1995). In the context of this role, the incorporation of and role-playing around a superhero theme, can assist a trauma survivor in experiencing thoughts and feelings contrary to and corrective of the impact of victimization. A sense of mastery replaces feelings of helplessness.

As a developmentally oriented clinician, my first task is the establishment of a relationship that mirrors as closely as possible the characteristics of a secure attachment. My goal is the search for and consolidation of the child's true self. I want to be responsive to the child, so that I can begin to establish a secure base from which my client will be able to explore his or her struggles and past trauma. With me as a secure base, my client can risk new behaviors, make important disclosures, and resolve trauma. They can reclaim their stolen childhoods.

THE ROLE OF NEUROSCIENCE

In my work with parents who must engage in interactive regulation activities with their children who are traumatized and have attachment disorders, an understanding of brain development has been an invaluable aid to treatment. Principles of neuroscience have also been helpful in soothing these vicariously traumatized parents, particularly those who are afraid that their children's histories have caused irreversible behavioral and emotional damage.

When parents better understand that the brain is organized hierarchically and is a social organ and therefore develops as a direct result of experience, they more fully comprehend the importance of incorporating touch, affect, and sensation into interactions with their children. This developmentally oriented play becomes important in helping to rebuild the connections to their children that have been compromised by abuse and neglect. These parents become better equipped to understand the relationship between trauma, the brain, and behavior, the result of which is deeper empathy and capacity to nurture these most challenging children.

Superheroes and Neuroscience

For clinical interventions to be most effective, particularly when applied to young clients with attachment disorders, they must be developmentally appropriate (James, 1989; Shelby, 2004). Trauma changes the brain and corrective parental and therapeutic experiences can undo the harm inflicted by trauma (Perry, 2005). Developmental science is clear about the remarkable plasticity and responsiveness of the developing brain to enriched interpersonal environments (Schore, 2003). Superheroes can be part of that enriching environment because they appeal to the limbic system due to their strong visual and emotional stimulus value. It is the limbic system that appraises facial expression, posture, tone of voice, and tempo of movement. Superheroes are rich in all of these cues. The relaying of sensory information to the limbic system allows incoming information about the social environment to trigger adjustments in emotional and motivational states, which in turn guide action (Schore, 2003). This can occur either by autoregulation or by relying on others for interactive regulation. That interaction begins between the child and the toys within the playroom, attaches to the child–therapist relationship, and finally expands to include the parents or caretakers.

In addition to the power of the superhero fantasy to contribute to the corrective experience, the dramatic self-presentation inherent in the superhero's costume functions much like the mother's face. In this context, the costume is associated with positive feelings as well as the promise of hope, rescue, safety, and trust. Equally important, the superhero's visual impact arouses strong emotion, which can evoke affect and contribute to self-regulation. During affective displays, different centers of the brain are engaged and the child is poised to make associations, to integrate past with present experiences as well as action, feeling and thought—the basis of healing from trauma.

As we observe the child confront his or her enemies through the vehicle of the superhero, we better understand the his perception of relationships. As we watch the child use the superhero to help others, we can develop hypothesis regarding the perception of the trauma they are attempting to heal from. As we observe the superhero balancing power and vulnerability, we can appreciate the child's level of fear-and his efforts to overcome it. Only after we can fully understand the child's "map" of the world, can we formulate a treatment plan.

From the perspective of neuroscience, the attractiveness of the superhero also speaks to his lack of integration. Self-doubt, fear, self-loathing, anxiety, and unmet dependency needs are all split off. To the extent that superheroes are invincible, they have no need to self-regulate. Without fear or anxiety, self-soothing, and relating become unnecessary. Their sense of mission becomes isolation.

It is in the early stages of treatment that my clients with attachment disorders more readily use superheroes. As these children accept dependency needs, risk expressing them, and redefine power, superheroes transform from loners into leaders, and then into friends. As I assumed the role of a superhero with one of my young clients, I proclaimed, "I have fear. I'm just the boss of it!" I was attempting to model self-regulation and integration, rather than invincibility.

THE THERAPEUTIC APPEAL OF SUPERHEROES TO THE CHILD WITH ATTACHMENT DISORDER

Often children who have been victimized and subordinated to the will of others have not had little opportunity to develop a "true self." These children seem to implicitly understand the notion of a "secret identity." One child I worked with described this dichotomy as "my inside self and my outside self." Of the people in her environment who had manipulated and scared her, she said to me, "It's scary when people's outsides don't match their insides." Such a situation makes effective communication between the child and those around her impossible because she can no more accurately read cues than the adult can send them. As a result of this miscommunication, the capacity for relationship building becomes severely impaired. Affect must be engaged for repairs in this area of development to be made, and the superhero can be an effective vehicle for affective engagement with the child, as well as between the child and adults.

In a similar manner, a superhero's external persona, appearance, and characteristics do not match his internal, or alter persona. This is typical of many of my clients with attachment disorders who have developed a false outer, or social self in order to survive neglect and abuse. These children also identify with particular elements of superhero stories, as well as with aspects of their powers or elements of their secret identity. Children who have been wounded by adults, long for a nurturing and competent care taker. This longing can be split off, hated, or openly expressed. I recall one little girl who cried as I made a comment about how lonely she had been. As she wiped at her tears she told me, "My eyes are leaking." Her mechanistic interpretation symbolized the detachment she experienced from her own affect. This little girl had no experience of nurturing. Unlike the incompetent and unavailable adults in their lives, superheroes arrive when they are needed and know exactly what to do. Unlike their battered mother, a female superhero is invincible. Unlike their drug-addicted caretaker or parent, the superhero is always alert and responsive. The child can experience the safety of being in the hands of an all-powerful, responsive adult who is always good. Unlike the wounded and quixotic parent, superheroes are predictable. Additionally, the fact that superheroes are magical and mythical allows the child to identify with and perhaps incorporate defenses he or she needs against his or her own vulnerability.

Attachment disordered and traumatized children share a fear of vulnerability. They associate it with danger and conceal it beneath a façade of invincibility and fantasies of omnipotence. The superhero's power is associated with protection, competence, and mastery.

Another unique aspect of the superhero myth is that, in many cases, superheroes have decided to channel their anger or need for revenge into good deeds. As a result of this choice, they have earned the respect and admiration of society. Batman and Spider-Man, although isolated from society, are compensated with admiration and emulation. The drama in their lives overshadows the lack of a family life. In fact, it is the repudiation of this normal human need that adds to their heroism. Insofar as they choose this life, they have power that is typically denied the child who lives in the foster care system, or who is torn from her/his family of origin by that family's failures. In fantasy play with superheroes such as Batman or Spider-Man, the foster child with an attachment disorder can defensively exclude his secret need for affiliation and nurturing and instead be a hero rather than a scapegoat or a reject. Like the hero with the secret identity, the child can split off needs he associates with pain. In his play the victims have all of the pain and the superhero has all of the resources.

Unique to superheroes is the notion of transformation, an additional characteristic that can assist the attachment disordered child. The fact that Spider-Man and Batman acquired their powers through their own efforts facilitates their usefulness. Likewise, Luke and Leah Skywalker of the Star Wars series have inherited something positive from their father—his ability to tap into the Force, which they use for serving others. In the end of the second trilogy, Luke transforms his father. I have not yet seen a child who did not wish to be able to transform his or her parent. One little girl whose father was in prison and whose mother was a prostitute, expressing her anger at the police because they couldn't "make her (child's mother) be good." Repeatedly, I have witnessed children devise strategies in their play to change a bad character into a good character. So many of these children perceive themselves as being bad. The belief in transformation is critical to maintaining hope for personal redemption. They must be able to see "a self different from the one reflected in the family mirror" (Rubin, 1996). Identifying with a superhero or part of a superhero facilitates this process.

Last, but perhaps most important, is the quality of resiliency that is displayed by characters such as Batman, Spider-Man, Princess Leia, and Luke Skywalker. Rubin (1996), in her discussion of the "transcendent child" identifies three characteristics of this population. These include disidentifying with toxic people, seeing beyond their own victimization and social relatedness. Superheroes engage in all of these behaviors. Like Rubin's transcendent child, they have a sense of mission—a commitment to something larger than themselves. The very fact of a child's attraction to a superhero bodes well for his or her prognosis. It speaks to the child's capacity for transcendence.

AN ORIENTATION TO TREATMENT

A developmental orientation begins with an assessment of the quality of a child's attachment to his or her caretakers. Because attachment is important to cognitive, affective, social, and moral development, impediments may reduce a child's resilience to stress, negatively affect self-regulation, and restrict or prevent the formation of attachment behaviors. Similar to human development, a clinical case is conceptualized in stages. If treatment proceeds toward healthy development, it begins with the formation of a therapeutic alliance built on a foundation of trust. As trust continues to grow and consolidate, the child's issues emerge and play themes change to reflect the appearance of new issues. In addition, more adaptive coping strategies evolve to replace dysfunctional patterns of emotion, thought, and behavior. Risks are taken. For traumatized children, hypervigilance decreases and exploratory play takes its place. Children in treatment begin to display a wider range of affect and previously split-off or hated aspects of the self, such as vulnerability and dependency, appear.

As assessment evolves into treatment, the child's map of the world emerges, and is transformed. With Damien, the child who will be described in the case study that follows, a treatment priority was to focus on his inner working model of the world as well as his mother's inner working model of him. It became important to provide corrective experiences to address the developmental deficiencies that stemmed from Damien's early history of abuse and neglect. "The brain's development is an experience dependent process, in which experience activates certain pathways in the brain, strengthening existing connections and creating new ones" (Siegel, 1999, p. 12). In order to create new connections, I needed to "replicate the healthy parent infant relationship by imitating the active, engaging, playful, and nurturing ways in which parents interact with their young children" (Jernberg & Booth, 2001, p. 33). I also had to evoke affect because "emotion serves as a central organizing process within the brain." (Siegel, 1999, p. 7). My approach to treatment in the first phase is nondirective. As therapy progresses, I become more directive, always making interventions or interpretations within the role the child has assigned to me.

CASE STUDY

Damien was diagnosed with reactive attachment disorder. His adoptive parents, Mary and John, made the initial contact after obtaining my name from Child Welfare Services. When I first met Damien, he was 5 years old, and he had been in his adoptive home for a year. I worked weekly with him and his family for a little over 2 years. Born the middle child of three, Damien was abused from infancy by his biological father, who both held his head under water and shook him violently when he cried because he "liked the way the baby's cry changed." The father would not validate what Damien had said about having hurt his penis. The biological family saw Damien as "messed up." Of his father, Damien told me, "He shooked me a lot . . . he throwed us in bed . . . we're not balls!" He complained to me, "I keep doing that feeling" (fear in the context of flash backs). Of life with his biological father, Damien reported, "I was scared living with him. He was the meanest to me. I hate the thing we're talking about." When I asked Damien to tell me the size of his anger, sadness, fear, and love, he said they were all the same size. Damien was filled with very strong emotions without the self-soothing skills he needed to manage them. Around this time, Damien drew a picture of his father shaking him (Figure 10.1).

After the sudden death of his biological mother when Damien was 4 years old, his father placed him and his siblings with relatives. Damien's response to this was anger. "We're not cats," he proclaimed. After

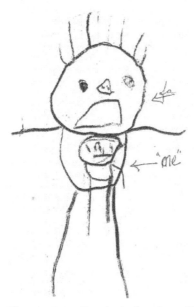

Figure 10.1   Damien's drawing of his father shaking him.

disruption in two of these placements, his grandparents' refusal to take the children, and the near drowning of his older brother, Damien was placed in foster care. When his current adoptive parents took Damien and his siblings into their home, they were informed by the state that he would probably need permanent institutional care because of a litany of disturbed behaviors. These behaviors included hiding food, pulling and scratching his penis until medical attention was required, resisting touch, tying himself up in his sheets, aggression toward his younger sister, sexualized behavior toward his mother, responding to authority with terror, violent play, and homicidal thoughts.

Treatment Planning Considerations

The focus of treatment was on improving the quality of interaction between Damien and his adoptive parents and siblings. To accomplish this goal, I needed to develop a therapeutic alliance with him and with his parents based on my own responsivity to their needs. To attune to Damien's parents, my first question was, "Which of Damien's behaviors are the hardest for you?" For the mother, it was Damien's rejection of her nurturing, his aggression, and his hurting his penis. For Damien, it was his intrusive memories. Attachment work addresses all of these. If Damien could feel secure and safe, he would be less intensely and less frequently triggered. His hypervigilance would be reduced, allowing him to take in positive and corrective experiences. Like all of the trauma survivors with whom I have worked, Damien's hypervigilance led him to attend almost exclusively to those cues in his environment, which he associated with danger. Positive experiences were often repressed from awareness because they were not relevant to personal safety. I also assumed that once he felt safe relying on adults, he would also stop hurting his penis. As the most vulnerable part of his anatomy, Damien's genitals were associated with vulnerability, which he hated to experience: "I hate what we're talking about."

I speculated that Damien's unintegrated trauma-related rage resulted in his self-destructive behavior. In this context, his parents questioned whether Damien's father had pulled on his penis as a punishment. I wondered whether at some level Damien knew that his birth mother's neglect was partly caused by her disappointment in Damien's gender. Significantly, the adoptive mother, Mary, had at one time confided that her original wish had been to adopt only Damien's sister. When she and her husband realized the traumatic consequences of that scenario, she changed her mind.

During the initial assessment phase, I saw Damien both individually and with his mother. Individual work with Damien was critical because his mother could not tolerate witnessing or participating in any violent play. Herself a witness to domestic violence as a child, she was terrified of the intensity of Damien's rage and was frightened by him. She was thus unable to soothe him when he needed it the most. Mary perceived Damien to be a highly complex child; she saw him as both a tragic victim and a predator. Interestingly, Damien's anxiety typically escalated in direct response to Mary's fear, creating a vicious circle. I also met with both parents at least monthly to focus on attachment games designed to encourage engagement appropriate to Damien's evolving tolerance for vulnerability and dependence.

Organization of Case Material

I have divided this case presentation into four parts, reflecting the phases of treatment—forming a therapeutic alliance, working through, consolidation–resolution, and termination (O'Dessie, 1997). It is important to consider that like development, the so-called stages of play therapy are neither fluid nor linear, bounded by observable and generalized change, rather than a passage of time. In the midst of therapeutic progress, relapse invariably occurs. As new issues emerge, children often regress. Furthermore, stages can overlap. For example, the formation of trust during the first stage is fragile and can be easily undermined or lost by failures in empathy or therapist absence or illness. The development, maintenance, and repair of trust is an ongoing process. The second stage consists of supplying corrective experiences, using the child's metaphor to address damages to development, introducing the concept of alternative behaviors, integrating split-off aspects of the self and replacing acting out with symbolic and controlled expressions of feelings and behavior. If there is success in the first two phases, the third phase is marked by the child beginning to risk new, more flexible and adaptive behaviors, as well as a broader range of affect. In this particular phase, I continued to build trust by accepting Damien's aggression, reflecting his feelings, and following his lead in play. The structure of sessions was predictable and consistent. I believed that fighting was the level of tactile contact that Damien could tolerate, and I therefore remained connected to him by honoring any means of self-expression he chose. The original neurological circuitry at the root of Damien's behavior problems was all encoded in the context of fighting for his survival in his birth family. As we fought, we were accessing that circuitry. During these fights, I consistently used affect language to describe his feelings and those of the character he assigned to me. This helped Damien to integrate information from his left and right brain, a crucial component in developing self-regulation and in the formation of an observing ego.

As I introduced a new concept, I carefully observed his responses to my words and changed or maintained my behavior accordingly (attunement). I did not depart from the role Damien assigned me, and I stayed with his power theme. When I introduced the issue of self-regulation in the face of frustration, I talked with Damien about making his "stand it muscle' stronger. I then checked with Damien regarding his resonance to the metaphor. The task of the fourth, or termination, phase is to say good-bye. With Damien, it was imperative that this process not duplicate the dynamics of prior losses. Collaboration and attuned planning ensured that the termination was therapeutic, rather than traumatic. Choices were agreed on, such as the number of remaining sessions, the length of time between them, and follow-up plans to meet with both Damien and the family. A transitional object—a Peter Pan figure—was chosen to give to Damien.

The First Stage of Therapy—Forming the Therapeutic Alliance

During the initial session, Damien's predominant play theme was danger and conflict between "bad guys and good guys"; he always assumed the role of good guy. As we engaged in sword fights, his affect was grim and his facial expression rigid. Any unexpected event in his life such as a chance encounter with his birth father in public or his adoptive father leaving town for a business trip, increased the intensity of his aggression, both at home and in session. In this first stage of treatment, Damien told me about "monsters under the bed that want people ... they want to kill them." Damien's hypervigilance was reflected in his constant concern that the bad guys would not stay dead, even after his repeated attempts to kill them in playroom. These "bad guys" were also very greedy, and typically depicted as Indians who "want all our stuff." Repeatedly, bad things, such as suffocation and car accidents, happened to the good guys.

In his second session, Damien incorporated my idea of an ambulance that could help the injured; however, he did not allow the policeman to protect his characters. Damien's crash scenes incorporated all of the vehicles in the playroom and expressed his intense feelings of vulnerability.

Luke Skywalker appeared for the first time during the fourth session. Damien chose the small rather than the large Luke figure as well as the small figure of Darth Vader, who was repeatedly vanquished. In the same session, Damien assigned to me the role of alligator and then fed me to Darth Maul. When I later reported on Damien's progress to his mother, she indicated that he had become more responsive during the attachment games that I had taught her.

During the latter part of this first stage, I coached Damien's mother in the basics of nondirective play therapy and asked that she attend attachment training. During her occasional visits into the playroom, we initiated a feeding activity. Her willingness to provide an emotional and physical space for Damien in her life indicated that she was beginning to recognize and develop the capacity to satisfy his needs. Paradoxically, she lost trust in me during the course of these training experiences due to concern that play therapy would not be enough to help Damien. As a result of her loss of trust, I spent considerable effort reassuring and soothing her, I had become a container for both mother and child. She subsequently reported renewed improvement.

Assessment and Treatment Planning Based on First Stage Progress

I concluded that Damien perceived the world as a dangerous place and as a result, had to be ever-vigilant for signs of danger. In the playroom, weapons were his only source of strength and protection. The inevitable fate of good guys made it clear that he did not place much faith in their ability to prevail. He could not yet trust others to protect him, and he felt powerless to manage his own rage and self-loathing. Damien's focus on dominance through violence mirrored what he had witnessed. On a hopeful note, Damien did occasionally allow victims to be rescued by ambulance. This mirrored his fantasies of being rescued from the abuse in his family of origin.

The appearance of a hero in Damien's fourth session, in conjunction with his mother's initial report of improved behavior, heralded early therapeutic progress and the beginning of the next stage of therapy. He was beginning to internalize enough nurturing to risk allowing the emergence of previously split-off dependency needs. Damien's play battles evolved from chaotic and generalized, with an emphasis on weapons and aggression, to fights between characters that personified his inner struggle. Although Damien identified with the damage Luke experienced at the hands of his father, he also represented the potential for healing and the controlled use of strength (the Force). Like Damien, Luke was permanently changed by his wounds, albeit for the better. I also assumed that Damien was attracted to Luke and his sister Leia because they, like him, had lost their mother. Luke's appearance in Damien's play also signaled movement toward considering relationships as a potential source of safety.

It was significant that I was given Darth Maul to eat. I assumed Darth Maul represented Damien's vengeful oral aggression and rage. Symbolically, he was giving me his rage and his badness to digest. Equally important, once eaten, Darth Maul was permanently gone. The elimination of Darth Maul was accomplished through an alliance between the crocodile (my role) and Damien. Again, Damien was using relationship to solve a problem. I complained I was hungry, and I got fed. Damien got rid of an enemy. Reciprocity, a key factor in relationship had emerged. Mary's continuing reports that Damien was more responsive during their therapeutic work at home validated that my role as bad guy altering Damien's map of the world.

Damien's sense of trust continued to grow. This was clear during the seventh session, when he disclosed the abuse he suffered at the hands of his biological father. Although Damien said that he "hated the thing we're talking about," he could nevertheless tell me what helped him to let love in (mommy) and what made it hard to let love in (being bad). He went on to explain to me, "I keep doing that feeling" (fear and intrusive thoughts). Damien's play fighting during that session consisted of my putting on a witch hat (at his direction) and him shooting me.

Damien's willingness to expose his vulnerability prompted an introduction of the subject of grieving; however, he did this simultaneously by recounting "mommy died." This synchronicity cemented my belief that we were about to enter the "working through" stage of treatment. I assumed that Damien's execution of the witch (me) expressed his anger at my role in bringing back a bad memory. This is always a delicate dance in the treatment of traumatized children. The risk of being perceived as a perpetrator is ongoing. Because I evoked the same feelings he associated with his maltreatment, Damien transferred the rage he felt toward his mother onto me. I also wondered if his growing attachment to and dependence on me scared him.

The Second Stage of Therapy—Working Through

Damien became very aggressive again after seeing his birth father. In the playroom, Luke and Han Solo repeatedly fought with Darth Maul who initially vanquished them but was in turn defeated. I assumed that Damien was working through painful feelings related to having been "throwed" by his father. In subsequent sessions, Damien fought against a dinosaur and an alligator; throwing and stomping them as I shouted at the monster to stay out of our lives. This play also came to represent Damien's metaphoric attempt to ward off intrusive thoughts, which we locked tightly into a "history box." This play was typically followed by the regressive and self-soothing activity of sucking on a bottle.

During the tenth session, Damien became very angry with me when after arriving early, he had to wait to see me. He fought with me, calling me "ugly, worthless, bad, and nasty." When I interpreted to him that he was mad at me because he had to wait, he agreed and settled down. Acting the role of victim, I then talked about how much I wanted friends so that I could be protected and cared for. Themes of family violence emerged. He repeatedly fought the "Beast" to protect Belle, stomping and throwing a menacing alligator. As he did this, I again told the alligator to stay out of our lives, and we put intrusive memories into a history box and closed the lid.

Damien began to spend less time fighting, expanding his play activities to include art and water. In a typical session during this phase, the theme of struggle and rescue predominated. All of the figures that he chose repeatedly sunk in the water table. When I introduced boats, he initially ignored them and only reluctantly included them, along with cars, to "save the people." As an example, Cat Woman appeared on a raft to offer assistance; however, Damien turned the tap on her, telling me, "She's going through it." Similarly, rescue boats, cars, and helicopters came to help, only to be turned away. Slowly, Damien began to experiment with the theme of floating.

Assessment and Treatment Planning Based on the Beginning of the Second Stage

During these sessions, Damien spoke to me in the same angry way his father had spoken to him. However, his ability to tolerate an interpretation of this behavior signaled to me that he was beginning to develop the capacity for self-reflection—an observing ego. He was beginning to connect behavior to feelings, and feelings to experience. Damien's regressive play clearly suggested that although he was anxious, he could ask for comfort and did not need to rely on rage as a defense against anxiety and vulnerability. His use of exploratory play during this phase also suggested tentative steps toward the development of security. Damien was beginning to feel safe enough with me to allow himself to be curious—a significant developmental accomplishment.

Middle Phase of the Second Stage of Therapy

During this portion of treatment, Damien introduced a "Princess of Power" into his play. She fought with swords that she referred to as "son," and it was through the use of these protective weapons that the bad guys were told not "to treat me that way." Although the Princess of Power was typically buried in a sandstorm, she was ultimately victorious. The Princess of Power play gave way to greater involvement with the art supplies, and Damien soon began to gravitate away from fighting and rescuing games. Instead, he began to enjoy creative artistic activities. He played games that had nothing to do with fighting, he drew, and he enjoyed making handprints. Damien's mother reported that at home, he was making eye contact, sharing his feelings, "molding to my body when we hug," and expressing concern for her welfare.

Assessment and Treatment Planning Based on the Previous Sessions

The appearance of powerful female figures demonstrated Damien's awareness of an alternative role for women to that of victim. It was intriguing to me that he named her sword "son." In wielding it, Damien seemed to be attempting to integrate the concepts of masculine–feminine and power–vulnerability. Within the home, Damien's mother created a "mad pad" for him on which they drew pictures, and he instructed her in what to write. This included drawings and a description of Damien's feelings about the abuse he had experienced. In addition to the nurturance-based attachment games that I had taught her earlier in treatment, she also enjoyed playing tug-of-war with him. Together, Damien and his parents engaged in "mirroring games" tailored to his ability to tolerate this level of intimate interaction. Mary would give Damien one minute to look at her and then ask him to close his eyes and attempt to describe such things as her clothing and hairstyle. She would then do the same with Damien. When he woke in the morning, she would say, "Did you change during the night, or are you still handsome, have brown hair, and have brown eyes?" In the context of this daily check-in, Damien's mother was certain to touch him by tracing his ears, his nose, and his mouth. In light of Damien's anxiety during aggressive play such as wrestling, his father played gently with him and role modeled appropriate physical contact with the mother. He also instructed Damien about how to take care of his penis.

Second Stage Crisis—Testing Behavior

Following the emergence of exploratory play, new play themes, and behaviors signaling more secure attachment, Damien and his brother announced that they were "running away" because they didn't "like the rules." Mary reported that during this incident, Damien slept in a nearby field during a rainstorm, without his coat. Another crisis quickly followed when Mary reported that Damien had committed a "sexual assault" on her. According to her, Damien, who was wearing a "demonic expression," put his hand down her blouse, and grabbed her breast and ignored her protests to stop.

In response to their running away, I suggested that Mary tell the boys that as opposed to being homeless cats, they were her "forever" children. Running away was not an option for solving problems, and they would work together as a family to solve their own. Damien cried and hugged her. Regarding the so-called sexual assault, I suggested to Mary that Damien was acting out what he had witnessed between his birth parents. I reminded her that Damien's play themes included the family violence that he had witnessed, and that his biological father had asserted power over his wife with violence. Damien's behavior, albeit inappropriate and disturbing to her, had simply reflected what he had earlier learned about intimacy. In a sense, Damien was staking his claim on Mary.

The Third Stage of Therapy—Consolidation of Therapeutic Gains

By the 22nd session, Damien expanded his repertoire of characters and created themes of transformation, such as Darth Maul becoming a good guy. As Prince Phillip killed dragons and serpents, he also gave them a heart. Peter Pan appeared more frequently in Damien's play, replacing Luke and other wounded figures. Damien also began integrating his masculine and feminine aspects by dressing up as Cinderella and later deciding that I would be her and that he would be the prince. Damien was most interested in the part of the story where Cinderella loses the slipper that is later found by the prince.

Around this time, Damien also began playing with the dollhouse, initially surrounding and filling it with soldiers. Although a huge, well-armed monster attacked the house, killing all of the protectors and attempting to destroy the roof, good ultimately triumphed. Following my suggestion, Damien offered flowers for those who had died in the battle. During this particular session, Damien reported a nightmare about being mean to his mother, being chased by guys, and being abandoned to them. Damien and I reenacted the nightmare, at the end of which he built a city—a transformation in its own right. Many of Damien's subsequent play themes involved threats from carnivorous animals or boys being eaten. I assumed this reflected his fear of annihilation, being destroyed by his own aggression, and being abandoned. I was able to use his drawing to address the relationship between his fear and his self-mutilating behavior.

It was at this point in Damien's treatment that, at his adoptive parents' request, Damien's biological father sent him a letter. I informed the biological father that we were not interested in prosecuting him and that together we would help Damien heal and have a successful adoption. In his letter, Damien's birth father stated that he was "sorry you got hurt" and explained that the "best thing I could do was give you a mother and father where you would be well cared for and safe." Following this letter, Damien gave colors to his feelings and was able to locate them in different parts of his body.

Assessment and Treatment Planning Based on the Previous Sessions

Damien's increased use of exploratory play and incorporation of a secure base suggested continued development of coping strategies. His movement away from aggressive characters to ones such as Cinderella indicated transformation through love, which mirrored his own experience. Something lost was restored—the motive for the search was now love, not rage or revenge. Peter Pan fought to protect the "lost boys." Through the role of Peter Pan, Damien was the little boy who lost his parents, and who in turn, created a family to protect other lost boys. For Damien, Peter was the brave and benevolent father figure whom he never had. The choice of Peter Pan also reflected Damien's wish to be rid of his intrusive memories as well as his rage and fear. Like Peter Pan who could fly out of Hook's reach, Damien was now out of the reach of his birth family. Damien was allowed to decide, if, when, where, and for how long he saw members of his family of origin. It was Captain Hook who lost a hand; Peter Pan was whole. It was Captain Hook who was vulnerable to the ever-lurking crocodile; Peter Pan was resilient, resourceful, and ultimately victorious. Interestingly, Damien's birth family feared the consequences of his disclosures. Perhaps Captain Hook represented the birth family as Damien currently saw them, with Captain Hook symbolizing Damien's vulnerability and aggression.

During this phase of treatment, the appearance of a king in Damien's play symbolized the development of executive functioning. Although not necessarily the most well-armed, the person in charge rules with wisdom and powerful observation skills. The king notices that some people are not what they seem and takes appropriate action. I suspected that Damien had consolidated his feeling of protection when Mary and John discontinued the visits with his extended birth family. Damien's willingness to place flowers on the graves of bad guys suggested that he was becoming more accepting of and compassionate toward his own unacceptable feelings—his shadow. Of equal importance, Damien may have been considering forgiveness. His birth father's letter reinforced Damien's growing understanding that it was his father's deficiencies rather than his own that caused the maltreatment, and it was his father's love that motivated placing his children for adoption. Themes of destruction followed by themes of building were symbolic of repair. Along with these transformative themes, Damien's mother reported that he was giving loving hugs, looking at her face, maintaining eye contact, and continuing to mold to her body during feeding activities.

The Fourth Stage of Therapy—Termination

During what were to be the last several sessions, Damien became increasingly playful as he engaged in a variety of play activities. His progress became even more evident following one particular playroom mishap. As he stood on a folding chair, it collapsed, hitting him in the diaphragm and knocking the breath out of him. As Damien lay on the floor, his face white and his eyes wide with fear, his mother and I rushed to his side. Mary was speechless as she held his hand. I told Damien that I knew it felt as if he were not getting enough air and that he was very scared because of that. In fact, we could tell that he was indeed getting enough air because his lips and skin were pink. We assured Damien that we would stay with him, and should he be unable to breathe, that we would help him with CPR. As he waited for the discomfort to pass, Damien was able to relax, and as soon as he felt better, he resumed his play. Damien expressed neither fear of retaliation nor anger over what had occurred.

Damien elected to have a party during our last session and chose both the time and the food. During that last session, I gave Damien the Peter Pan figure that we had played with and watched attentively as I put Peter's sword in a special place so that no one else could use it. We reminisced, and I told Damien that I would think about him on the date and time of his appointment and I would be available for phone calls, letters, or a follow-up appointment should he need it.

Outcome and Follow-Up

I met with Damien 15 months after his last session. He chose knights to fight against Godzilla who, along with a shark, was easily defeated. A friendly alligator gave us rides, while an initially threatening snake protected her eggs. Toward the end of the session, he transformed me from a villain into a "good-guy." Damien's parents reported that although still occasionally oppositional, he was also demonstrating healthier independence, connectedness, playfulness, and the ability to negotiate conflict resolution, both at home and at school. They were grateful that I had been was a calm and soothing teacher, who gave them skills and helped them to better understand Damien's strengths and potential.

At the next follow-up, when Damien was 9, his mother reported that he had become indifferent to visits with his paternal birth family and successfully continued to self-regulate both at home and at school. Around the time of that last visit, the family was remodeling their home, perhaps an externalization for the remodeling that had transpired within its walls. Around this time, Damien created a miniature city.

Reflections and Consideration of Parallel Process

The stages of play therapy with Damien paralleled the course of healthy development, moving from the establishment of trust to exploration, risk taking, and ultimately more mature levels of cognitive and affective processing. This process was evident in the progression of use of action figures—from the maimed survivor Luke Skywalker, to Peter Pan, Prince Phillip, and finally, the King. The very fact that he used a greater variety of figures and play media reflected resiliency and growth. Aggressive battles gave way to playful confrontations, and these battles took up less and less of both his inner and outer worlds. Damien's attachment to Peter Pan was rooted in his newly found and hard-won enjoyment of power and happiness.

The heroes and villains who populated Damien's early treatment had their parallel in the real-life characters in his life. From the outset, Damien's adoptive parents felt both threatened and undermined by the social worker, who believed that he was too damaged to survive in a family that already included his two traumatized siblings and his adoptive siblings. Subsequently, this social worker suggested placing Damien in a therapeutic foster home. When she also recommended that Damien have regular access to his birth parents, his adoptive parents worried that his growing sense of security would be undermined. It was clear from Damien's behavioral changes upon return from these visits that he was indeed being retraumatized. When he subsequently complained, "why do you make me be nice to the people who hurt me?" these visits were curtailed.

Even though this initial threat to Damien's early adoptive adjustment was resolved, parallel process continued. Just as he needed to learn to contain and appropriately express his rage, so, too, did his parents and I need to resolve our own strong emotional responses surrounding the visitations. My fantasy of transforming into a superhero and obliterating those who threatened Damien's well-being signaled both the risk of over-identifying with his revenge fantasies as well as our mutual wish for omnipotence. Assuming a rescuing stance would have clearly undermined the quality of the attachment and reattachment work that had to be done—Damien's parents were the rightful heroes. Relying on my treatment model, rather than Damien as my secure base, I could assure and soothe myself in the face of the emotional turmoil that permeated the treatment. In the language of neuroscience, I activated my frontal lobes so that my limbic system did not overpower my executive functioning.

REFERENCES

Deaton, W., & Carsel, J. (1995, Summer). Therapists out of court: Part I of II. *The Consultant*, 2–7.

James, B. (1989). *Treating traumatized children: New insights and creative interventions*. Toronto: Lexington Books.

Jernberg, A., & Booth, P. (2001). *Theraplay: Helping parents and children build better relationships through attachment-based play*. San Francisco: Jossey-Bass.

O'Dessie, J. O. (1997). *Play therapy: A comprehensive guide*. Northvale, NJ: Jason Aronson.

Perry, B. (2005). *How the brain develops: The importance of early childhood*. Arcata, CA: Humboldt State University.

Rubin, L. (1996). *The transcendant child: Tales of triumph over the past*. New York: Basic Books.

Schore, A. (2003). Experience dependent maturation of the regulatory system in the orbital-prefrontal cortex and in the origin of developmental psychopathology. In A. Schore (Ed.), *Affect dysregulation and disorders of self*. New York: Norton.

Shelby, J. (2004). *Developmentally sensitive post-traumatic play therapy*. Monterey, CA: Alliant International University.

Siegel, D. (1999). The developing mind: Toward a neurobiology of interpersonal experience. New York: Guilford Press.

CHAPTER ELEVEN

Luke, I Am Your Father! A Clinical Application of the Star Wars Adoption Narrative

Lawrence C. Rubin

"A long time ago, in a galaxy far, far away." As did those that preceded it, so begins the as yet unfinished latest installment in the Star Wars saga. Although penned by an 11-year-old, this particular episode will be no less epic in scope or mythic in its significance than those that came before. Just as in the original saga, there will be heroes and villains who fight glorious battles. Old regimes will fall to new alliances built on bonds of tenuous trust and security. There will be trials, tribulations, unfulfilled longing, and a poignant search for identity. This will be episode VII in the unfolding drama—not of Luke Skywalker, but of a boy who is adopted and who seeks to understand the circumstances of that adoption, who he is, and whom he is to become. To understand this particular boy who chose Star Wars as his therapeutic vehicle, we must first better understand Luke Skywalker, the character he directly identified with.

ADOPTION, SUPERHEROES, AND STAR WARS

Star Wars, beyond an entertaining high-tech, science fiction/fantasy, has been likened in its social, political, and religious scope and relevance to classical mythology (Campbell & Moyers, 1988; Geraghty, 2005;

Henderson, 1997; Lawrence & Jewett, 2002). According to Champlin (1992), "Lucas devoured the great [classical mythological] themes: epic struggles between good and evil, heroes and villains, magical princes and ogres, heroines and evil princesses, the transmission from fathers to sons of the powers of both good and evil" (p. 41). In addition to these grand mythic elements, Star Wars addresses, sometimes resolving but other times not, equally poignant societal issues including the clashing voices and actions of aggression and resistance, as well as between the will of the majority and the power of the minority. At a more individual level, protagonists, chief among whom are Luke Skywalker and his father, Anakin (aka Darth Vader), struggle with the very personal issues of redemption, loss, legacy, loyalty, and the importance of family. And in no small way does Star Wars address the issue of adoption and the search for personal identity in its aftermath.

In a volume centered on superheroes, Star Wars protagonist Luke Skywalker may appear oddly out of place. His name is not usually associated with the likes of Superman, Batman, and Wonder Woman. In many ways, his story more closely resembles the classical hero's journey (Campbell, 1949) than it does the typical American superhero myth. For the purposes of this discussion and the case that follows, however, the reader is asked to suspend the distinction between the (classical) hero and (modern) superhero and instead consider Luke Skywalker to be a member of both universes—a superhybrid, as similar to Superman, Batman, and Wonder Woman as he is to Moses, Hercules, and Ulysses. Lawrence and Jewett (2002) reminded us that

> The [American] monomythic superhero is distinguished by disguised origins, pure motivations, a redemptive task and extraordinary powers. He originates outside of the community he is called to save, and in those exceptional instances when he resides therein, the superhero plays the role of the idealistic loner. His identity is secret, either by virtue of his unknown origins or his alter ego: his motivation is a selfless zeal for justice. By elaborate conventions of restraint, his desire for revenge is purified. Patient in the face of provocations, he seeks nothing for himself and withstands all temptations. He renounces sexual fulfillment for the duration for the mission, and the purity of his motivation ensures his moral infallibility in judging persons and situations. When he is threatened by violent adversaries, he finds answers in vigilantism, restoring justice and thus lifting the siege of paradise. In order to accomplish this mission without incurring blame or causing undue injury to others, he requires superhuman powers. The superhero's aim is unerring, his fists irresistible, and his body incapable of suffering fatal injury. (p. 47)

True to this superheroic narrative, Luke Skywalker's birth is concealed from his father, as well as from the Empire. He is raised, as is often the case with superheroes, by those other than his biological parents. Luke is endowed with the (super)powers of telekinesis and strength by virtue of the Force that flows through him, which he uses to redeem his father and save society (the Federation). He continually, yet unswervingly, wrestles with internal conflicts that are inherent in the greater struggle between good and evil, often using his powers and vigilantism as means of defeating the Dark Side. Although his identity as a Jedi warrior is not a secret, per se, neither is it fully actualized and integrated until he saves his father at the end of the saga. Although he is part of what could be considered a superteam (along with Han Solo and Princess Leia), Luke forfeits the chance of romantic attachment; he is married to the job, so to speak. Last but not least, Luke's militaristic wardrobe, light saber included, is consistent with the image we have come to associate with superheroes.

Luke Skywalker's (super) heroic trajectory is clearly the primary textual element of the initial Star Wars trilogy (episodes IV–VI). Equally compelling; however, particularly as it relates to the case described later in this chapter, is the narrative surrounding his adoption and its aftermath. Luke, along with his twin sister (Princess) Leia Organa, are the children of Senator Padme Amidala and Anakin Skywalker, both of whom are embroiled in the battle between the Federation and the Empire for galactic control. After Padme's death during childbirth, the twins are separated for their own protection. Luke is subsequently raised by his aunt and uncle, and upon their death, he joins the Federation to fight the Empire, ultimately discovering that his arch enemy, Darth Vader, is really his biological father. Throughout his journey, Luke is guided by Obi-Wan Kenobi and Yoda, benevolent guardians who represent the "light side" of the Force. It is not until Luke resolves the conflicts in himself between good and evil, strength and weakness, and love and hate that he can reconcile with his father and become whole. Along the way, Luke discovers that Princess Leia is actually his sister, and in doing so, he reclaims his family, and thus his identity along the road to becoming a hero.

Interestingly, the narrative of Luke Skywalker's father Anakin, which forms the primary text of the second Star Wars trilogy (episodes I–III), is also rooted in early childhood loss, adoption, and its aftermath. Although we know that Anakin was raised (until age 6) by his mother, Shmi, the identity of his biological father is never revealed. Subtext suggests that his birth was, in a scientific rather than religious fashion, if not immaculate, then miraculous! Along his road to becoming an adult, Anakin is also mentored, at least initially, by benevolent caretakers, Qui-Gon Jinn and

Obi-Wan Kenobi. However, as the forces of good and evil fight for control of the galaxy (and his soul), Anakin's need for nurturance, confusion,
and ultimately anger are manipulated by the evil parent figure—Senator
Palpatine, aka Darth Sidious/the Emperor, and he is slowly yet irretriev-
ably lost to the Dark Side.

Clearly then, both father and son each struggle in many similar ways
to reconcile early losses, connect with meaningful parent substitutes and
actualize their destinies in the light of adoption, albeit one in the service
of good and the other in the service of evil.

It was earlier suggested that Luke Skywalker could be considered, if
not a superhero per se, a hero–superhero hybrid. He and his story share
many elements characteristic of both the classical (hero) and American
(superhero) mythological narrative. The element most relevant to this
chapter is the fact that both he and is father are adopted, although their
outcomes are very different. This particular element of Luke's narrative
joins him in yet another significant way to other traditional superheroes
of popular American culture.

Some of the most historically prominent superheroes are adopted.
The most well-known of these superadoptees is Superman, who as infant
Kal El, was sent to Earth by his parents Jor El and Lara as their home
planet of Krypton exploded. The superinfant was lovingly raised as Clark
Kent by adoptive parent Jonathan and Martha, who nurtured both his
mortal and his super soul as he experimented with his emerging godlike
powers. Peter Parker, son of murdered American spies Richard and Mary,
was adopted by his paternal uncle and his wife, Ben and May. After the life-
changing radioactive spider bite during adolescence, Peter's adventures as
Spider-Man and his perilous road to adulthood and identity began. Bruce
Wayne, son of Thomas and Martha, was orphaned following the brutal
murder of his parents. He would be pseudo-adopted and protected by the
loyal family butler, Alfred, while he honed his crime-fighting skills as the
vigilante Dark Knight known as Batman. And then there are the X-Men,
each as unique in their origins as in their mutant abilities. Ostracized
by society, each of them, including most prominently Wolverine, Storm,
Cyclops, and Rogue, are taken in and fostered by Professor Xavier in his
School for Gifted Youngsters.

An immense number of other superheroes have come and gone over
the years, and it is more than likely that many of them share in the adoption narrative with Superman, Spider-Man, Batman, the X-Men—and
Luke Skywalker. At this point, however, the discussion moves out of the
realm of the fantastic and fictional into the real-life impact and trajectory
of adoption. This discussion will be followed by the case of Alex, whose
identification with Luke Skywalker was therapeutically directed toward
working through issues related to his own adoption.

THE REALITY OF ADOPTION

Much has been written about adoption, from the deeply personal stories of adoptees, birth parents, and adoptive parents (the adoption triangle); to the clinical and empirical work of mental health professionals and social scientists respectively. The American adoption narrative has been influenced by the depictions in and interests of the mass media—sometimes for the better, other times for the worse. And the issues surrounding adoption have become part of the national discourse on the volatile associated topics of race, culture, genetics, and homosexuality. Yet regardless of the scope of adoption-related issues, the most powerful voice in the narrative is that of the adopted child (Ryan & Nalavany, 2003).

It has been estimated that since the late 1980s, close to 125,000 children are adopted annually, and of these, the percentage of domestic interracial and international placements has steadily risen (National Adoption Information Clearinghouse, 2004). Growing up in contemporary U.S. society is challenging, even in the best of circumstances; however, growing up adopted is, for many, doubly so. It is not that adopted children are maladjusted per se, for in actuality, empirical and meta-analytic studies have suggested that they are generally well adjusted (Smith & Brodzinsky, 2002). Certainly, too, nonadopted children experience a variety of disturbing events including illness, parental divorce, and abuse. Nevertheless, the challenge of mastering each of life's obstacles is compounded along the adopted child's developmental trajectory by the emerging reality and implications of their adoptive status. Two prominent themes emerge in the journey of the adopted child—the search for identity and loss. According to Brodzinsky, Schecter, and Henig (1992):

> The struggle to understand who you are, where you fit in and how you feel about yourself is universal; it is a unique part of being human. Adoptees go through the search for self in some unique characteristic ways and many of the differences [between them and nonadoptees] can be explained by the fact that adoption cuts off people from a part of themselves. To understand the psychology of adoption from the perspective of the adoptee is [also] to recognize and appreciate the unique role played by loss in the search for self. (p. 3)

So potentially profound is the loss associated with adoption that it has been referred to as a "primal wound" (Verrier, 1993). As the adoptee grows better able to cognitively appreciate loss, she comes to realize that no matter how wonderful it was to be "wanted" (by the adoptive parents), someone, somewhere, for whatever reason, "gave her away" (the birth parents). Loss becomes potentially fused to the adopted child's narrative and search for identity and self invariably becomes a search, in one form or another, either literal or figurative, for the birth parent. According to Verrier, "the search for self is a mission for many adoptees [and] seems to be intimately connected to the search for the birth-mother [or birth-father]" (p. 33). In addition, the unfolding narrative of loss in the child's life is compounded by the real, felt, or imagined losses experienced by the other members of the adoption triangle, the birth and adoptive parents.

The challenges of loss and the search for self are compounded in the cases of domestic interracial and transnational adoption. In each of these, the adopted child is reminded, typically by virtue of her appearance, that she came from another family, particularly in the case of non-White children adopted into white families. According to Pertman (2000), "children who look nothing like their parents [or extended families] are more deeply steeped in reminders that they are adopted" (p. 121). In addition to the dissimilarity in appearance with her adoptive parents, the transnational adoptee may experiences a "genealogical bewilderment," which is "the feeling of being cut off from your heritage, your religious background, your culture and your race" (Brodzinsky et al., 1992, p. 108). Importantly, and as in the case of adoption outcome research in general, there is little empirical support of the long-term adverse impact of interracial or transnational adoption (Brodzinsky, Smith, & Brodzinsky, 1998).

Regardless of the nature and circumstances of their adoption, research suggests that adoptees express curiosity about and search for their birth parents. It has been estimated that in countries that provide access to birth records (after the age of majority), "50% of adoptees initiate a search for their birth parents at some point in their lives" (Muller & Perry, 2001a, p.31). The search is more often for birth mothers than it is for birth fathers, has initially positive outcome, and typically follows a period of internal struggle over issues including identity and genealogy (Muller & Perry, 2001b). Although children in families more open to adoption-related communication freely ask questions about their origins, it is during late adolescence that the questions increase and early adulthood that adoptees more actively search for and contact their birth parents. As the following narrative suggest, adoptees do not have to leave the confines of their home to search for their birth parents or origins. Alex is one such adoptee, and he chose to work on his issues by exploring and expanding the Star Wars adoption narrative.

THE CASE OF ALEX

Alex, age 11, was seen over the course of several months in outpatient counseling by the author, who is a clinical psychologist and registered play therapist. The case was conceptualized from an Eriksonian–life-cycle perspective and the therapeutic approach, which is largely play oriented was client-centered. This orientation allowed the therapist to frame Alex's struggles in the context of Erikson's life cycle uniquely adapted to adoptees (Brodzinsky et al., 1992), providing leeway to express himself in any fashion and with any play media he saw fit.

Intake and Background

Alex's parents initiated counseling, indicating during the intake that he had been having difficulty adjusting socially and emotionally to his fifth-grade public school placement where there were reports of bullying. Previously an ostensibly happy and easygoing child, Alex had become more petulant both at home and at school, sensitive to criticism either real or perceived and prone to tantrums when he did not get his way. Of even greater concern, particularly to his mother, was that Alex had begun questioning the circumstances of his birth, the identity of his birthparents (particularly his birth father) and had made comments including "it's so sad to be adopted." The only seemingly significant change in Alex's life at the time of intake was his mother's return to full-time employment outside of the home. His father, who was ill, and considerably older, remained in the home.

As was his older brother, Alex was adopted at birth; but unlike the brother and his adoptive parents, Alex was dark-skinned and of Asian descent. Soon after his adoption, Alex's adoptive parents fought a long and highly publicized custody dispute. Alex's birth father was allowed to visit with him and the family over the next several years; this man was simply introduced as a friend. Although Alex's adoptive parents reportedly made no subsequent efforts to conceal his adoptive status, neither did they solicit him on the topic, choosing instead to answer adoption-related questions as he brought them up.

Alex was described as an affectionate, engaging, creative, and relatively healthy infant and child, who suffered only with occasional headaches. Although somewhat small for his age, he nevertheless developed friendships and was athletically competitive. He was a highly creative and imaginative child who grew to enjoy history, geography, reading, and video games. He was particularly drawn to Star Wars.

First Contact

From the outset, Alex was a warm, engaging, and expressive child, both verbally and artistically. Almost immediately, he shared his fascination with Michelangelo, whom he proclaimed was misunderstood by those around him. Like Michelangelo, Alex was interested in art, architecture, and sculpture, as well as astronomy and the physical sciences. Alex was also a child fascinated by opposites—peace and violence, past and present, men and women. He often wondered what it would be like to travel in time. Without prompting, Alex volunteered his adopted status, wondering out loud what it would be like to travel back in time to witness his adoption. He lamented, "I look so different from everybody else in my family!" Toward the end of the session, Alex shifted to his favorite topic, Star Wars, and mused that if he could change his name, he would choose to be called Michelangelo Skywalker, son of Luke and grandson of Anakin. He decided at that moment that he would like to write the next episode in the Star Wars saga. Given his interest in history, time travel, great men, and, of course, his adoption, this decision made good sense and would set the stage for the remainder of the therapeutic work.

Alex's Narrative

Over the next several sessions, Alex, with the assistance of the therapist as interviewer and transcriptionist, refined the following narrative, titled "Star Wars Episode VII: The Search for Luke":

> Luke is sad that his father is dead. Since he cannot get married because he is a Jedi Knight, Luke adopts a son named Michelangelo Skywalker from a space adoption agency on the moon of IV Yaven. And since Luke does not have a relative because they all died because they were old, he loses it (he goes crazy) and runs away!
>
> Michelangelo goes to another family. He lives with them on the ice planet of Hoth. As a child, he has been a Jedi Knight longer than anyone else in the universe. He went through harder training than any other Jedi and he likes wearing black clothes, which is like his father's (Luke) old uniform. He knows that he is adopted because he has already been with his father until he was eleven. Michelangelo becomes a Jedi from Master Mace Windue (the one with the purple light saber) because he wants to join the police, help his father and help other people. He feels depressed about two things ... kind of depressed because he lost his father, and happy because still has his dream. His dream is to become a Jedi Knight.
>
> To become a Jedi Knight, he had to train, which meant he had to go long distances and fight little droids by blocking himself without seeing them. He also had to pick up large things with his Force. On the inside, he just felt helpful and couldn't help but do good. Michelangelo has to go into a dark tree and Luke says, "If you think it's scary, the only scary thing is what you bring with you!"
>
> He becomes one of the finest fighter pilots and Jedi Knights and Commanders. Since the Empire lost, they want revenge—the Revenge

of the Empire. During the middle of the war, which is called the Second War, Michelangelo finds his father (Luke), leading the Empire. They fight for days and days and both are almost equally matched. But, Michelangelo has more power and confidence than any other Jedi in the Universe. He gets his confidence by everything around him (he has a lot of friends and because his stepmother and stepfather didn't die, who are also fighting in the war).

Commentary

Using Star Wars as a vehicle, Alex's creatively blended elements of both classical hero and American superhero mythology. It is replete with epic clashes between good and evil, heroes and villains, as well as the themes of loss, searching, redemption, and reconciliation. Luke is immediately depicted as a sympathetic character who loses his own father (Anakin), "goes crazy," and for these reasons, must place his son Michelangelo for adoption. Therefore, the adoption is due to his own, rather than his son's, deficiencies. Although the child grieves the loss of his father (raised on the ice planet of Hoth), he also identifies with him through both attire and pursuit of "Jedi Master" status. Michelangelo undergoes many perils over the next several years as he grows into a man. Although the two remain separated until their reconciliation at the end of the saga, Luke manages to guide his son benevolently from the "other side." In the end, Michelangelo grows into manhood, becoming, in a sense, one with his father.

Subsequent Treatment

In the remainder of the sessions, Alex and the therapist worked together to draw out similarities and differences between his Star Wars narrative and his own real-life story. Although he clearly enjoyed spinning the fantasy, it was equally important for him to be able to separate those elements from reality. Alex acknowledged that in the Star Wars universe, anything was possible, and that characters could have unlimited lives and power. Although not as rich in possibilities, Alex did indeed have two lives that underscored his narrative—the one before he was adopted, complete with a full cast of characters, and his present one. In the Star Wars universe, figures such as Yoda and Obi-Wan Kenobi guided him from the "other side"; however, his birth parents could only guide him through his own thoughts and fantasies about what they might be like. The seemingly unlimited power available to his on-screen heroes was offset by the very real limitations imposed on him by not being able to know his birth parents. Alex began to appreciate that in both his Star Wars and real universes, history, particularly the future was an as yet, unwritten chapter and that anything could happen.

The fantasy of Episode VII was helpful for Alex in working through some of his adoption issues; however, it also left him with still-unanswered, and perhaps ultimately unanswerable, questions; this is part of the legacy of loss in adoption. Throughout his fantasy play and the therapeutic conversations that surrounded it, Alex generated a list of questions. His adoptive parents, particularly his father, still had some difficulty discussing adoption with him, reasoning, "I don't bring it up because of the circumstances." He was referring to the earlier mentioned contentiousness and publicity surrounding Alex's adoption. Nevertheless, Alex composed the following questions for his biological parents:

- Why did you put me in an adoption agency?
- Why don't I know you?
- How many [biological] relatives do I have?
- Will I be a powerful man in the future?

Alex attempted to answer some of these questions himself but was of course, limited in information to only that which his adoptive parents had provided him. Some of this information was true; other parts of it were romanticized or simplified for him as he grew through childhood. He was able to express the sadness, anger, and confusion these questions, and some of the answers he had been provided, generated; he was encouraged, as were his parents, to continue conversations about adoption over the summer vacation. This is when the family would be traveling to spend time with extended family, most of whom, according to the mother, were fair skinned and blond (very different from Alex). In the last session before summer vacation, he generated answers to some of these questions. He reasoned that

- If I can imagine myself not adopted, I can look like everybody else in my family.
- If my [birth] parents didn't have money to keep me, I would use the Force to travel back in time to give it to them.

Postscript

In what was to be the final session (as Alex's parents neither made contact after summer vacation nor responded to the therapist's contacts), Alex's parents expressed relief that he had used his time in therapy to address issues related to the adoption. However, they remained ambivalent about proactively addressing the issues with him, contending that "If we do bring it up, we talk about it, and will answer questions." Alex's father remained relatively adamant about bringing up the issues—fearful perhaps of where that would lead and the emotions it would engender. Nevertheless, they reported that at least Alex was discussing adoption issues more openly, that his moodiness and outbursts had subsided, and he seemed more comfortable with himself, both at home and at school.

CONCLUSION

If life is an adventure, adoption is an epic. Adoption makes unique and additional developmental demands on all members of the triangle, particularly the child (Brodzinsky et al., 1992). Although Alex's adoptive parents were able to provide a secure base of attachment for him during infancy and toddlerhood, their own anxiety about the adoption and its aftermath lingered and made it difficult for them to be as open about it as they otherwise could have been. An intuitive and observant child, Alex became poignantly aware of the differences between himself and adoptive family. According to Brodzinsky et al. (1992), during middle childhood, the family should be deepening the adoption narrative so that the child can begin to create his or her own story that includes himself (or herself), and both the birth and adoptive parents. In many ways, Alex was denied this and began to create a subnarrative based around his interests in science, storytelling, and history. His emerging passion for Star Wars and his identification with Luke Skywalker was no coincidence. Although still very connected to his adoptive parents, Alex was silently grieving, and this most natural process was denied validation because his birth parents had not done their own psychological work around the adoption. By the time he was seen for counseling, Alex was beginning to wrestle with typical adolescent issues, which were compounded by the loss and search for identity that adoptees must address during this period. His childhood resilience and family's denial ran headlong into the inescapable questions that his adoption now made unavoidable.

The counseling helped Alex to deepen his narrative but only scratched the surface of the communication gap between him and his adoptive parents. The therapist can only hope that the family will continue to adapt to the lifelong journey that is adoption, each doing his or her own important work to integrate the experience into a shared narrative. May the Force be with them!

REFERENCES
Brodzinsky, D., Schecter, M., & Henig, R. (1992). *Being adopted: The lifelong search for self*. New York: Doubleday.

Brodzinsky, D., Smith, D., & Brodzinsky, A. (1998). *Children's adjustment to adoption: Developmental and clinical issues.* New York: Sage.

Campbell, J. (1949). *The hero with a thousand faces.* Princeton, NJ: Princeton University Press.

Campbell, J., & Moyers, B. (1988). *The power of myth.* New York: Doubleday.

Champlin, C. (1992). *George Lucas: The creative impulse.* New York: Abrams.

Geraghty, L. (2005). Creating and comparing myth in twentieth-century science fiction: *Star Trek* and *Star Wars*. *Literature/Film Quarterly, 33,* 191–200.

Henderson, M. (1997). Star wars: The magic of myth. New York: Bantam.

Kuiper, K. (1988). Star wars: An imperial myth. *Journal of Popular Culture, 21,* 77–86.

Lawrence, J. S., & Jewett, R. (2002). *The myth of the American superhero.* Grand Rapids, MI: Eerdmans.

Muller, U., & Perry, B. (2001a). Adopted persons' search for contact with their birth parents I: Who searches and why? *Adoption Quarterly, 4*(3), 5–37.

Muller, U., & Perry, B. (2001b). Adopted persons' search for and contact with their birthparents II: Adoptee-birth parent contact. *Adoption Quarterly, 4*(3), 39–62.

National Adoption Information Clearinghouse. (2004). *How many children were adopted in 2000 and 2001—highlights.* Retrieved December 20, 2005, from http://naic.acf.hhs.gov/pubs/s_adoptedhighlights.cfm

Pertman, A. (2000). *Adoption nation: How the adoption revolution is transforming America.* New York: Basic Books.

Ryan, S., & Nalavany, B. (2003). Adopted children: Who do they turn to for help and why? *Adoption Quarterly, 7,* 29–52.

Smith, D., & Brodzinsky, D. (2002). Coping with birthparent loss in adopted children. *Journal of Child Psychology and Psychiatry and Allied Disciplines, 43,* 213–223.

Verrier, N. N. (1993). *The primal wound: Understanding the adopted child.* Baltimore, MD: Gateway Press.

Nontraditional Therapeutic Applications of Superheroes

Becoming the Hero: The Use of Role-Playing Games in Psychotherapy

George Enfield

> If more people would play war games perhaps there would be fewer wars ... little wars leave neither widows nor orphans.
> —(Wells, 1913)

Role-playing, therapeutically defined as an "attempt to simulate or replicate significant portions of the extra-therapy environment for observation and manipulation in the therapist's presence" (Kanfer & Phillips, 1966, p. 120), has long been recognized as means of treating a range of clinical problems, including low self-esteem, anxiety, depression, and social and interpersonal skill deficits. Role-playing games (RPGs), the logical extension of role-playing, are face-to-face or virtual (Internet) experiential activities in which players take on the roles of specific predetermined or self-created characters who embark on either a pre-scripted or spontaneous adventures that are controlled by the game players. RPGs may comprise simple unidimensional characters such as the inspector in *Clue*, the complex characters found in multilayered games such as *Dungeons and Dragons* and *Warhammer*, or virtual universes as in MMORPGs (massively multi-played online role-playing games). The appeal of RPGs is in their utilization of constructed narratives in the form of game characters, which allows for experimentation along the boundaries separating reality from fantasy and "limited me" from "possible me" (Waskul & Lust, 2004). Within a therapeutic context, RPGs also "provide an experience of a virtual [and/or live] community, ameliorate social anxiety and loneliness, allow the trying on of new identities, and assist in the developmental task of forging a sense of identity apart from one's family" (Ellison et al., 2006, p. 384).

Role-playing games vary in their complexity, from simple board games such as *Marvel Hero Clicks, Heroscape*, and *Hybrid,* to very elaborate venues in which players either develop their own unique individual characters or a complete casts of characters, such as *Dungeons and Dragons, Monsters and Mutants*, and, most recently, *Truth and Justice*. Role-playing games can be equally broad in subject matter and time frame, ranging from early-history battles of Romans and Barbarians, to distant-future post-apocalyptic games such as *Shadow Run*. They may also consist of actual historical events such as a particular Civil War battle or documented showdowns from the American Frontier or pure fantasy and fiction adventures, such as *Star Wars*. This degree of flexibility can provide the therapist with an infinite number of possible combinations that allow individuals or groups of clients to practice a variety of skills in a simulated role-play situation. Through engagement in the role-playing activity, clients may express conscious issues, such as those that brought them into counseling, or they may symbolically express and play out unconscious struggles.

ROLE-PLAYING THE SUPERHERO

Over the past several years, I have observed that preadolescent boys in my psychotherapy practice express a preference for, and gravitate toward, action figures that are part of popular, cartoon, and comic book culture. Heroes and their unique journeys of discovery seem particularly appealing to this population who enjoy play-acting and role-playing. Through identification with superheroes and their heroic quests, clients can venture beyond everyday constraints and the mundane to vicariously act out alternate personality or interpersonal styles. As metaphors, heroes and superheroes can assist clients in accessing some of their own unconscious fears and desires, as well as experiment with the behavior at the bounds of their comfort level or that of their defenses. For example, superheroes such as Spider-Man with his strong sense of responsibility or the Beast or Maul who as they grow in strength or size lose the ability to reason, have particular appeal to clients who struggle with similar dilemmas. In the role-playing game, the client and the superhero work together as allies to take control and work through their issues. The questions are thus whether a strong interest in heroes and role-playing can be effectively channeled during therapy and how can a therapist explore challenging clinical issues that are typically avoided by clients. There is also the question of whether role-playing activities can be used in more concrete ways with younger clients to practice and then generalize social and esteem-building skills.

HEROES AND THEIR JOURNEYS

Joseph Campbell's (1972) conceptualization of the mythological hero's journey can be a useful starting point for understanding the appeal of role-playing games that in one way or another, involve a hero (or superhero). The popularity of the hero motif is evident in the story lines of the more popular figures in popular literary and movie culture. These include to name a few, Harry Potter, X-Men, Superman, Spider-Man and both Luke and Leia from the Star Wars films. The journeys that these characters make involve challenges and obstacles that may be relevant to the clinical work that preadolescent boys often need to perform, such as working on self-esteem, self-regulation, interpersonal communication, and boundaries.

From a child's perspective, the hero of fiction is that person outside of the nuclear family whom they can look up to and emulate in their day-to-day lives. It is not at all uncommon for me to hear boys in my waiting area discussing the latest episode of *Naruto* or *Dragon Ball Z*. Although these may be today's passing fads or the latest in a long line of quickly fading popular-culture characters, the seemingly fundamental need for the role they play in the lives of this preadolescent population remains constant. Hero's have a challenge or burden placed on them. In response to this calling, they undertake a journey to explore or seek out the solution to these challenges. In the process, their body is changed in some way, and through the course of the journey, their fundamental beliefs are also altered. They are brought to a point of greater enlightenment. Through identification with the hero and his journey, role-players can complete themselves by filling in the parts of their identity and vicariously acting out those that were missing in early childhood or that made them stand out as different. Many of the preadolescent clients I have treated perceive themselves as being out of touch with their peers and desperately want to feel as if they are part of a system. That is, they are willing to embark metaphorically on a journey to discover who they are, how to relate to others, and to acquire a sense of focus or direction.

From the perspective of play therapy, metaphor is the language of change. Clients learn and practice new skills through the course of play. The preadolescent is often in the position of still wanting to play but not feeling comfortable doing so. Because they are physically larger, these clients perceive playing with toys to be beneath them and worry that they will be perceived by others as immature. The role-playing game allows the preadolescent the opportunity to play without having to sacrifice their pride—after all, they are not really playing with toys. Boys in particular are attracted to the role-playing games for several reasons. First there is the vicarious adventure inherent in playing the role of, or along with, a hero. The adventure, in turn, is a vehicle through which the clinician can explore issues of power, control, popularity, perceived importance, and the belief that they can be bigger, stronger, smarter, or more popular than they actually are. Another attractive aspect of the role-playing game is that clients are able experiment with and master elements of an alternate identity—the person they would like to become.

MATCHING THE RPG TO THE CLIENT

As previously noted, RPGs are as varied as the people who play them. Before deciding what kind of RPG to use in a given clinical situation, it is important to consider the needs of the population with which one is working with. Such considerations include the age and developmental level of the client, their interests, whether they prefer the historical or the fictional, and how easily they can enter into as well as and step away from the metaphor or role they chose. It is also important to consider whether the game in question will be played with two or more players, what gender best fits the particular chosen game, the level of aggression that is appropriate, and what type of medium to apply. In this latter context of medium, it is important to consider whether clients are more comfortable with concrete, easily represented games such as the *World of Warcraft* and *Hybrid* or those with greater levels of complexity and abstraction such as *Truth and Justice*. Finally, it is crucial to match the game to the client's specific treatment needs.

When considering treatment planning, it is also important to determine client goals. In this way, the therapist may facilitate incorporation or exploration of the interpersonal interactions in the game into the treatment. For example, if the therapeutic goals is it to regulate feelings of inadequacy, it becomes important to choose a game that provides the client with a greater degree of control and power, such as a superhero-based genre. If the therapy is to address impulse or anxiety-based behaviors, a game containing opportunities for planning and sequencing would be useful. If instead, the client is struggling with tantrum behaviors stemming from feelings of powerlessness, a game in which he confronts formidable opponents might be called for.

In the nondirective treatment, it is the client who charts the course of treatment (Landreth, 1991), even if that particular client is struggling with anger control problems. However, there is also evidence that more directive forms of treatment, including anger-management-based group therapy, can be an effective modality of intervention with this population. Superhero role-playing games that directly address and provide clients the opportunity to express themselves as well as engage in problem solving around anger issues abound in the gaming industry. Recently, there has been an influx of these games, heralded by the introduction of Milton Bradley's combat game, *Heroscape*. In this game, two or more players construct a game board, select heroes to fight for them, and attempt to achieve specific objectives. These objective might include eliminating an opponent, capturing or collecting goods, holding a position, or rescuing an ally. Other manufacturers have either entered or reentered the RPG market through their introduction of RPGs such as *Dungeons and Dragons* by Wizards of the West Coast, *Mutants and Masterminds* by Green Ronan, *War Machine* by Iron Winds Publishing, and *Truth and Justice* by the Atomic Sock Monkey.

The RPG industry, which for some includes tabletop combat games such as *Warhammer, Warhammer 40K, War Machine, Confrontation, Gangs of Mega City*, and *Rezolution2175*, appear to have found a relatively large niche population. The population that plays these games is mostly male, beginning with the 8-year-old who plays the "click-type games," to the adult who engages in the full-scale and more complex role-play and battlefield games such as *Warhammer Fantasy* and *Confrontation*. In the very simple hero click game, the player enters basic identifying information into the base of the given figure, the clicking of which establishes the various behaviors and attributes of that character, including adjustment to injury or mutagenic power. In the more complex games such as *Dungeons and Dragons* or *Mutants and Masterminds*, the player can act as a hero or general in a heroic situation, or use the miniatures more strategically or for the purpose of full character or plot development. Miniature gaming, although relatively unknown to the general population, is a form of play that gained some prominence in the works of H. G. Wells, who wrote two books on the subject, *Little Wars* (1913) and *Floor Games* (1911). *Floor Games*' influence, in turn, can be seen in the works of both Margaret Lowenfeld and Dora Kalff, in their development of sandplay (Turner, 2004).

APPLYING THE RPG IN CLINICAL PRACTICE

In a discussion of superheroes, it is compelling to limit ones thinking to only those characters with an ostensibly "super" attribute such as flight, X-ray vision, telepathy, strength or speed. In this context, traditional supercharacters would include, among many others, Batman, Thor, Wonder Woman, Phoenix, Hulk, and Spider-Man. In the gaming world, the hero or superhero is not necessarily the one who has a superpower but one who must overcome the odds and remain true to their beliefs and values. The hero of an RPG may take the form of a general controlling a vast army, similar to those that H. G. Wells discussed in *Little Wars*. Similarly, the individualized characters in *Dungeons and Dragons*, although not possessing super skills per se, struggle no less than do superheroes with moral and ethical dilemmas. Like Spider-Man who attempts to balance great responsibility with his great power, and the legendary likes of Hercules, Jason, and Arthur; characters in the *Dungeons and Dragons* world struggle to understand their origin, their destiny, and everything in between. Complex, fantasy-based, multilayered and character-driven, role-playing games like *Dungeons and Dragons* provide the very medium that appeals to preadolescent boys wrestling with issues of identity, power, and connection.

Dungeons and Dragons is a role-playing game in which a group of players share a "quest" to accomplish a specific common goal. There are three primary roles in the game; one is that of a player character (PC), the other is the game master (GM) or dungeon master (DM), and the third is the NPC (nonplayer characters). The role of the PC is taken by all the members of a group, who in turn, develop characters to represent themselves—complete with attributes such as strength, intelligence, wisdom, charisma, dexterity, and constitution. They further develop the character by endowing it with physical characteristics, personality traits, temperaments, and an occupation. The PCs then agree on and follow a particular storyline. The singular role of the GM or DM entails that of a judge and jury who presides over questions pertaining to rules, the mediation of conflicts, and the development of maps. The remaining populace is identified as the NPC who can be either allies to the group or adversaries, whether humanoid or monster. *Dungeons and Dragons* games can be single events or campaigns lasting weeks or months, depending on the involvement of the players. During the playing of the game, journaling the adventures is possible; however, some games can be played mentally, which requires a table of papers that hold vital statistics and dice, representing the element of fate involved. More highly detailed games come complete with figures and terrain to represent the physical environment.

CASE STUDIES

In the following section, I present two cases. The first focuses on a therapeutic application of a *Dungeons and Dragons*-like game with a group of 11- to 13-year-olds. The second reflects the course of individual treatment with an 11-year-old boy who explored his impulsivity and boundary problems with a superhero RPG. In each of the cases, the prominence in the relation between metaphoric role-playing and the client's behavior, both at home and at school is evident. Through initial assessment, it was determined that the boys in the group preferred the fantasy motif, whereas in the case of the individual client, preference was given to the superhero model—specifically, the Beast and Maul.

Dungeons and Dragons RPG Group

I expanded on H. G. Wells's notion of "little wars" to create a role-playing game in an outpatient group setting that would help clients improve communication, social skills, problem solving, and sequencing. This group was based on the Jungian and client-centered notions that although unconscious issues (both individual and collective) shape our behavior, the client can also guide the course of treatment. It is the role of the therapist to be present to facilitate the process by providing the feedback and tools that will help clients to generalize what they have learned into their outside world.

The focus of the group was to develop a character and, in turn, use that character as a conduit for work on both intra and interpersonal interactions. Before the commencement of the group work, each child met with the therapist to develop his individual character and select his own playing piece from a miniature gaming series. Once the child developed a character profile and selected a playing piece, they painted their piece(s). Painting of the figure is one more step in the process through which the player connects with their individual character in order to personalize it, and to increase investment in the success of the group. Initially, a loose version of *Dungeons and Dragons* was chosen because that was the game most familiar to the clinician. Once the group began, it became apparent that the structure of the activity was such that each of the clients could, and did, modify their characters, thus changing the original structure to fit their needs as both individuals and as a group. Although the game was therefore dramatically revised from its original form, it was considered far more clinically useful because it was tailor-made to the needs of the participants.

Background of Dungeons and Dragons Group

For the purposes of clarity and flow, this discussion follows the initial four clients in the *Dungeons and Dragons* therapy group who ranged in age from 9 to 11, and were enrolled in the fourth and fifth grades. Tommy, a 10-year-old was a long-time client of the agency who had received previous therapeutic services. He was the middle of three siblings who was described by his parents as the "black sheep." Tommy was previously diagnosed with attention-deficit/hyperactivity disorder (ADHD)—combined type, and although likable, he was impulsive and disruptive in school as well as aggressive and oppositional at home.

At nine years of age, David was the youngest client in the group. While also diagnosed with ADHD, he was experiencing symptoms of posttraumatic stress disorder related to physical abuse by his father. This resulted in a custodial change to his mother's and maternal grandmother's care, where he subsequently became the focal point of their criticism.

Tony, age 10, was referred due to a history of abuse and neglect in the nuclear family, as well as sexual abuse by someone outside of the home. As a result, he was placed with his maternal grandmother, whose home caught on fire soon after he was referred for treatment. Although Tony and his older brother remained with their grandmother while her home was rebuilt, they experienced numerous failed attempts by the biological father to regain custody. The boys had some subsequent contact with their mother during this period; however, her own mental health problems undermined these visits.

The fourth member of the initial group was Larry, a biracial 11-year-old who was referred by his school because of "unusual" and impulsive behaviors. Larry, who had a history of aggression toward peers and siblings, was also very talkative and prone to interrupting. Larry was highly impulsive, distractible, and disruptive, and made numerous negative self-comments.

Group Format

A *Dungeons and Dragons* role-playing group format was chosen to explore and assist the boys with the social difficulties they were having at home and at school. It was structured so that they could work together to accomplish a common goal: rescuing the princess from the clutches of the Evil Ogre. The quest to save the princess was considered relevant because each of the boys also struggled in relationship to a key female figure in their lives: their mothers. In addition, I decided to make the ogre female to allow several of the boys to work on enmeshment issues with their parents

The group process consisted of several stages. First, the boys individually developed and carefully hand-painted a character to represent themselves in the game. Next, they were asked to populate their dungeon. These two steps took several weeks because it required one session to develop the character, one to paint it, and several to make and populate the dungeon. The cardstock structure that they constructed, called *Chunky Dungeon*, created a unique room that each of the boys designed and populated with a monster that the rest of the group would have to confront. A group leader was chosen who would then be responsible for guarding the treasure against wandering monsters. This leader would also help the rest of the group members to organize the story line of the game.

The structure for each of the sessions followed a consistent pattern. The boys would gather in the waiting room and await the arrival of the group leaders. The group would then move to the treatment room where the game was set up. The initial 10 minutes of the session were allocated to a discussion of what had occurred during the preceding week, and each of the boys was asked to adhere to a Code of Chivalry (see Appendix A). When these introductory comments were completed, the roles for the day's activity were assigned.

The boys were assigned various roles including the scribe (the note taker of the day), the leader (the person who organized the group, developed the final solution, and helped maintain the flow of interactions), the dice holder (for the most impulsive member), and the party member (who offered possible solutions and who moved figures in and out of the dungeon). The game was played for approximately 40 minutes with the remaining time spent in wrap-up, review, grounding discussions, checking the code of chivalry, and developing personal goals for the following week.

Game Modifications

The initial justification for group treatment was to provide a venue that would help the boys work on issues that might be difficult to address effectively in individual counseling. *Dungeons and Dragons*, however, is a potentially complex and highly detailed game with several volumes of rules and ways to handle almost every detail of daily life, from sleeping to combating monsters. Although these details lend themselves to limitless possibilities, the concern was that the complexity would get in the way of the boys working on the issues at hand, that is, enhancement of social skills, frustration, tolerance, and cooperation. Therefore, many of the accessories, rules, and roles of the game were simplified, so as not to detract from the therapeutic mission of the group. The only aspects of the original game that were left intact were basic stats, armor, weapons, bonuses, spells (if any), gold, and health.

Illustrations of Sessions

A typical session began when the boys came together for a snack. During the course of the snack, they discussed the events of the week and took turns listening to each other. When members attempted to top the other's stories, the group leader reminded the others in the group that each of them saw the world differently and that what may appear easy to one person might be quite challenging for another, and vice versa. This was followed by the weekly assignment of group responsibilities and planning the activity for that meeting.

At times, it was necessary for the group members to illustrate what they were doing, so that the group leader was clear about the process. For example, when the boys were confronted with a locked door in the dungeon, their initial efforts included seemingly random efforts at pushing, pulling, or prying it open. When the leader of the group was asked to reflect on the unfolding process, he quickly commented that there was writing above the door that stated, "Only the biggest to the smallest may pass." The GM's initial idea was to have the boys organize themselves by physical size; however, they worked it out among themselves, deciding instead to organize from the eldest to youngest. Believing this to be a positive solution that had been reached by cooperative consensus, the GM unlocked the door, only to encounter another behind it. This time, the boys pushed, pulled, and pried for a far shorter period of time

Another activity placed the boys in a swampy area where a mysterious cloud descended on the group, with each member becoming afflicted with a problem. On this day, David, who was designated a "pure and noble paladin," was selected as the group leader, whose task it was to guide the members through the swamp. However, David was the only person in the group who could foresee the pitfalls. Unfortunately for the rest of the group, he was only allowed to share this information with Tony, to whom he had provided directions for navigating the swamp. Making matters more challenging, Tony, Tommy, and Larry were able to use only one leg and one arm. Larry was further impaired by his prescribed inability to speak. The process of navigating the swamp lasted the entire session, which ended with the boys reviewing the experience and praising each other for their efforts.

Outcome

The initial group, consisting of Tony, Tommy, Larry, and David met for two consecutive school semesters before taking on new players. By this time, the "original four," as they came to be called, were coming to the end of treatment. In each case, reports from both home and school indicated improved social functioning and diminished impulsivity. In general, there was a significant decrease in reported detentions, from an initial level of two to three per week to a final level of two per month. Additionally, the boys' communication skills had improved. During group time, they remained engaged in conversation for longer periods of time, asked each other more questions and cooperated more extensively in planning activities such as confronting obstacles and monsters. As each of the boys took turns playing the leader, they were increasingly effective in designing and implementing strategies for the others. Initially working in a single room of the dungeon, the boys progressed to moving through multiple rooms of increasing complexity and challenge.

Individual improvements were also noted. Tommy, initially the clown who enjoyed provoking others, increasingly demonstrated leadership skills and was far more focused than when he began group. Although academics remained a constant struggle for Tommy, he fought less at home with his siblings and was able to maintain his grades, which in turn allowed him to participate in school sports. This was a dramatic change from the preceding year, when he spent several weekends a month in Saturday detention.

When David began group, he was disruptive, continually sought attention, cried easily, rejected the other members, and left the room when he became upset. By the time the group ended, David was an active group leader who was also an effective problem solver who could easily confront obstacles and help others in need. There was an accompanying increase in his ability to express himself to others in the group as well as plan before acting. This improvement was also observed at school, where David's grades improved. At home, his family began to recognize that David was capable of taking on more responsibilities and had significantly decreased the negative self-talk that had characterized his behavior prior to treatment.

When Tony began in the group, he was shy, talked minimally, and even then, inaudibly. Over the course of the group he became more vocal, was increasingly willing to risk discussing his ideas, and could redirect the others when they got off task. Tony's most impressive gains were noted in the courtroom. When group started he was submissive to both his father and elder brother. His grandmother reported that he complied with all of their requests and demands without challenge. Seven months into the group, Tony was summoned once again by court order to participate in the custody hearings. This time, he was able not only to address the judge directly, but could now express the desire to remain with his grandmother and not have further visits with his father. The judge granted his request.

Larry, who attended the group less consistently than the others, demonstrated improvement both in school and at home. By the time he finished in the group, Larry's grades had improved significantly, and he demonstrated a greater degree of impulse control and planning ability.

Individualized Application of a Superhero Role Playing Game

Role-playing games and tabletop adventure games can be used in an individual treatment as well in group therapy. Game that can be more readily adapted to an individualized format include *Hero Clicks*, the *Star Wars Miniature Game*, *Marvel Hero Clicks*, or combat games such as *Heroscape*. These games are less complex than those used in group format and can be played almost entirely in a single session. These games also provide players a closer connection with the character, freed from the distraction of other players. Because tabletop adventure games do not provide for complex character development, players are not as heavily invested in them, and thus their defenses may not be as easily threatened. This detachment is further strengthened by the predetermined story lines, which in turn, provide the client more of an opportunity to use simple metaphors. As the illustration that follows will demonstrate, clients using individualized tabletop RPGs can more directly explore and process issues of fear, power, and control.

Marvel Hero Clicks

I typically leave game selection to the client. In my office, I have numerous games displayed on my shelves, much like a sandtray therapist displays miniatures. Darren, the client who I discuss in the following section, selected *Marvel Hero Clicks*, which contains a miniaturized Marvel Comic universe, complete with the traditional superheroes, including among others, Spider-Man, Thor, Captain America, the Fantastic Four, the Incredible Hulk, and Maul. The base of each of these figures contains statistics required to play the game, including special powers, affiliation (either good or evil), as well as defensive and offensive capabilities. Each of these characters is on a revolving base, so as the game progresses, the player can accomplish the necessary strategic tasks by turning the base to the left or right. When the base is turned in this manner, it "clicks," and thus the name, *Marvel Hero Clicks*. The game is played on a grid table system that allows the player to monitor play carefully and measure distances. A basic set comes with several superheroes, with most players expanding the ranks through additional purchase. Expansion packs contain random new heroes, which may include duplicates, and thus ardent players usually make selective purchases at a gaming shop, convention, or online.

Client History

Darren was the eldest of three children of mixed descent, who along with their mother, experienced domestic violence by their father. As the eldest, Darren was often the recipient of the greatest abuse and had witnessed violence against his mother. During a particular 2-year period, the family was imprisoned in the home by the father, who had nailed shut the doors and windows. Following their eventual escape, the father was incarcerated. Darren, however, was continually plagued by nightmares and frequent violent tantrums. When not acting out, Darren was described as a shy, constricted, and distractible boy. Following a brief hospitalization, he was referred to me for treatment. At the time of the referral, he was exhibiting aggressive behavior both at home and at school.

Treatment

Soon after meeting Darren, I determined that he was locked into an aggressive means of resolving conflicts and expressing feelings, and a more directive intervention would provide the necessary therapeutic structure. After explaining the various RPGs in my office, Darren seemed particularly interested in *Marvel Hero Clicks*. Using the sample in the game pack, Darren and I were able to explore the various superhero characters and how they related to him and his life.

Following the initial sessions during which Darren explored the various characters, he gravitated to Maul, a Wildcats comic figure who has the ability to grow in size and strength so that he could combat his opponents, the Deamonites. We opened the game by fully exploring Maul's abilities and mission, as well as those of his opponents. We also discussed the circumstances in which Maul transformed and his capacity to regulate this power. We further discussed Mauls relationship with his teammate, Voodoo, who has the ability to regulate Maul and provide him with a conscience.

In the course of watching Darren play the game, we discussed how unfortunate it was that we could not all have friends like Voodoo to help us control our feelings when we were angry or feeling out of control. Together, we also wondered how to reach out to others when we felt angry or isolated with our feelings. As the sessions progressed, Darren became interested in the X-Men archrivals of Saber Tooth and Wolverine, each of whom, although highly competitive and aggressive, healed quickly from his wounds. Darren quickly recognized the similarities between himself and these characters. In this context, Darren and I were able to explore his own anger around the abuse and disruption of his family and how he could better express these feelings around others.

OUTCOME AND REFLECTIONS

Darren was seen for 12 sessions before the family relocated in order to be closer to relatives. At the time of termination, the frequency of Darren's tantrums had diminished, and his mother described him as being more relaxed, engaging and cooperative both at home and at school. Although he continued to experience occasional nightmares, Darren was unwilling to address these either in therapy or at home. Darren's ability to work metaphorically through some of his conflicts with the superheroes provided him with a sense of mastery and control that he was able to transfer into his life. I hope his healing adventure will continue.

REFERENCES

Campbell, J. (1972). *The hero with a thousand faces.* Princeton, NJ: Princeton University Press.

Ellison, S., von Wahlde, L., Shockley, T., & Gabbard, G. (2006). The development of self in the era of Internet role-playing fantasy games. *American Journal of Psychiatry, 163,* 381–385.

Kanfer, F., & Phillips, J. (1966). Behavior therapy. *Archives of General Psychiatry, 15,* 114–128.

Landreth, G. (1991). *Play therapy: The art of the relationship.* New York: Bruner Routledge.

Turner, B. (2004). *H. G. Wells floor games: A father's account of play and its legacy of healing.* Cloverdale, CA: Temenos Press.

Waskul, D., & Lust, M. (2004). Role-playing and playing roles: The person and persona in fantasy role play. *Symbolic Interaction, 27,* 333–356.

Wells, H. G. (1911). *Floor Games.* London: Frank Palmer.

Wells H. G. (1913). *Little Wars.* New York: Macmillan.

ONLINE GAMING RESOURCES

- http://www.thewarstore.com
  An online site that carries many of the games mentioned in this chapter, as well as other gaming and sandtray materials.
- http://www.theworldofhobbies.com
  A regional hobby shop that carries many of the click and miniature games.
- http://www.theatomicsockmonkey.com
  Maker and distributor of Truth and Justice, the least expensive hero game.

- http://www.worldworksgames.com
  Creator and distributor of the Chunky Dungeon system, a three-dimensional tabletop game of inexpensive paper construction.
- http://www.hirstarts.com
  Distributor of three-dimensional molds with which to produce dungeons, dragons, and other buildings suitable for RPGs and sandtray play.

APPENDIX A

Code of Chivalry

Date:___/___/20___
Group member's name_____

1. Members will participate.
2. Members will listen to each other.
3. Clowning around will be limited.
4. Provoking of peers is not accepted
5. Members will remain in the group room.
6. Members will respect their peers.
7. Members following the code will be rewarded.

1. Quality of participation
   Poor 1 2 3 4 5 *Great*
2. Amount of listening
   Bad listening 1 2 3 4 5 *Great listener*
3. Amount of clowning
   Lots of goofing off 1 2 3 4 5 *No goofing off*
4. Amount of provoking
   Lots of provoking 1 2 3 4 5 *No provoking*
5. Participated in the group discussion
   No 1 2 3 4 5 *Yes*
6. Members will respect their peers
   Very disrespectful 1 2 3 4 5 *Respectful of others*

Total: ___ average score of 25 needed for reward.

CHAPTER THIRTEEN

To Boldly Go! Star Trek Superheroes in Therapy

Jeffrey Pickens

The primary reason for examining the world of the Star Trek superheroes is because of its enormous, if not incomparable, popularity in contemporary media culture. Gene Roddenberry created the original *Star Trek* science-fiction television series in 1966; the show was canceled a mere 3 years later. Since that time, Viacom Inc. (owner of Paramount Studios and the UPN Network), along with the support of millions of fans worldwide, has made the Star Trek enterprise into one of Hollywood's most profitable properties (Satzman, 2002). Star Trek's television incarnation began with the "original series" (ST-TOS; Butler et al., 1966) in 1966 and continues to date in reruns. Its sequels and spin-offs have included *The Next Generation* (ST-TNG; Bole et al., 1987); *Voyager* (ST-VOY; Frakes & Williams, 1995); *Deep Space Nine* (ST-DS9; Dorn, 1993); and the most current prequel, *Enterprise* (ST-ENT; Livingston & Vejar, 2001). These five television series have aired continuously in primetime for 25 of the past 35 years (this does not include syndicated reruns, cartoons, or other spin-offs). Within the Star Trek movie universe, *Nemesis,* the tenth motion picture released by Paramount, is part of a theatrical series that has netted more than $1.25 billion in domestic box office receipts, trailing only Star Wars, Jaws, and James Bond as all-time serial movie franchise leaders (Hoffman & Rose, 2005). This amazing popularity suggests that the themes and characters of the Star Trek universe are appealing to fans both young and old. (See Appendix A)

Star Trek's popularity and appeal, which is based on it uniquely accessible themes and characters, make it an unlimited therapeutic resource. Gene Roddenberry's original *Star Trek* television series was, in many ways, a western that just happened to take place in space—in the future. Dramatic plots involving a cast of heroes led by Captain James Tiberius Kirk, offered potent metaphors for many psychosocial issues of the day. Few other popular television series offer as many opportunities for fantasy play. It is not surprising that many authors have employed Star Trek as a theme for exploring physics, neuropsychology, philosophy, and more. The various heroes of the Star Trek universe provide unique screens onto which we may project our own fantasies and aspirations. By identifying with the ST characters and their quests, we may also become more aware of our own dreams and desires. Working with these superhero characters and exploring personal and shared superhero mythologies in therapeutic settings can help us better understand our clients and ourselves. Star Trek offers particularly helpful metaphors for therapeutic and educational work with young people, such as the teen discussed later in this chapter, who struggled with severe anxiety and an undiagnosed learning problem.

"MAKE IT SO!" THE POSITIVE OUTLOOK OF STAR TREK

Star Trek provides a glimpse into a special category of heroes, who rely on their humanity rather than physical prowess or science to solve problems. Star Trek challenges us to project ourselves into a future, which although seemingly ideal, is fraught with age-old conflicts. Very "human" characters such as captains James Kirk and Jean Luc Picard, often struggle with their with their machine-like side kicks, Mr. Spock and Commander Data, who rely exclusively on logic and reason to solve problems. Although exotic alien creatures are often endowed with superpowers, the human protagonists are provided with the tools of science and technology to enhance their power and elevate them to the level of true superheroes. This is not to say that Star Trek reifies technology. Quite the contrary; many of the television episodes demonstrate the ultimate supremacy of people and mind over machine and science. Spock from the Original series, Data from the Next Generation, and female Vulcan science officer T'Pol of the new *Enterprise* series, continuously exemplify the absolute power of the rational mind. Interestingly, and despite the strength of reason to solve problems, Captains Kirk and Picard often successfully employ basic human emotions to circumvent the logical recommendations of Mr. Spock and Data, who remain baffled. Instead, it is often the brash, heroic, and impulsive efforts of the all-too-human captains that save the day and prove that it is individualism, intuition, emotion, and the power of will that prevail. The message of Star Trek is that the human mind and spirit solve difficult problems. Despite these tensions, Star Trek heroes were and are positive and optimistic, modeling a healthy diverse team boldly exploring space and solving problems together.

Heroic Captain Kirk does not "beam down" to alien planets to conquer, as do his villainous nemeses, the Romulans and Klingons. The crews of the Star Trek *Enterprise,* in all incarnations, set out to explore and discover, not to subjugate, control, or convert. Star Trek instills a sense of competence and a message that says, "if I apply my human ability diligently, then I can and will overcome adversity." Few shows that are popular with adolescents portray this level of humanism or optimism. The audience is compelled to wonder "if this is what humans can do in the future, maybe there is something I can do right now." Although life aboard the U.S.S. *Enterprises* is organized around a military model, themes of individualism dominate those based on collectivism (see ST:TNG episode 123;-*I Borg*). Star Trek depicts a utopian future populated by a diversity of individuals working toward, rather than subjugated to a common good. The "prime directive" of noninterference compels the crew to preserve, rather than change, alien societies.

Superheroes in Outer Space

From a psychosocial perspective, most superheroes are flawed by the circumstances of their origins. As discussed elsewhere in this book, many of the traditional superheroes are fragile loners whose struggles emanate from either early adversity or the burden of power (Brooker, 2001; Fingeroth, 2004; Lawrence, 2005). Popular figures such as Superman, Batman and Robin, Spider-Man, Luke Skywalker and Daredevil, grew up without the benefit of parents. Many superheroes had to rely on extrafamilial mentors who helped guide them along the path to righteousness. Superboy had Ma and Pa Kent, Spider-Man had Uncle Ben and Aunt May, Batman had Alfred, and Luke Skywalker had Obi-Wan Kenobi. In sharp contrast, most Star Trek heroes are remarkably functional, well-integrated, and resilient individuals notable for making their own decisions to leave behind both family and mother earth so that they might "boldly go where no human has gone before." However, they do surround themselves with surrogate family of their own, traveling together through space (Lawrence & Jewett, 2002), working efficiently and cooperatively side by side. Roddenberry's positivistic vision of the future includes racial harmony, interspecies cooperation, freedom from mundane stressors, mastery over both matter and energy, and even an interactive virtual-reality "holodeck" for recreation. Although this utopia is frequently interrupted by emergencies of galactic proportion, the crew of the *Enterprise* typically rises to the challenge to reestablish harmony.

Like all superheroes, Star Trek protagonists work for the benefit of others—so much so that they have been referred to in scholarly circles as being Christian in their outlook (Caprio, 1978). In contrast to comic book heroes who have been condemned as corruptive and mind-poisoning role models who rely on brute force (Lawrence & Jewett, 2002), the Star Trek heroes, although combative, are inherently conflict avoiders. Although they have the capacity to set their phasers to kill, they more routinely use these weapons to stun their enemies. This discretion was not available to the Lone Ranger.

In many respects, the heroes of ST are akin to both the American Monomythic hero described by Lawrence and Jewett (2002), and the heroes of antiquity who "ventured forth from the world of common day into a region of supernatural wonder; fabulous forces are there encountered and a decisive victory is won" (Campbell, 1956, p. 30). Table 13.1 provides an overview of the superpowers of several of the ST characters.

Table 13.1   Superpowers of Star Trek Superheroes: What They Do, and How They Do It

Superpower	Tool or Technique
Ability to travel rapidly to other planets (Faster than light space travel)	Warp drive
Ability to move massive objects	Tractor beam
Ability to instantly scan the inner body	Medical tricorder
Ability to scan an area for life forms	Tricorder
Disintegrator ray, stun ray, other weapons	Phaser and Photon Torpedo
Matter-to-energy transfer of people and things from one location to another	Beaming from one location to another
Energy-to-matter creation of food, medicine, interactive environments, and characters	Food synthesizer, drug synthesizer, medical hologram, Holodeck
Expert knowledge	Spock (science) McCoy (medicine and xenobiology) Uhura (language and communications) Data (information) Mr. Scott (engineering)
Super-strength	Spock, Data, Worf
ESP "mind-meld"	Spock
Immobilizing neural neck pinch	Spock
Able to function in lethal environments	Data
Super-empathy, lie detection	Counselor Troi

CREW REPORT: THE STAR TREK CHARACTERS

The characters and themes of Star Trek, particularly the superhero subnarrative, offer a limitless range of possibilities for exploring the psychological issues of young people. These Star Trek superheroes have distinctive and predictable *emotional valences* that emerge in each episode. To begin, we have the quintessential hero embodied in the personages of Captains Kirk, Picard, Janeway, Sisco, and Archer. Although each is arguably a superhero by virtue of wielding the tools of science and technology, they are first and foremost heroes—and very human. All of these leaders exude confidence, intellect, cunning, benevolence, wit, sex appeal, and power. These team leaders strategize through problems and effectively push their crews to perform beyond their potential. Although they manage to find romance throughout the universe, they always remain faithful to ship, crew, and mission. It is she (the ship) to whom the captain is most securely attached (Lawrence & Jewett, 2002). Decisive but rarely impulsive, emotional but never out of control, these captains balance leadership with dependence and are key roles models at the epicenter of the each episode.

These captains, although rugged individualists, rarely stand alone. They are joined and counseled by calm, reassuring, and loyal command officers extolling the virtues of logic, wisdom, and science. The captains rely on these sage alien counselors (Spock, Data, Counselor Troi, Tuvok) who are physicians and therapists, robots and aliens, and who typically model and preach moral reflection before action. In many ways, these are *superego* characters. In contrast, Star Trek also offers many highly emotional and volatile characters that consistently call for action or try to spur the captain to lash out in the name of revenge or loyalty. These hotheads (villains and antiheroes) see the universe in simplistic good and evil terms and are quick to stereotype their enemies and tend to act first and think later. They inhabit the *id* of the Star Trek universe. Teens find hotheads humorous (Worf: "I am Klingon. If you doubt it, a demonstration can be arranged") but also can identify well with the contrasting emotional valences portrayed by the mix of supporting characters in relation to the pivotal captain superhero in each episode.

Captain Janeway, the female captain of *Voyager*, is just one of many strong female characters that populate the Star Trek universe. The television show has long pioneered the depiction of women in strong, positive leadership roles, as well as being very empathetic, nurturing, sexy, and in control. Janeway's character offers an excellent venue to explore the often competing demands placed on girls and women in society. Female adolescents may find an interesting contrast between Janeway's strong, stoic, and steely-eyed style, and the compassionate, empathetic, and nurturing ways of Counselor Deana Troi. These characters and their contrasting emotional valences can stimulate discussion of "What does it mean to be female or feminine?" and other explorations of gender roles and expectations.

Mr. Spock, the logical Vulcan science officer of ST-TOS, is cool, unemotional, and logical; in many ways he illustrates the cognitive–behavioral capacity to use our rational thinking to control our emotionality. Spock typically models high-level abstract formal reasoning, thinks three-dimensionally, and brainstorms with others to overcome problems. An excellent example is how Kirk and Spock together outthink and foil Ricardo Montalban's Kahn character in ST-II: *The Wrath of Khan* (Meyer, 1982). Many of the original *Star Trek* episodes depict an unemotional Mr. Spock calming hotheaded crewmembers, such as ship surgeon Leonard McCoy, who lusts for action or revenge—a more "human" response. The character of Mr. Spock is extremely self-confident, capable of contending with threat, and masterfully in control of science and technology to do his bidding (Lichtenberg et al., 1975).

Similarly, Commander Data of ST-TNG is an android who has no emotions at all; but like Pinocchio, wishes he could be more human. When he serendipitously meets his twin, who gives him an emotion chip for his positronic brain, Data is soon overwhelmed by emotions and must disable the device. Yet, this character is truly a superhero with superhuman strength and intellect. Data offers many useful metaphors for therapeutic contexts and the concept of turning off an overloaded "emotion chip" can be very appealing for teens.

Just as Spock and Data provide a useful vehicle for exploring emotions, many interesting opportunities exist in the Star Trek series for exploring gender issues. For example, during one of the early episodes (*The Trouble with Tribbles*), Communications Officer Uhura (an African American command officer) wanted to adopt cute little fuzzy aliens called Tribbles. However, Captain Kirk refused to allow them on the ship. This plot offered an excellent contrast between nurturing and authoritarian approaches to parenting, often attributed respectively to women and men. Other episodes of both the original and subsequent series offer additional opportunities to explore gender-based and relationship issues.

The cast and crew of ST offer many opportunities to explore diverse personality types. If ST is a shared interest, then therapists may consider assigning ST episodes as enjoyable "homework" assignments for later discussion. The Star Trek characters offer personality and emotional patterns that can be referenced when exploring a client's temperament, emotional control, interests, and choice of role models. Table 13.2 shows how popular ST characters can be placed into personality and emotional categories. This offers an opportunity for exploring how we are both

Table 13.2 "To Boldly Go!": StarTrek Hero Characteristics and Therapeutic Uses

Series/Film	Captain Leader, Strategic Thinker, Moral	Command Staff Brains, Logic, Loyalty	Counselors Caregiver, Empathic	"Hothead" Prone to Acting Out with Strong Emotions	Sidekicks Comic Relief, Humor, Emotive
TOS	James T. Kirk (emotive)	Spock—alien (unemotive)	Dr. Leonard McCoy (empathic)	Mr. Scott (Scotty) (emotive)	Chekov (emotive) Sulu (emotive) Uhura (emotive)
TNG	Jean Luc Picard (unemotive)	William T. Riker (emotive) Data—android (unemotive)	Deanna Troi—alien (empathic) Dr. Beverly Crusher (empathic)	Worf—alien (emotive)	Geordi LaForge (unemotive) Barclay (emotive)
Voyager	Kathryn Janeway (unemotive)	Tuvok—alien (unemotive) Chakotay (emotive)	Dr. Schweitzer (medical hologram) (Emotive, empathic) Kes—alien (empathic)	Tom Paris (emotive) B'Elanna Torres—alien (emotive)	Harry Kim (emotive) Neelix—alien (emotive)
DS9	Benjamin Sisko DS9 (emotive but very controlled)	Kira Nerys—Alien (emotive) Dax—Alien (empathic)	Dr. Bashir (empathic)	Odo—alien (emotive) Quark—alien (emotive)	Miles O'Brien (unemotive)
Enterprise	Jonathan Archer (emotive)	T'Pol—Alien (unemotive)	Dr. Phlox (empathic, emotive)	Charles "Trip" Tucker (emotive) Malcolm Reed (emotive)	Hoshi Sato (emotive) Travis Mayweather (emotive)

DS9 = *Star Trek: Deep Space Nine*; TNG = *Star Trek: The Next Generation*; TOS = *Star Trek* (original series).

similar and dissimilar to these characters. They may thus serve as role models who appeal to both male and female adolescents.

Mirror, Mirror: Teen Identification with Star Trek Characters

The various Star Trek characters possess unique psychological and physical characteristics that can be useful when exploring clients' temperament, interests, and emotionality. Many of the Star Trek characters are physically attractive (Cunningham et al., 1995; Gilbert et al., 1998), engage in flirtatious relationships with each other, and have (implied) romantic attachments. It has been argued that sex and sexuality, coupled with fast-paced action and special effects, function as a lure for teen audiences (Chapin, 2000; Ward & Rivadeneyra, 1999), From the overt sexual escapades of James Kirk to the simmering ties between best friends Kira and Odo or between Janeway and Chakotay, the Star Trek universe has always been tinged with, if not underscored by romance. As such, teens can give voice to sexual fantasies and sexual identity issues and struggles.

Some would argue that the characters and story lines of the Star Trek series appeal mostly to children and teens. Although cultural critics may not consider Star Trek to be high art per se, this is not necessarily a disadvantage. With the advent and widespread popularity of violent, banal, and antisocial reality television, the positive messages and morality plays of Star Trek offer a potentially corrective experience for young viewers. Rarely do the ST characters seem motivated by self-indulgence or self-preservation; they are basically polite, deferring, and prosocial. Only rarely do the protagonists become stressed, and when they do, crises are handled, and peace is ultimately restored. Although the occasional life and death struggles raise the tension level, violence and aggression often surrender to the cool and collected power of these attractive space heroes.

The peculiarly sophomoric presentation of the future in the Star Trek universe may also be appealing to teens, who are just beginning to consider abstractions and alternative realities. Painfully self-absorbed, these young viewers may be able to readily identify with some of the more pensive and introspective characters who struggle with deeply personal and moral dilemmas. By identifying with some of these futuristic heroes, teens can create alternate solutions on a holodeck of their own making, communicate with an empath, or simply slip away into the future to work out problems of the moment. Finally, there is the ubiquitous element of humor that permeates the dialogue and relationships on Star Trek. This serves as an excellent icebreaker and rapport builder for self-conscious young clients.

"To Boldly Go!" Tips for the Therapeutic Use of Star Trek Themes and Characters

As was earlier noted, Star Trek is a familiar component of adolescent popular and media culture. Its many characters and themes provide a universe of metaphors and symbols that can be incorporated into both the process and content of therapy with adolescents. Star Trek–related discussions with the interested adolescent can lead to an exploration of gender, racial, identity, and relational issues. Counselors may engage their clients through discussions of particular television and movie scenes that are relevant to their lives or may address issues through metaphoric conversation and problem solving. As most social and personal dilemmas in the Star Trek universe are resolved peaceably, counselors can assist their clients in learning effective ways of self-regulation and interpersonal peacemaking. Following are some tips for accomplishing these objectives. A discussion of Blake, a fascinating young man who allowed me to enter his universe with the assistance of the rich and diverse metaphors of Star Trek, follows as well.

- Mr. Spock's ongoing struggle to control his emotional human side through the use of logic is a vehicle for adolescents attempting to contain and direct their impulsivity. Use Spock's mind-quieting exercises and autohypnosis to help clients learn to self-regulate. (ST:TOS episodes 45- *A Private Little War* and 50-*By Any Other Name*)
- Commander Data has an electronic emotion chip that can be turned on and off at will—a metaphor for self-control and self-restraint. Therapeutic discussions around hypothetical questions such as, "How would you use an emotion chip if you had one?" can be productive. (ST:TNG episodes 152 and 153-*Descent*, 13-*Datalore*, and 77-*Brothers*)
- Navigator Ensign Sulu's job is to monitor the viewing screen on the bridge of the *Enterprise*. Ask a client to pretend that he or she is Mr. Sulu, and use the screen into deep space as a projector for fantasies.
- In an early ST:TOS episode, Kirk and crew transport to an Eden-like world where their light and dark fantasies come to life. Ask clients, "What would you conjure up if you could go to that planet?" (ST:TOS episode 17-*Shore Leave*)
- In an early episode of ST-TOS, alien telepaths called the Talosians capture several of the crewmembers and bring to life their most concealed memories. Ask clients, "If the Talosians looked into your memories and changed them into reality, how would your life be different?" (ST:TOS episode 16-*The Menagerie*)

- Discussing the personalities of the various Star Trek heroes and the dilemmas the client was experiencing, ask them to consider "What would ____ do in this situation?" Engage clients in a discussion of their favorite and least favorite of the Star Trek characters with questions such as, "What makes that person your favorite?" "How would your life be different if you were ____?" and "Is there a character you find attractive?"
- The mind-over-muscle conflict permeates Star Trek. Kirk and Picard constantly battle to outsmart much more physically adept opponents. Ask clients to imagine solving some of the social dilemmas in their life in each of these ways and then compare the possible outcomes. (ST:TOS episode 19-*Arena*)
- As the first female captain in the Star Trek universe, Janeway models strength, compassion, and resilience for her female (and male) audience. Ask clients to consider the stereotyped ways that both men and women are depicted in both media and society, and how they can break through these in their own lives.
- In contrast to Janeway, Barclay is a nervous, imperfect character—a loner lacking in confidence and locked in his own world of anxiety. As a result, he becomes addicted to the escapism made possible on the holodeck. Use this character as a focus for discussions of addiction, defenses, and unhealthy and healthy coping. (ST:TNG episode 128-*Realm of Fear*, 69-*Hollow Pursuits*, ST:VOY 130-*Pathfinder*)
- In the premier episode of ST-TNG, the viewer is introduced to the holodeck, a bigger-than-life-sized virtual-reality stage on which crew members can be anyone they like or travel anywhere they choose. Ask clients to imagine having a holodeck with which they could be anyone they chose or travel throughout history. (ST:TNG episode 1-*Encounter at Farpoint*)

SHIP COUNSELOR'S LOG: THE CASE OF BLAKE

This is the rather unusual case of an adolescent male with anxiety episodes associated with an undiagnosed reading disorder. Blake was 17 years old when he first came to my attention. His mother contacted me to ask whether I would tutor him for the Scholastic Achievement Test (SAT). He was subsequently referred to a clinical psychotherapist, assessment specialists, and other members of the team. The case was reconstructed from notes obtained from Blake's the lead therapist. Because dialogue was not tape recorded, parts of the case are reconstructed from notes.

Blake was a remarkable teen—robust, healthy, smart, imaginative, talkative, outgoing, and confident. However, he experienced episodes of panic related to academic performance. Blake was preparing to graduate from high school the following year and stated from the outset that one of his goals was to attend Harvard University to major in mathematics or physics. On the other hand, Blake seemed high-strung as he tapped his foot incessantly and seemed uncomfortable in his chair. He stood over 6 feet tall and was a very muscular student athlete who had participated in wrestling since ninth grade. Blake was now a junior and the captain of the high school wrestling team. His mother Emily was a divorced woman in her mid-40s and lived with Blake and his 13-year-old sister, Hannah. Blake's mother explained that he was "stressed out about school and the SAT" and that he had recently experienced several panic episodes in school. She was familiar with his strong desire to attend Harvard, and that as a student he excelled in some courses (such as math and science), but performed poorly in English and history. Blake's mother said that he was "bored with some of his teachers because he was so exceptional."

Blake was very animated whenever we discussed scientific concepts. He was a formal operational thinker who could discuss abstract and complex matters. Blake told me that he was "stressed" preparing for the SAT test and that a lot was riding on that exam. He told me of two occasions when he suffered anxiety reactions at school, which included hyperventilation, flushing, feeling faint, and nausea.

Blake and I shared an interest in Star Trek television shows. He came to share with me through play and conversation some of his fantasies about Star Trek superheroes. Blake particularly identified with characters from Star Trek. He saw himself as a starship science officer with a dream of conquering Harvard and the business world and perhaps even going into space someday. He persuasively argued that as a physically fit person with a physics degree from Harvard, he could someday patent inventions and build successful companies. His conviction and earnest, albeit rehearsed, defense of this grandiose scheme suggested that he had given it much thought.

During one of our conversations, Blake saw some Star Trek paperbacks on my bookshelf and commented that he did not think someone like me would be into Star Trek. I offered to lend him a book, but he declined saying he was "too busy to read right now." I soon discovered that Blake could not read well. This would be a seemingly insurmountable challenge for someone who was Harvard bound. Subsequent psychological testing revealed that while his comprehension, memory, problem-solving, and general intellectual skills were above average, his verbal skills were uneven, and he had significant deficits in reading comprehension and vocabulary. One of my earliest thoughts was "How had Blake gotten through high school so far?" I came to learn that he was an amazing word memorizer, who could recognize many words without sounding them out. This allowed him to read at the elementary to middle school level and was sufficient for moderate success at his public school. His grades allowed him to remain on the wrestling team, an important activity in Blake's life. He agreed to work with me to prepare for the SAT test, so that he could pursue his dream of going to Harvard. Blake was initially resistant to feedback about his reading problems.

I was unsure whether Blake would respond to therapeutic play. Some adolescents resist play therapy because it seems juvenile to them at a time when they are desperate to project a grown-up image. Blake was sufficiently mature that we could work within a cognitive–behavioral approach. The cognitive goals were to help Blake understand his limitations in reading, and to rewrite his internal dialogue, which centered around making excuses for his poor performance on verbal tests. I also thought it would be important to help Blake consider that, despite his difficulty with reading, he was otherwise a strong student. We would explore his perspective about the unduly high importance he attributed to SAT scores and how this was driving his anxiety. We would examine his fixation and dream of "going to Harvard" and work to develop diverse, realistic additional goals. On a behavioral level, I planned to help Blake recognize anxiety symptoms and reduce his stress response with imagery, breathing, and relaxation techniques.

Studies suggest that many children show a discrepancy between overall IQ and school achievement as the result of difficulties in reading (Shaywitz et al., 1990). As many as 25% of poor readers have very high IQs and reading scores well below their grade level. Researchers have examined the way children read including their errors and the various aspects of the reading process that are particularly difficult for them (Ehri, 1998; Fletcher et al., 1994; Francis et al., 1996; Shaywitz et al., 1990; Stahl & Murray, 1998; Stanovich & Siegel, 1994). These authors have consistently demonstrated that most children move through a series of stages, becoming increasingly sophisticated at using letter-sound knowledge to identify words. As in Blake's case, readers who have not developed this orthographic knowledge, have other language skills that can enable them to read without phonological awareness (Perfetti et al., 1987).

It Is Cold in Space: Using Star Trek to Break the Ice and Build Rapport

T: So you said you like Star Trek? Check out these figures.

BLAKE: Oh yeah. I have watched all the old shows and the *Next Generation* on TV. Those are cool [picks up some action figures].

T: These are fun. Which do you know?

BLAKE: "This is Superman, Batman, and Darth Vader. This is the captain."

T: Do you know his name?

BLAKE: Yeah ... sure ... Captain Picard. Jean Luc Picard.

T: That's right!

[Blake picks another figure from shelf.]

T: Who's that?

BLAKE: The Klingon guy who works for Picard. He's called Worf. He's cool. He's a bad ass.

T: What do you like about these characters?

BLAKE: I like Kirk. He is the big star of the original *Star Trek*.

T: Oh so you know about Captain Kirk?

BLAKE: Oh sure—everyone knows about Kirk and Picard. They're cool. They have phasers and tractor beams and stuff like that. They travel faster than light. Stuff like that is awesome.

T: Captain Kirk has Mr. Spock, and Captain Picard has Mr. Data and Worf.

BLAKE: Yeah ... Data has like superstrength and genius brains and stuff.... Picard always has him to help out.

T: Do you have any special friends who help you out?

BLAKE: No. But well, sort of. I guess "Cosmo" is my friend. His name is actually Raphael, but I call him Cosmo ... he is on the team. I can count on him to watch my back.

T: What do you mean "watch your back?"

[Blake remains silent.]

T: How do you think it helps to have Cosmo on your side?

Blake [Looking away and into the distance]: Cosmo's my "bud" ... he and I might open a company some day. I plan to open a company after Harvard. I was going to get a PhD in physics first, maybe double major with chemistry or engineering so I can build and invent stuff. I figure then its better to start up a company to sell my inventions and ideas and stuff. I can be the head of a big company, and that's like being Picard because you lead people, tell them what to do, have people on your team. Other people try to mess with you or bring you down. They, like, talk behind your back and stuff. There are a few on the team who don't really care about the team and stuff, so Cosmo usually lets me know what's up, even if I am not there, and he lets me know what people are saying. I can count on him so that's cool.

I had now heard about Blake's dream of a career as an entrepreneur and inventor. He had confessed to some social insecurity (despite trying to portray a macho image). This sports-based peer rivalry and close bonding with protective friends is considered "normal" for teens, particularly school athletes (Adler & Adler, 1998; Messner, 1992). I thought his comments were grandiose and narcissistic, which is also not uncommon among adolescent males (Bleiberg, 2001; Kohut, 1977; Lapan & Patton, 1986). I was intrigued by Blake's identification with the character of Captain Picard—he seemed to have an internal script of himself as the hero and captain. I had asked Blake whether he would consider other alternatives such as going to the state university. He was adamant that he needed to go to Harvard and no place else. We talked about his feeling of pressure to do well at school and how he needed friends like Cosmo to "watch his back." We had established a nice rapport, using ST as a common interest. I lent Blake a DVD of a *Star Trek* episode so we could discuss it next time. He seemed pleased with this type of homework.

When we next met, Blake and I explored his current feelings of anxiety about school. He was concerned that he would not do well on the verbal portion of the SAT. I asked if this would effect his decision to apply to Harvard. He said, "No, because my dad knows someone there who will contact admissions for me."

T: So you are confident you will go to Harvard?

BLAKE: Yes, my dad has a connection, so he will help me when I apply.

T: But won't you have to perform well on the verbal SAT?

BLAKE: Well, I would like to, you know, get a high score. I am going to do well in math. I just don't know what I can get on the English parts. I know I have to break 500 or even my Dad's contact can't do anything for me. I will be able to go for a wrestling scholarship if I can just break 500 on the verbals.

T: Tell me about the Verbal part.

BLAKE: English is fine. I have lots of vocab down pat. No problems there. I don't do well on some of the other parts.

T: So you are feeling good about vocabulary, that's great! But you are not sure about some of the reading parts?

BLAKE: Yup, pretty much.

T: You know those doctors in Star Trek? If I could just use one of those tricorders on you, what do you think it would tell me Blake? [I wave an imaginary tricorder over Blake.]

BLAKE: [Laughs] It would say "red alert" to reading because that is the problem, sort of that I freak when I see those long reading questions.

T: OK. So you are worried you won't do well on the reading comprehension items . . . is that right?

BLAKE: Yes, I guess so. At least the harder ones. Those are tricky.

T: OK. Let's see if we can figure out what's going on.

We didn't have a "tricorder" so I asked Blake to read for me from a Star Trek book. He looked solemn as he began to read slowly. He read until he got to a word he did not know. He reached the word *incongruous* and stopped. He said "in- . . ., in- . . ." and he pointed at it for me to see. I said "incongruous," and I was going to define it for him, and he said, "Oh yes, incongruous, things that are not conforming to expectations." This response seemed odd to me. Blake continued to read and came to another word he did not know. This time it was *continuum*. I took the book, flipped to some other pages, and selected another paragraph. His body language became tense and anxious. He said, "I don't want to read out loud like a baby, that is not why I am here. Can we work on some vocab drills or something?" It was an abrupt change in his tone. We stopped reading to reduce his anxiety. I showed him an SAT preparation book. He seemed pleased to have something else on which to focus. He did not wish to work on math because he asserted, "I will do fine on the quantitative part." We worked on vocabulary words, and he offered to make some flashcards of the ones he missed. I again asked if he wanted to borrow a Star Trek book. Blake squirmed in his seat and provided elaborate excuses about pressure on his time and how he had no time for pleasure reading. I asked him about reading tests.

BLAKE: Yeah, I guess that is the part of the SAT that I'm worried about.

T: Tell me about what it feels like when you take these reading tests.

Blake I get tensed up . . . I start to feel upset.

T: You feel tense?

BLAKE: Yeah . . . I know this is the part I screw up . . . and it frustrates me because the questions are just so stupid and just a lot of reading.

T: When does it start to get you upset?

BLAKE: It can start whenever I even think about the [expletive] SAT . . . this verbal test is [expletive]. I guess I am not a great reader.

T: Blake, you are a smart person, and you can learn to do this. But you have to work at it. It's just like anything else. Were you good at driving the first time you tried it?

BLAKE: Ha, not really.... I was like all over the place ... kept stopping short and stuff. It made my dad nervous to drive with me.

T: But now how is your driving? I notice you drive here to see me.

BLAKE: Oh, I am good at driving now ... its fine. It's like I practiced and just got better.

T: Well, I think it's going to be the same with reading. You need to practice and you get better.

BLAKE: I have been trying to read. I am just not good at it.

T: Maybe no one has taken the time to show you the trick to doing it better?

BLAKE: What's the trick?

T: I think the trick is just being able to sound out the words, but you were never really taught how. I know someone who can show you. Right now, reading is difficult for you, and it makes your feel stressed.

BLAKE: I am not in the mood to take more classes or sit with babies who don't know how to read. It's boring. I don't want to be in a rejects class.

[At this point, a decision was made to supportively confront Blake's unwillingness to commit to his own stated goal of improving his situation.]

T: I can see what you mean. In the past, when they asked you to take a reading class, it seemed like special education and marked you as not doing well. I can't blame you for feeling too embarrassed to partici-pate in that. But this is different. This is not for babies Blake. you are not being left back or given remedial work at school. This will be at a private company, and you will be working with someone privately. There will be no one other students to be compared with. No ba-bies and no rejects, I am sure. Plenty of adults need to improve their reading. That's all this is.

BLAKE: I really don't have time for this right now. We have wrestling season and I am kind of busy. [pause] I know, you are going to say I am procrastinating again. But really, I am swamped.

T: Blake, I remember when I was in college and the stress was getting to me, too. I really know how you feel. But one reason you feel so swamped might be that you have to work extra hard. It could become easier for you once your reading improves. Blake, let me ask you something. What would Jean Luc Picard do when there is a problem on the *Enterprise*? Does he say he is too busy to deal with it?

BLAKE: No, Picard always takes charge ... makes the decision and just says, "Make it so!" He is cool that way.

T: Why don't we try to ask what Picard would do in your situation?

BLAKE: [Pauses, thinking] Well ... he would find some way to solve this. I don't know. No one seems to have a reading test on Star Trek

T: Yes, but what would Picard do, or what might he tell a crewmember with this problem to do?

BLAKE: If I was on the crew, I guess he would order me to take care of the problem. Get the training or whatever it took.

T: And what if Picard had a problem ... would he avoid it?

BLAKE: No ... he would probably try to fix whatever the problem was.

T: Let's try to follow Picard's advice. Let's try to fix the problem. What do you say?

BLAKE: OK. I can try

T: I am sending you to a pretty high-tech place. They use computers. It's very futuristic, maybe it is like what they would use on the Enterprise.

BLAKE: "OK I guess that might be cool."

T: That would be great Blake. I'd appreciate it if you give it a try.

I was pleased that we used Blake's favorite Star Trek character (Captain Picard) as a role model and that this had helped to motivate him to take charge of his problem. He was referred for reading help. I also gave Blake a DVD to borrow with holodeck episodes (ST-TNG episode 13-*The Big Goodbye*, in which a stressed out Captain Picard blows off steam as Detective Dixon Hill, and ST-VOY episode 79-*Concerning Flight*, in which Captain Janeway meets Leonardo da Vinci, who helps her to solve a mystery).

Report to the Holodeck! Star Trek Play Therapy

In another session, I confirmed that Blake had begun his tutoring with a reading specialist. He continued demonstrating some agitation and anxiety, usually associated with a perceived pressure to excel. The pressure seemed to come from within, when his dream of going to Harvard was thwarted by his below-par reading. He persisted in saying he wanted to go to Harvard to become a physicist with the help of his father's "special contact."

T: Did you watch any of the episodes about the holodeck? Tell me about
that.

[We discussed the two holodeck episodes.]

T: Did you find that realistic? Does a captain get to be fooling around like
that on the Holodeck?

BLAKE: Yeah, I guess even Picard needs to chill out sometimes! [laughs]

Blake then spoke at length about the importance of sports in his
life and how he was captain of the wrestling team. Blake explained that
"Captains are under a lot of stress" and that they need to "blow off
steam." He said there was no harm in Picard doing so on the holodeck,
and his crew would call him if they needed him. Blake seemed to identify
with Captain Picard. I drew a parallel between play therapy and the ST
holodeck.

T: [referring to action figures] This is kind of like the holodeck, Blake,
because we can make up any kind of stories we want. It's not as cool
as the holodeck, but are you willing to give it a try? [pause, Blake
thinking it over.] After all, Blake, even Captain Picard allows himself
fun time in the holodeck.

BLAKE: OK . . . but it still seems kind of lame.

I asked Blake to reenact the part of the episode with the holodeck
to help me to remember it. Blake overcame his resistance and narrated
the sequence using several voices. I praised his talent at doing this, and
in response, he was beaming. The use of the holodeck metaphor and
Blake's superhero, Captain Picard, was helpful in introducing the process
of fantasy play. The episode modeled recreational activity as therapeutic.
This allowed Blake to play with me, as something that "even Captain
Picard needed to do sometimes."

Blake showed me how Captain Picard could dispatch some of the
Borg—a predatory cyber civilization. He used chess pieces to represent
Borg, and he knocked them over. He showed me how Picard would stun
them but not kill the enemy, but Blake said he would probably kill them
because "the Borg are like evil, dude, you have to just kill them or they
keep coming back like zombies." I resurrected the chess pieces and moved
them toward Captain Picard and called in reinforcements from the assem-
bly of action figures. Blake enjoyed this and soon allowed himself to play
in this way with me for several minutes. It became clear to Blake that by
using Star Trek, we could have some fun while at the same time, doing
some serious work. I also found it very appealing to use a favorite pastime
to build rapport and strengthen my empathy—without being judgmental.
I was fascinated by Blake's idealization of Captain Picard, as a symbol

of strength, drive, and ambition. As the session ended, I once again gave Blake a Star Trek episode to watch for homework and suggested that we could discuss it during our next meeting.

Star Date Mind Meld: Blake's Healing Trance

Blake again spoke of his plans for attending Harvard University. He was fixated on this singular goal, and although he was an exceptional student of science and mathematics, his language grades were poor. This grandiose fixation on attaining entry to Harvard was unrealistic, and certainly Blake seemed to be putting all of his goals in one basket. Blake was internally driven and hard on himself, and I was mindful to try to monitor how much he was taking on as we went forward. Nonetheless, so far, we had a nice rapport going, and he was willing to continue working with me on his stress and anxiety. Still, he seemed to be a very driven and intense young man.

I showed Blake some stretching exercises, and he responded well. He even taught me some movements his school wrestling team used to limber up. I then showed Blake a video clip from ST:TOS episode 45-*A Private Little War*. This featured Mr. Spock who has gone into a "healing trance." I felt this metaphor might be useful for Blake to develop some relaxation and mind–body techniques, especially when he became anxious at the prospect of reading tests. Blake was riveted by the show.

Blake and I also worked on a "healing trance" similar to the one used by Mr. Spock. First I talked him through a relaxation procedure, and he responded well. I reminded him that this relaxation technique combined with an instruction to "imagine you are Mr. Spock and you can control all of your emotions," could help him reduce anxiety. We worked on visualizing ourselves as Mr. Spock entering his "healing trance." After that, Blake took about 20 minutes to complete another assessment, and I then turned on the gaming console as a reward while I scored his test. While playing the game, Blake was more animated and uninhibited than I had seen. He enjoyed the game, and he liked that I was watching him and asking the occasional question. I praised his good marksmanship, and after a period of game time, we ended the session.

Fire Phasers! Video Game Incentives and Exploring Academic Skills

Blake showed interest when I introduced a video game system. The game allowed the player to chase down and "shoot" aliens on a strange oth-erworldly landscape. Blake had previously resisted working on practice academic achievement tests for me. He agreed that SAT preparation was one goal of our working together. Blake's anxiety about testing was un-derstandable and test anxiety is a well established problem for motivated teens at this level (Samson, 1980; Spielberger & Vagg, 1995). In the spirit of desensitizing Blake to the testing context and to give us a chance to practice our stress management skills, I felt it was appropriate to rein-troduce practice testing into our time together (Dendato & Diener, 1986; Kennedy & Doepke, 1999). In response to my suggestion, Blake agreed to take a practice test for me, and in exchange, he would get to "check out the game system." I reminded Blake that the test did not count for anything—it was just a practice test, and he should do his best, but to try not to become upset. The video game was used as a reward to motivate Blake to work on some testing to desensitize him.

Red Alert: Turning off Blake's Emotion Chip

In another session, Blake told me about his panic attack at school. This was a particularly embarrassing and sensitive subject for him. Because he was familiar with the Star Trek shows, I asked if he knew about Mr. Data and his emotion chip. He said he was not sure. This time, I showed Blake part of two episodes of ST:TNG (ST:TNG episode 13-*Datalore*, and ST:TNG episode 77-*Brothers*). These are episodes that explain how Commander Data was built as a robot who initially did not have an "emotion chip," and thus no emotions. Data's twin brother Lore, who has an emotion chip, implants it into Data to destroy him. When Data receives the emotion chip, he suffers from an excess of emo-tional reaction that literally shuts him down. I used this material as a metaphor to discuss with Blake how emotional reactions can some-times overload and disable us. Following this, we would try to con-trol our own "emotion chip" by using techniques like turning it off, or combined with the Vulcan healing trance to calm our minds and turn off excess emotions. Blake understood why I had selected these episodes.

BLAKE: "You think my emotion chip is malfunctioning like Data?"

T: Well, you are not a robot, so you don't have an emotion chip, but yes, there is something similar about the way your emotional reaction overwhelmed you at school.

BLAKE: Yeah, I guess you could say I went into overload mode.

T: Does anyone really have total control of our emotions?

BLAKE: No, not really. Humans are not Vulcan. We cannot help being emotional.

T: Right, we are human and so try not to be so embarrassed about that. It happens to all of us.

BLAKE: I bet it doesn't happen to you.

T: Not true! In fact I can tell you about a time when I really overloaded. [I proceeded to self-disclose to Blake a time when I was extremely upset about some work I was doing and that I had snapped at people because I was so stressed out and lost control. I said, I'm a psychologist, but I am also still a human, and this is what happened to me].

BLAKE: Yeah ... I guess we have to accept that sometimes we just get freaked out.

T: Do you sometimes still feel freaked out?

BLAKE: I was mostly freaked about the SAT thing, but now that I am doing something about it ... I still don't love to read or anything ... but I don't feel like I am going to hurl every time there is a test.

T: How are you able to control your human emotions, Blake?

BLAKE: Like we have talked about ... you just have to realize what is happening. When I get butterflies in my stomach or start feeling weird, I realize I am stressed out. I take deep breaths and do the muscle thing (I had shown Blake progressive muscle relaxation). I just do the Vulcan mind trance, and like Data.... I could tell myself to "turn down my emotion chip so I won't seem to go into a freak-out mode."

T: Do you think you will be able to take a practice test for me today?

BLAKE: Yes ... I can do it. Not sure how good I can do, but I am willing to try it

T: Excellent Blake ... just having a positive attitude like this is going to help you do better.

We practiced inducing his relaxation response before beginning a practice test. I praised Blake and summarized the positive skills he was developing.

Resistance Is Futile: Termination of Therapy

Blake stopped working with me soon after the preceding conversation. He had also stopped visiting the clinical psychotherapist but was continuing with his reading tutor. I spoke to both him and his mother to discourage them from discontinuing therapy, but both seemed to have reached the consensus that therapy was no longer needed. I did not resist because their tone was positive, optimistic, and forward-looking, and I had to admit that good progress had been made. Blake had not had another panic attack since the original episodes. According to his mother, Blake's work at the Learning Center (reading tutor) was very helpful to him. Within just a few weeks, he had improved his reading scores. His mother even remarked that he was reading more at home, something she rarely noticed him doing before. I suggested she purchase Star Trek comic books to encourage this behavior and sent her an e-mail with links to Star Trek Web sites that are popular with teens. Apparently, by providing some basic phonetic reading skills, Blake quickly integrated them into his repertoire of other reading skills and showed good progress in his reading and comprehension. Blake ultimately took the SAT college board and scored exceptionally well in the quantitative area, but poorly in the verbal. Blake was aware that higher scores were needed for Ivy League college admission. What came as a surprise was that in my last conversation, Blake's mother told me that he decided to forgo applying to college for awhile. He was working for his father and apparently doing quite well. He planned to earn some money, take the SAT again, and then apply to colleges the following year. He had not yet given up on his dreams, and we all hoped he was still college bound in the future.

CONCLUSIONS: CAPTAIN'S LOG—BEAM ME UP!

I have explained how Star Trek provides a unique blend of supercharacters, utopian futuristic ideals, and science fiction stories with moral dilemmas and strong psychoemotional content. The use of Star Trek themes, as suggested in this chapter, is just one more way that superheroes can be used as symbols and metaphors in therapeutic work. Perhaps adding Star Trek action figures to your collection of play objects or revisiting the old episodes now available on DVD may offer a shared context for building rapport and exploring issues with adolescents and perhaps adults who are familiar with Star Trek. The series of television programs and films offer a unique diversity of characters and characteristics that lend themselves in a particularly useful way to working with teens and children. The heroes are easily identified with, have specific personalities and emotional valences, and, although many key characters are human, they nonetheless have superhero qualities. Star Trek characters employ technology, alien friends, and superior reasoning to overcome adversity and in so doing, present a positive image of the future for mankind.

From the alien Mr. Spock, whose emotional control can be an effective model for clients with anger control problems, to Mr. Data's "emotion chip" that can be turned on and off at will, Star Trek provides powerful messages about emotionality. These examples can be employed as an adjunct to relaxation or other cognitive–behavioral techniques to reduce anxiety reactions. On a similar note, there are projective tools, such as using a tricorder to "read" your client, employing Mr. Spock's Vulcan mind meld for a "look" into a client's mind, or using Mr. Sulu's viewing screen for a look into the future (or past).

The therapeutic application of Star Trek with adults has been documented, albeit minimally (Forrest, 2005). However, no such documentation exists for the use of Star Trek with adolescents. The case of Blake demonstrates how rapport could be built around a common interest in Star Trek and how one teen's identification Captain Picard paralleled his own personal struggles. Blake looked at himself as a captain and hero of his own *Enterprise,* but became anxious when his reading problem came to the surface, and he realized that his grand plans for attending Harvard might need to be amended. Nevertheless, it was his strong identification with a future such as that presented in Star Trek and the idea that heroes do not give up, that were among his most positive assets. Blake remained motivated by his dreams and showed excellent promise to maintain his momentum to overcome his reading challenges. This underlying confidence, which was reinforced during Star Trek discussions, will serve him well as he moves ahead.

Blake was not open at first to therapeutic play until he was reminded that even Captain Picard would engage in fantasy play on the holodeck. This idea was enormously appealing to this teen and may be a helpful way to introduce adolescents to therapeutic play techniques. The holodeck, like some of the planets that Star Trek heroes visit, is a place where fantasies become real. This again is a useful way to elicit projective responses to explore the fantasies of a young client. After sharing the holodeck episodes with Blake I could ask, "What would you make happen on the holodeck?" Our shared interest in Star Trek not only enabled the building of rapport but provided many therapeutic reference points to facilitate insight and growth. It is unlikely that Blake would have felt comfortable entering into this working relationships were it not for our common bonds with the Star Trek stories of the future.

Star Trek offers many additional opportunities for introducing, discussing, and role-playing a wide range of psychosocial themes. As shown, there are many ways to use the material—from jargon to video clips to use of action figures in play. From issues of war and prejudice, to personal issues of love, friendship, and duty, the Star Trek teleplays provide a wide range of useful therapeutic and educational metaphors. The positive outlook portrayed in the Star Trek future offers healthy models for adolescents, in contrast to many other media products that are popular with teens but may offer few redeeming characteristics. Roddenberry's dream of a diverse utopian future continues not only to entertain but to inspire. Greenwald (1998) documented how Star Trek has inspired

NASA astronauts and jet propulsion scientists to pursue their careers and counts notable visionaries such as Stephen Hawking and Arthur C. Clark as fans. It is this popular familiarity, Star Trek's positive optimism for the future, and a rich tapestry of humanistic characters and story lines that can provide a unique vehicle for working with adolescents.

Star Trek's diversity can offer a bridge into teens' unique culture. Unlike many media depictions of racial tension and divide, Star Trek offers a positive integrated view of humanity's future. This is a powerful message of tolerance and forgiveness for those working with racial and ethnic or cultural issues. If humans and Klingons can get along, certainly humans should be able to do so as well. So, enter the wormhole into another universe. Enter the playful fantasy world of Star Trek and boldly go into psychotherapy with the Star Trek superheroes.

REFERENCES

Adler, P. A., & Adler, P. (1998). *Peer power: Preadolescent culture and identity*. Piscataway, NJ: Rutgers University Press.

Bleiberg, E. (2001). *Treating personality disorders in children and adolescents: A relational approach*. New York: Guilford Press.

Bole, C., Carson, D., Chalmers, C., Compton, R., Landau, L., & Legato, R. (Directors). (1987). *Star trek: The next generation* [Television series]. United States: Paramount Television.

Brooker, W. (2001). *Batman unmasked: Analyzing a cultural icon*. New York: Continuum Publishing Group International.

Butler, R., Chomsky, M., Daniels, M., & Wallerstein, H. (Directors). (1966). *Star trek* [Television series]. United States: Desilu Productions.

Campbell, J. (1956). *The hero with a thousand faces*. New York. Meridian Press.

Caprio, B. J. (1978). *Star trek: Good news in modern images*. Riverside, NJ: Andrews McMeel Publishing.

Chapin, J. R. (2000). Adolescent sex and mass media: A developmental approach. *Adolescence, 35*, 799–811.

Cunningham, M. R., Roberts, A. R, Barbee, A. P., Duren, P. B., & Wu, C. H. (1995). Their ideas of beauty are, on the whole, the same as ours: Consistency and variability in the cross cultural perception of female physical attractiveness. *Journal of Personality and Social Psychology, 68*, 261–279.

Dendato, K. M., & Diener, D. (1986). Effectiveness of cognitive/relaxation therapy and study-skills training in reducing anxiety and improving academic performance of test-anxious students. *Journal of Counseling Psychology, 33*, 131–135.

Dorn, M. (Director). (1993). *Star trek: Deep space nine* [Television series]. United States: Paramount Television.

Ehri, L. C. (1998). Grapheme-phoneme knowledge is necessary for learning to read words in English. In J. Metsala & L. C. Ehri (Eds.), *Word recognition in beginning literacy*, Mahwah, NJ: Erlbaum.

Fingeroth, D. (2004). *Superman on the couch: What superheroes really tell us about ourselves and our society.* New York: NY: Continuum International.

Fletcher, J. M., S. E. Shaywitz, D. P. Shankweiler, L., Katz, I. Y., Liberman, K. K. et al. (1994). Cognitive profiles of reading disability: Comparisons of discrepancy and low achievement definitions. *Journal of Educational Psychology 86*, 6–23.

Forrest, D. (2005). Consulting to Star Trek: To boldly go into dynamic neuropsychiatry. *Journal of American Academy of Psychoanalysis and Dynamic Psychiatry, 33*, 71–83.

Frakes, J., & Williams, A. (Directors). (1995). *Star trek: Voyager* [Television series]. United States: Paramount Television.

Francis, D. J., Shaywitz, S. E., Stuebing, K. K., Shaywitz, B. A., & Fletcher, J. M. (1996). Developmental lag versus deficit models of reading disability: A longitudinal, individual growth curves analysis. *Journal of Educational Psychology, 88*, 3–16.

Gilbert, D. T., Fiske, S., & Lindzey, G. (Eds.). (1998). *The handbook of social psychology*. Boston: McGraw-Hill.

Greenwald, J. (1998). *Future perfect: How star trek conquered planet earth*. New York: Viking Press.

Hoffman, L., & Rose, L. (2005, June 15). Most lucrative movie franchises. *Forbes*. Retrieved September 20, 2006 from http://www.forbes.com/2005/06/15/batman-movie-franchises-cx_lh_lr_0615batman_2.html

Kennedy, D. V., & Doepke, K. J. (1999). Multicomponent treatment of a test anxious college student. *Education and Treatment of Children, 22*, 203–218.

Kohut, H. (1977). *The restoration of the self*. New York: International Universities Press.

Lapan, R., & Patton, M. (1986). Self-psychology and the adolescent process: Measures of pseudoautonomy and peer-group dependence. *Journal of Counseling Psychology, 33*, 136–142.

Lawrence, J. S. (2005). Superman on the couch: What superheroes really tell us about ourselves and our society (Book Review). *Journal of American Culture, 28*, 453–456.

Lawrence, J. S., & Jewett, R. (2002). *The myth of the American superhero*. Cambridge, England: Eerdmans. (See cited chapter 11, "Star Trek's humanistic militarism"; and chapter 12, "Star Trek faith as a fan-made religion").

Lichtenberg, J., Marshak, S., & Winston, J. (1975). *Star trek lives!* New York: Bantam.

Livingston, D., & Vejar, M. (Directors). (2001). *Star trek: Enterprise* [Television series]. United States: Braga Productions.

Messner, M. A. (1992). Boyhood, organized sports, and the construction of masculinities. In M. A. Kimmel & M. A. Messner (Eds.), *Men's lives*. New York: Macmillan.

Meyer, N. (Director). (1982). *Star trek: The wrath of Khan* [Motion picture]. United States: Paramount Pictures.

Perfetti, C. A., Beck, I. L., Bell, L., & Hughes, C. (1987). Phonemic knowledge and learning to read are reciprocal: A longitudinal study of first grade children. *Merrill-Palmer Quarterly, 33,* 283–319.

Samson, L. G. (1980). *Test anxiety: Theory, research, and applications.* Hillsdale, NJ: Erlbaum.

Satzman, D. (2002, January 14). Star Trek saga bringing galaxy of profit to Paramount: Sci-fi series and films provide steady income. *Los Angeles Business Journal; Media and Technology.* Retrieved March 13, 2006 from http://www.findarticles.com/p/articles/mi_m5072/is_2_24/ai_81862137

Shaywitz, S. E., Shaywitz, B. A., Fletcher, J. M., & Escobar, M. D. (1990). Prevalence of reading disability in boys and girls: Results of the Connecticut Longitudinal Study. *Journal of the American Medical Association, 264,* 998–1002.

Spielberger, C. D., & Vagg, P. R. (1995). Test anxiety: Theory, assessment, and treatment. Washington, DC: Taylor & Francis.

Stahl, S. A., & Murray, B. A. (1998). Issues involved in defining phonological awareness and its relation to early reading. In J. Metsala & L. C. Ehri (Eds.), *Word recognition in beginning literacy.* Mahwah, NJ: Erlbaum.

Stanovich, K. E., & L.S. Siegel (1994). Phenotypic performance profiles of children with reading disabilities: A regression-based test of the phonological-core variable-difference model. *Journal of Educational Psychology, 86,* 24–53.

Ward, L. M., & Rivadeneyra, R. (1999). Contributions of entertainment television to adolescents' sexual attitudes and expectations. *Journal of Sex Research, 36,* 237–249.

Star Trek Episodes Mentioned in Text

ST:TOS episodes: 16-*The Menagerie,* 17-*Shore Leave.* 19-*Arena,* 42-*The Trouble With Tribbles;* 45-*A Private Little War;* and 50-*By Any Other Name;* ST:TNG episodes: 1-*Encounter at Farpoint,* 13-*The Big Goodbye,* 13-*Datalore,* 69-*Hollow Pursuits,* 77-*Brothers,* 123-*I Borg,* 128-*Realm of Fear,* and 152 and 153-*Descent;* ST:VOY episodes: 79-*Concerning Flight,* and 130-*Pathfinder.*

Star Trek II: 'The Wrath of Khan.' Star Trek © Paramount Pictures.

APPENDIX A

The Star Trek Canon and the Popularity of Star Trek

Star Trek represents one of the most popular media phenomena in history. An Internet Google search with the phrase "Star Trek" produced more than 17 million hits. Venders list more than 3,000 Star Trek book titles and more than 100 musical recordings for sale. Many adolescents are familiar with Star Trek, and this presents an opportunity to use the series heroes in therapeutic discourse and play. From serious scientific ramifications, to its continued place in the popular culture, Star Trek is an enduring social phenomenon. But you do not have to be a Trekker, Trekkie, or a Star Trek expert to use these themes and heroes in discussions. Star Trek media are familiar and available, and Web sites provide essentials of Star Trek. For example, see the following resources:

- www.startrek.com
- www.stwww.com
- www.trektoday.com
- www.gateworld.net/startrek/characters/index.shtml

Star Trek Television Series

Star Trek: The Original Series (ST:TOS), 1966–1969
Star Trek: The Animated Series, 1973–1974
Start Trek: The Next Generation (ST:TNG), 1987–1994
Deep Space Nine (ST:DS9), 1993–1999
Voyager, 1995–2001
Enterprise, 2001–2005

Star Trek Motion Pictures

I: The Motion Picture (1979)
II: The Wrath of Khan (1982)
III: The Search for Spock (1984)
IV: The Voyage Home (1986)
V: The Final Frontier (1989)
VI: The Undiscovered Country (1991)
Generations (1994)
First Contact (1996)
Insurrection (1998)
Nemesis (2002)

Scholarly Analysis

Professors Robert Sekuler of Brandeis University and Randolph Blake of
    Vanderbilt University present a synthesis of Star Trek, psychology,
    and neuroscience, exploring mind and brain with anecdotes from
    Star Trek episodes and movies. (Sekuler., R., & Blake, R. (1998). *Star
    Trek on the brain: Alien minds, human minds.* New York: Freeman.)
Professor Lawrence M. Krauss, a theoretical physicist, wrote *The Physics
    of Star Trek,* exploring the factual and fictional aspects of Star Trek

technology—from antimatter to phasers to tractor beams. (Krauss, L. M. (1995). *The physics of Star Trek*. New York: Basic Books.)

Judith Barad, PhD, a professor of philosophy at Indiana State University, along with author and journalist Ed Robinson explore the ethics of the Star Trek series in relation to the world's great philosophers and their theories. Moral dilemmas presented in the Star Trek series raise questions about good and evil, right and wrong, power and corruption. Barad, J., & Robertson, E. (2000). *The ethics of Star Trek*. HarperCollins.

Pop Music Based on Star Trek

Title: The Picard Song "Make It So"
Artist: Dark Material
Released: March 1, 2001
Available online: http://tborgax.homepage.dk/audio.html and http://tborgax.homepage.dk/index.html

Star Pilot on Channel K (SPOCK)
"Never Trust a Klingon" and other hits
This Swedish band "S.P.O.C.K." is dedicated to Star Trek, with song and album names from the original series. Available: http://www.subspace.se/spock/

Religion/Philosophy of Star Trek

Lawrence, J. S., & Jewett, R. (2002). Star Trek faith as a man-made religion. In: *The myth of the American superhero*. Cambridge, England: Eerdmans.

Porter, J. E., & McLaren, D.L. (1999). Star Trek and sacred ground: Explorations of Star Trek, religion and American culture. (pp. 245–270). Albany, NY: State University of New York Press.

Kraemer, R. S., Cassidy, W., & Schwartz, S. L. (2003). *The religions of Star Trek*. London: Westview Press.

Hanley R. (1998). *Is Data human? The metaphysics of Star Trek*. New York: Basic Books. An excellent list of academic works on Star Trek and religion and philosophy was developed by Dr. Jennifer Porter, available onlinehttp://www.ucs.mun.ca/~jporter/startrekbiblio.htm

Star Trek Action Figures

www.StarTrekToys.com

CHAPTER FOURTEEN

Hypnosis and Superheroes

Jan M. Burte

From the time we are very young, fantasy is a crucial part of our development. We are taught and intuitively seek out fantasy characters after whom to model ourselves. It is part of our character formation and part of our self-image. As we get older, however, we also get the message that overt behaviors, such as running (flying) with a towel pinned around our neck through the house as Superman is no longer acceptable and so we take it under cover and hide our superhero abilities beneath our more mortal disguises. We create covert fantasy to maintain those identities a little longer. In essence, we become legends in our minds. This is where hypnosis becomes such a powerful tool. In hypnosis, we are again returned to using fantasy as a coping mechanism and for character development. We give ourselves permission to be both Superman and Lex Luthor. Interestingly, hypnosis patients who are caught in their own negative self-hypnotic statements, find it easier to identify themselves as the supervillains such as Darth Vader or with superheroes with negative characteristics, such as the Hulk. After all, in hypnosis you are "not responsible for what your mind chooses." Because of this, I have found in my hypnosis practice that using superheroes and supervillains represents an incredible resource for fostering self-examination, change, and growth.

In this chapter, I hope to detail some of these areas, offer suggested techniques, provide a few caveats, and include vignettes of cases in which superheroes have been especially helpful. I intend to discuss how hypnosis using superheroes has been shown to be an effective tool in treating pain (Burte 2002a, 2004), enhancing psychoneuroimmunological interventions (Burte, 2002b), bolstering ego strength, and overcoming trauma.

I focus this chapter on these three areas of pathology though the use of superheroes in hypnosis can encompass a much broader scope of clinical issues. For children, any condition treated with hypnosis can use super-heroes as part of the metaphorical or storytelling techniques' employed. For adults, a range of conditions such as performance anxiety, insomnia, panic, and anxiety disorders, to name a few, have shown their amenability to using superhero characters in treatment. For adults, superheroes may at times include those we typically identify from contemporary literature or those from more biblical or classical sources of literature. Mythological superheroes are an ingrained part of adult self-concept.

ABOUT HYPNOSIS

Before introducing the use of superheroes in hypnotherapeutic interventions, it may be helpful to provide a brief discussion of hypnosis, especially with regard to how it applies to patients who are experiencing pain and various other medical conditions.

The induction of hypnoidal states via breathing exercises, yoga, and chanting has historical as well as, most likely, prehistoric roots. Were our earliest ancestors entranced by the wall paintings and stories told before the flickering lights within the inner recesses of their caves? Clinical hypnosis, however, can be directly traced back to John Elliotson (1792–1869), an English surgeon who used hypnosis for pain management (Bassman & Wester, 1992). Milton H. Erickson (1966, 1986) used hypnosis with acute and chronic pain patients, and later Hilgard & Hilgard (1975), Hilgard & LeBaron (1982), Melzack & Wall (1965, 1983), and Barber & Adrian (1982) broadened its clinical applicability in pain management. More recent researchers have continued to understand the applicability and mechanism of action of hypnosis in the clinical, medical, and psychological arenas.

A LEGEND IN THEIR OWN MINDS

To face the challenges of life, people must believe in themselves. When the task or challenge before us appears insurmountable, it is our faith in ourselves and not reality-based facts or data that get us through. We need to believe that we are more than the sum total of our past experiences if we are to be able to take risks. What is it that enables us to be a risk-taking species? Perhaps it is that we can envision ourselves as more than we are at any given moment in time. In superheroes, we can conceptualize and quantify these images. In this way, the superhero becomes the animated embodiment of our inner strengths and weaknesses. Through the use of hypnosis, the individual's internalized strengths can be brought out. Through the use of superheroes in conjunction with hypnosis, they can be integrated into the patient as viable identifiable character traits.

The superhero selected by the patient is a symbolic metaphor. It is wise for us as therapists to minimize interpreting the patient's choice of character to best understand the client's metaphorical meaning. A character may represent power or some other attribute. To the client, the presence of that attribute may have a positive, negative, or neutral meaning. One might see Superman as a control freak using his superabilities to throw off the balance of nature by preventing necessary natural disasters. Indeed, questioning a child about superheroes often leads to as many disliked as liked characters. Some superheroes are preferred for their flaws as much as for their strengths.

As Erikson might argue, using hypnosis may represent a more respectful way to work with clients than direct confrontation of their conscious beliefs. The use of metaphor, especially via representation of superheroes, helps patients to express unconscious feelings, self-perceptions, and desires. They can embrace and internalize desired traits while rejecting undesired ones. Does every fan of superheroes know that the Flash is full of himself? It is, therefore, imperative for the clinician using superheroes in hypnotherapy to respect the patient's unique connection to the character and not interpret the character selected based on stereotypes. Through the use of metaphors and indirect suggestion, deeper meaning can be conveyed. The etiology of superheroes, as well as how they live their lives conveys messages that take on greater significance when a superhero is presented in a story. In some cases the superhero represents only an anchor to draw the patient into the "indirect messages" relayed in the hypnotic storytelling technique. Children are primed by fairy tales and later by stories of their first "superheroes," their parents. Lessons about life and "experiences" not personally experienced help to educate. The superhero in hypnotherapy becomes a powerful medium for focusing and learning new behaviors, skills, and emotions within the subconscious. The use of metaphors in daily language creates a common story or denominator we all share. We all know the fairy tale or the superhero, and in sharing it we engender trust and rapport from our clients, which in turn enhances our ability to do hypnotic work. I have often found that creating hypnotic stories of a pleasant nature initially for children such as all the superheroes playing baseball, is a way of encouraging them to engender and embrace superhero storytelling techniques in hypnosis. Then moving on, more difficult themes (loss or separation), complicated issues or behaviors (symptoms) that motivated their seeking therapy, can be addressed with less anxiety.

Dissociation as a hypnotherapeutic tool when united with superhero imagery can allow for pain control and new ways of processing information as well as for experiencing events without actually being there. Dissociation via superheroes offers a variation on the many uses of inducing a dissociative state as illustrated in the hypnotherapeutic literature.

In this approach, patients are age-regressed back "to a time before they can remember" (a confusion technique) and then progressed slowly. During the age regression, they are reminded of how their mind and their body continued to heal them and take care of them even though they were too young to consciously understand. "When you were born your body and your mind knew how to heal your wounds and fight infections ... and you didn't understand but your mind did ... and it took care of you. You needed to do nothing at all ... and your mind and your body took care of you ... just as they will take care of you now." The focus is on allowing the individual to trust his or her unconscious mind to allow healing and to support it. From this point forward, images the mind may want to introduce to help in the process can be suggested. "The mind may remember (for adults) images that help you to feel very strong in helping you heal. These images or feelings may be real or imaginary or anything your mind creates but you know that you can allow these sensations to occur so you can continue to heal. Perhaps there is a character or memory that made you feel super (disguised suggestion) in the past. Take your time and see what your mind presents to you."

MANAGING PAIN WITH HYPNOSIS

Pain has been viewed as evolving from either physical or psychological causes (Fordyce, 1976; Sternbach, 1978). Indeed, even the most recent edition of the DSM, offers diagnostic categories for a "real–organic" or "functional–imagery" basis for pain. In this context, Sellick and Zaza (1998) found that in randomized controlled studies of hypnosis in managing cancer pain, substantial evidence of improvement exists when nonpharmacological pain management approaches are sought.

A constructionist view was proposed by Chapman and Nakamura (1998) who suggested that hypnosis alters the learned pain experience by interacting with feedback processes that prime the associations and memories tied to pain. This associative learning process shapes the formation of pain experience and expectations, ultimately reducing the experience of pain. What then is the pain response when a posthypnotic suggestion with associated superhero imagery (Superman) is triggered in response to anticipated or actual pain? Indeed, the response I have observed is a type of induced dissociative experience in which the individual reports significantly reduced levels of anticipated pain or, rather, that the discomfort is tolerable and controllable.

From a neurocognitive perspective, Gruzelier (1998) noted the significant role of the interior cingulate cortex in managing sensory input in conjunction with the frontolimbic inhibitory processes allowing patients to suspend reality testing and critical evaluation. In addition, the amygdala is inhibited and the hippocampus is activated. Suspending reality may be exactly what is needed if one is to become Wonder Woman or Superman in dealing with his or her pain. Hypnosis represents the means by which the superabilities of superheroes can be experienced in an unobstructed cognitive and physiological manner. In addition, patients may be more susceptible to hypnosis (and induced superhero qualities). Pain patients may spontaneously shift to an altered state of awareness and rapidly enter trance as a means to escape pain (Araoz, 1985).

Applications

Pain comes in myriad forms too numerous to delineate, ranging from acute to chronic, trauma and burn-related, illness, and postsurgical. Pain reduction in acute burn victims (Wright & Drummond, 2000), those undergoing acute procedural pain or chronic pain conditions (Patterson & Jenson, 2003) and burn patients requiring debridement (Ewin, 1986) as well as pediatric patients (Foertsch et al., 1998), can benefit from hypnosis and superhero strengths. In these populations, clinical experience has demonstrated that superhero imagery may represent a powerful means to assist in the dissociative and regressive patterns reported by Patterson & Ptacek (1997).

Hypnosis has also been applied to preoperative, operative, and postoperative procedures (Deefochereux et al., 1999; Howard, 2003; Meurisse et al., 1999). Chronic pain has been shown to have both a physiological and psychological component. It has been shown to result in lowered self-esteem, hopelessness, and despondency, which can be alleviated, in part, by hypnosis (Turk & Holzman, 1986) via empowerment and pain management. Acute pain is frequently associated with an increase in anxiety through which the patient seeks to escape the pain and has not yet developed "neural pathways" (Melzack & Wall, 1983) or strong emotional associations to the pain. If these associations and pathways can be circumvented by empowering the patient with superheroic levels of physical and emotional strength, can the acute pain pathology be prevented from becoming chronic pain pathology? I believe that in many cases it can. Anbar (2000) found that children with recurrent abdominal pain in the absence of an identifiable or physiological cause, respond positively following a single hypnotic session. Traditional approaches may use glove anesthesia with transference of the pain off the body and various forms of dissociation and suggestion (Burte, 1999). Carlson, Broom, and Vessey (2000) reported on the effectiveness of hypnosis in helping patients to reinterpret painful experiences and reduce negative associations.

A key term commonly using in the hypnotic process is *transformation,* the process whereby individuals can alter their sense of self and, in so doing, engender alternate qualities and traits, either covertly (self-perceived limitations) or overtly (habit changes). Hypnotic intervention enables patients to experience the qualities of superheroes in overcoming a multitude of emotional and physical limitations. By becoming that character while in trance and maintaining the ability to call on that character via posthypnotic suggestion, the person can, at will, transform into the character regardless of the place in time. Character traits can be "locked in" and become viable parts of their selves.

Adults and children alike are capable of using multisensory experiences to enhance their trance experience (Burte et al., 1994). In this way, the incorporation of the unique physiology of the superhero as well as the imagery of the abilities superheroes possess can be used in treatment. For example, patients may use the self-healing powers, the ability to see inside the body, and the ability to separate parts of their body—qualities that various superheroes possess—to manage pain and to promote healing. Because superheroes always eventually get better, the use of superhero identification in hypnosis can also provide encouragement and promote positive self-hypnotic statements. The literature on hypnosis in pain management is prolific, yet in none have I found specific references to using superheroes. Although I am sure many of the pain practitioners I know employ metaphors and storytelling techniques that may incorporate superheroes, it is an underrepresented technique in the published literature. In what follows, I hope to give specific examples of techniques employing superhero imagery that I have found especially helpful with pain patients.

Case Study

One such case was that of George (Burte & Araoz, 1994; Burte, 2002a; Burte, 2004), a 12-year old-boy brought to my office after being diagnosed with cancer. George was on multiple medications and was experiencing pain from annoying needlesticks and Broviac catheter changes, as well as pain directly attributable to his illness. In addition, he experienced nausea and discomfort secondary to his medication regimen.

Individual tests of suggestibility indicated that George was a good hypnotic subject. He was taught how to relax his mind and body. Then, using superhero metaphors, George was taught to draw on his favorite character, He-Man, who like many superheroes, feigned fearfulness in his disguised state, but was all-powerful, albeit mortal, in his superhero state. Once in trance, George was encouraged to feel the transformation from Prince Adam (the ordinary character) into He-Man (the strongest man in the universe). What was extremely relevant to George's case, was his ability to identify with his fears of cancer and pain in the mortal state, yet face them with reduced fear, head on, in his superhero state. An interesting note, He-Man's arch-enemy was a supervillain named Skeletor (a skeletal-looking villain). George's illness had metastasized to his bones, so that was where the battle was to take place.

Trance logic is the ability to suspend reality. In George's case, not only did he suspend reality by transforming from himself to Prince Adam and eventually He-Man, but he could then, as He-Man, enter into the body of Prince Adam and fight Skeletor (his cancer) while feeling less pain. Pain became a dissociated discomfort that he could shake off. Unfortunately, in the real world, Skeletor ultimately won the final battle but via hypnosis and superhero transformation, George fought until the end with less pain.

The approach chosen involved having George first learn how to enter a trance. Once there, he began to experience the feelings and senses of being Prince Adam. It was important to engage all five sensory modalities (sight, hearing, taste, touch, and smell) as well as kinesthetic (place in space) in his experiences. Once he was Prince Adam, George could then transform into He-Man. He would raise his imaginary sword and recite, "By the power of Grayskull and He-Man" and transform. Once He-Man, he would imagine that he had been transported to a new world that existed inside the body of Prince Adam. Trance logic allows this to occur—he would feel no pain and defeat Skeletor time and again. Also as He-Man, pain associated with needlesticks and Broviac catheter changes were reduced, and bone pain and medication side effects were also diminished. It was critical to teach George how to induce trance for himself, and at one point he developed his own rapid induction. He would raise one of his crutches and recite the transformation phrase, "By the power of grace go I and He-Man," and on returning his crutch to the side of the chair, he became He-Man. (For girls, a similar character named She-Ra, the strongest woman in the universe, can be employed.)

In George's case, two goals were sought. The first was direct control of his illness-based pain, as well as the pain and discomfort associated with the medical procedures and medications involved in his treatment. The second goal was to empower George to fight his illness via a psychoneuroimmunological imagery approach.

TRAUMA

The use of hypnosis for treating trauma is well represented in the literature. Prewritten hypnotherapeutic scripts in which experienced hypnotherapists provide an induction, a series of suggestions, posthypnotic suggestions, or a combination of these for a range of disorders is readily available for the novice hypnotherapist. In many instances the therapist can read the monologue-like story or script to the patient. Scripts for recovery from trauma (Havens & Walters, 1989) and working through ongoing emotional consequences of trauma for adults (Yapko, 2003) and children (Mills & Crowley, 1986) are also helpful and readily available. For more experienced hypnotherapists, writing their own scripts unique to patients' needs or generating a story or metaphorical script from information the patient brings to each session is more common. In the *New Hypnosis* (Araoz, 1985), it is often a matter of following and leading patients into their own internal representations of the trauma that is most effective. At these times, calling on superhero images can assist in helping the patient feel either safely removed from the trauma or more capable of confronting it. Prior trauma also lends itself to the hypnotic application of superheroes. Patients can be induced to use an approach known as New Hypnosis (Araoz, 1985). In this technique, in the course of conversation, the patient's self-talk or negative self-hypnotic statements are investigated to determine the underlying language that maintains the symptomology. Individual traits of superheroes can then be imposed onto their symptoms. Using this model in the course of conversation, patients discussing anxiety, for example, are asked to focus on their psychosemantics—the descriptive language used to describe their emotions (i.e., sick to my stomach, a pain in the neck)—and their somatopsychic behaviors—the physical behaviors and physical manifestations they express while describing their emotional state (i.e., clenching and unclenching their hands, a hand motion). The patient is then led into focusing on the phrase or emotion as part of their induction.

Through a progression of observing, leading, discussing, and checking (OLD-C), the therapist guides patients' experience toward a hypnotic state via the symptomology, while circumventing the need for inducing a relaxed trance state. During the subsequent discussion phase, the patient presents unique associations and imagery. By permissively suggesting supports (superhero abilities), the therapist can guide the patient away from the negative self-hypnotic statements toward strategies of greater control and mastery. The role of incorporating superhero imagery becomes relevant as the patient produces negative self-hypnotic associations and experiences in any of the five sensory modalities. Both superheroes and supervillains can be associated with the negative self-hypnotic statements and self-perception.

A situation in which hypnosis using superheroes is helpful is seen when the negative self-hypnotic language places challenges before patients that they believe they cannot overcome with their own perceived abilities. Some of the advantages of using superhero imagery in this instance include (a) specific traits unique to a particular superhero can be incorporated; (b) the process of becoming a superhero often engenders a certain degree of anonymity, with which comes an ability to take risks with a reduced fear of failure; (c) superheroes can be brought in to assist in situations without patients necessarily having to become that character or even identify with him or her—hypnosis has been used to get in touch with the inner child or to allow overt communication with loved ones who have died to resolve unfinished business; (d) hypnosis can also call on superhero characters to assist in facing fears. As noted earlier, facing anxiety-provoking situations or facing fears may be made easier if first addressed in trance with the assistance of a superhero and then later overtly with posthypnotic suggestions with which the superhero will be there to assist.

In this technique, the patient is asked to discuss which qualities he or she needs in to face a given task or past trauma and is then asked which superhero could be of the most help to them. This technique without the use of a superhero is often employed in ego-strengthening exercises, as well as when increased physical stamina (as in physical rehabilitation) is required. Rather than getting in touch with an inner child, the patient is encouraged to get in touch with an inner superhero. Research has supported the use of hypnosis, improving rates of rehabilitation and recovery for trauma victims. For some individuals, using superheroes as role models can be effective in developing coping skills for facing fears and physical challenges. Superheroes always get up, even when facing defeat or despair. Luke Skywalker sought out Yoda to become a Jedi. Batman overcame the loss of his family to become a hero.

I have found that rehabilitation patients often go into a spontaneous trance by way of becoming another character, and can often push their abilities beyond that of mortal men. Hypnosis to reduce perceived pain intensity allows patients to become more compliant and able to withstand physical rehabilitative interventions (Mauer et al., 1999) as well as promote increased rates of anatomical and functional healing (Ginandes & Rosenthal, 1999). I have also observed that some individuals, while in trance, call on others to assist them through the process. Superheroes become the coach, the physical support to increase endurance and stamina.

Especially with children, avoidance of addressing issues can be better faced with the support of superheroes and hypnosis. Boredom also can be reduced by using superhero imagery to increase attention and endurance. A child pretending to be his favorite sports hero can often engage in a repetitive activity such as throwing a ball against a wall for hours, long after he would have been otherwise bored or fatigued. Wayne Dyer once said, "You'll see it when you believe it." A variation on that might be, "You'll be it when you experience it." Hypnosis, through its power to provide a multisensory experience, allows for the transformation from ordinary self to superhero to occur.

The use of superheroes as a tool during hypnotic intervention is illustrated by a patient who could "not even imagine" accomplishing a given behavior or overcoming a given emotion. Hypnosis can be described as a state of Focused Internally Directed Experiential Learning-FIDEL (Burte, 2004). Patients often have difficulty spontaneously imagining symptom reduction or the desired behavior or emotion occurring. It is difficult to have individuals imagine behaviors in which they have not engaged or that are so anxiety evoking they are avoided at all costs.

Case Study

Prior trauma, even of a seemingly minor nature can have a significant impact on children's future functioning. From an early age, Sam had been eneuretic. Consequently, on multiple sleepovers, he had wet the bed, resulting in peer ridicule. Subsequently, when coerced to continue to attempt sleepovers, he became highly anxious and attempted to control the situation by staying awake all night. Fatigue and fear of falling asleep resulted in the development of panic attacks and an urgency to go home in the middle of the night when he felt he could no longer keep himself awake.

Sam became a phobic child who was afraid to sleep at other children's homes. The result of these repeated failed attempts was multiple late-night embarrassments. Sam came to therapy because as he approached his 14th birthday, his school was planning an eighth-grade two-night trip to the nation's capital. Sam greatly wanted to go on the trip but feared the embarrassment of being unable to sleep out overnight.

Medication and psychotherapy had been to no avail, and his prior therapist suggested that hypnotherapy be tried. Sam was eager to try anything to be able to go on the trip. During the first few sessions of hypnosis, Sam was hypervigilant and resistant to trance. He also avoided approaching any imagery associated with sleeping out of his home. Sam had a history of attention-deficit/hyperactivity disorder and was currently being treated with psychostimulants. As noted, he also had a history of enuresis, which had been resolved some 4 years earlier. Sam was asked to focus on his body image and to imagine himself at home in his own bed. He was asked to focus on any sensations, images, sounds, and smells of which he became aware. He was gradually led into a state of focused self-awareness. Once in that state, Sam was asked to imagine a superhero who could endure emotional stress. He was asked to try to recall any superheroes who had to endure separation from family to become stronger. He was able to create images of Anakin Skywalker leaving his mother behind, as well as Luke Skywalker going to a distant planet to train to become a Jedi Knight. Sam was then directed to imagine himself at his friend's house once again, trying to reexperience the feeling that he had previously described as "depressed but ten times worse" and to listen to the negative self-hypnotic statement, "I just want to go home," that he repeated to himself at those times. Then once he was able to feel the upsetting feelings, he was asked to introduce the imagery of the superhero and to feel the strength of this character. "Hear the voice inside telling him to endure, because in the end he would be stronger." He stated that he was able to feel strengthening. He was then directed further into the experiential learning experience. He repeated to himself frequently, "Feel the force." This proved helpful to him as he learned how to feel stronger. The induction proceeded with him describing himself on a planet with Yoda from the Star Wars series, of having to go to a place to face his greatest fears and calling on the power of the force to remain calm. This experience had a profound impact on him as he described in detail the scene with himself now as the character. It is likely that he had unconsciously internalized the scene, which in hypnosis, he could now call on to help him address his deeper fears. He could be both dissociated and yet learning a new skill at the same time.

Another quality of superheroes is that they do not die at the end of the day (or movie). By allowing the superhero to merge with him, it assured Sam that he would ultimately succeed and endure, and further ensured that his irrational fear of dying (associated with panic) would not come to pass. In my many years of doing hypnosis, I have learned that patients often look to their therapist to give them new or different skills or to offer them opportunities to explore things in ways they would not condone on their own. The therapist is the catalyst and permissive agent, "to go where no man has gone before," and thus even adult patients are much more willing to embrace fantasy in hypnosis. Children, of course, go there with little or no prompting. I would urge therapists not to be afraid to ask patients to attempt using superhero imagery in hypnosis as a means of bringing about profound changes in their patients. Erickson often used metaphor and symbolic imagery to enhance specific behaviors, cognitive self-interpretations or noncritical judgments of the symptoms to bring about change in his patients. Metaphorical superhero ego strengthening stories provide patients with patterns they can readily call on.

As part of another hypnotic induction, the individual is guided into visualization of favorite superheroes. Generally speaking, I have found that with adults and teens, it is helpful to take a very nondirective approach when doing this due to the sense of silliness that many patients experience at this point. We are taught to see ourselves as we really are (whatever that means) and to put aside illusions of ourselves. By embracing a very permissive approach in treatment, patients are encouraged to envision a favorite superhero, to experience the world via his or her extended powers and abilities. By using age regression—bringing the adult back to their childhood—we can dissociate them from their rigid adult beliefs, self-images, and fears of looking foolish, thereby giving them permission to engage in fantasy, to restore their belief in their abilities (superhuman or otherwise) that have been lost in time. Such a dialogue might include, "as you go back to the age of 10, perhaps you can recall a favorite comic book or cartoon superhero. Can you recall a favorite . . . superhero? Good . . . Try to recall as much as you can about how you felt as you watched his adventures occur. What do you see or hear happening as you observe him or become him?" The goal here is to engage the adult in childhood memories and use new hypnosis techniques of OLD-C to deepen their experience.

EGO STRENGTHENING AND SELF-PERCEPTION

Patients often seek hypnotherapy for alleviation of specific symptoms and habits. For some patients, however, what is sought is to explore past issues that have resulted in damage to their sense of self and self-perception relative to others. For these patients, ego strengthening via hypnosis can be a powerful tool. Unlike some other forms of psychotherapeutic intervention, ego strengthening by means of hypnosis and self-hypnosis offers the patient the opportunity to examine "alternative selves" and to experience and not just verbalize "what if" and "if only" scenarios.

Patient can also question negative self-hypnotic statements that may be damaging their self-definitions and learn to reframe them into more positive self-statements and images. Ego strengthening, then, is the process by which hypnosis is used to help patients develop new self-empowering definitions in an experiential multisensory manner. They get to try on new personas and discard old ones that eventually no longer fit.

Many times, the patient has no prior model to draw on when attempting to create these new personas. Role models have either been absent or discarded, and consequently fantasized characters may often fill the void. Superheroes provide ideal archetypes for some of these personas, both positive and negative. Eventually for some individuals, the "as if" becomes the "I am." Examples of this are the children or adults who have convinced themselves that they cannot accomplish a task (face a socially stressful situation or quit smoking) or have defined themselves in a negative manner ("I'm fat or I'm ugly"). For many of these individuals, the ability to visualize themselves as something different from their current self-definition seems impossible.

One patient recently explained how at age 15, her mother suggested to her that if she lost 5 to 10 pounds, she would fit into a size 7/8 dress and not be fat. From that moment on, the woman (now 47) defined herself as a fat person. Through hypnosis, she was taught to alter her ego-dystonic image as a fat person who wanted to be thin, and instead see herself as a thin person with excess or surplus layers (even Shrek has layers). No one wants to lose any part of their identity, even layers of fat, but ridding oneself of excess or surpluses is often easily accepted. For some individuals, the metamorphosis can be even more profound as illustrated by the following case.

A standard age regression in which a patient is brought back to specific events and memories until a desired age is reached was used in this scenario. An alternative technique is presented in *Hypnotic Realities* by Erickson et al., (1976) patients can be regressed to a time before they can remember and then progress slowly, all the while endowed with superhero abilities or identities.

Case Study

One such case is that of a teenage boy I treated who had Marfan's syndrome and who was bitter and angry. He was the brunt of jokes due to the elongated limbs symptomatic of the condition, and he also suffered from the cardiac vulnerability commonly associated with Marfan's syndrome. Consequently, he was prohibited from engaging in contact sports or getting into fights. John was asked if he had ever been hypnotized before, and he indicated he had not. It was suggested that he might try. After two sessions of learning how to enter into trance, he was ready to attempt applying his abilities to achieving transformation.

John was asked to talk briefly about his favorite television shows and movies, and eventually conversation was informally brought about to any movies he saw with superheroes. He could identify quite a few cartoon, comic book, and movie superheroes. He stated that he especially liked superheroes who could change their appearance including Reed Richards (the stretchy character of the Fantastic Four). Interestingly enough, he stated that it was the intellectual component that he found attractive. He had difficulty admitting to the idea that Reed Richards could change his body shape and have extended limbs, which might also have attracted him to the character.

John was regressed back to his own birth "to a time before you can remember" and then slowly progressed back. But as he grew, he was to watch his body develop to learn to see what was unique about his body and what he could accept about being unique. For children, especially teens, the ability to accept their physical limitations or differences at a time when they are starved for acceptance is critical.

John described observing his arms and limbs as being disproportionate, his hands as being ugly. Slowly the image of himself and that of Reed Richards were merged and he was asked to describe his unique physique if he were to see himself as Reed Richards to understand his ability to see himself in a more acceptable way. Interestingly, though, and perhaps typical of "trance logic," John switched to a different character stating "I'm not Reed Richards anymore, now I'm the Thing. When asked why he had become the Thing, he stated it was because he truly saw himself as the Thing because, like that superhero, he couldn't change back to being normal whenever he wanted and that the Thing was always angry and bitter about his physical appearance. Once this was brought out, work began on him being the Thing and coming to explain this. We focused on the emotions being felt and the perceptions of how the world viewed him. At the conclusion of the session, I asked John if he had ever thought of himself as the Thing, and he said it had not occurred to him until the moment he recognized it while in trance. This is relevant because John had used Reed Richards with whom to identify overtly, but it was only once in trance that his sense of self-shame came forward with regard to his personal self-loathing. His anger rapidly dissipated in therapy, and John's academic performance and social functioning at school improved. He began to speak to girls more and develop through imagery ways of seeing himself as a positive being like the Thing whom girls could be attracted to and in whom he could trust his feelings without a fear of rejection. Self-acceptance is a metamorphosis that the Thing goes through as he comes to value his unique attributes.

For young children, the superheroes with which they identify are usually not the same ones with whom we commonly associate. Commonly young children do not find themselves drawn to the adult or even teen superheroes. To them, other, more lovable characters often take on the superhero qualities with which we identify. As early as 1986, Mills & Crowley pointed out how some children like the Hulk, who can take on protective roles for a child by allowing them to identify with powerful characters. They went on to point out how for younger children, Scooby-Doo, an unlikely superhero, takes on superhero proportions by scaring away the ghosts. A melding of this can be seen in cartoons where typical leading-man-type superheroes are paired with comic superheroes with whom children more comfortably identify.

Psychoneuroimmunology

Psychoneuroimmunology, in its simplest form, is a reciprocal communication among the psyche (mind), central nervous system, and immune system. Yang & Glasser, (2000) noted that stress via bidirectional interactions between central nervous system, endocrine system, and immune system, affects the hypothalamic–pituitary–adrenal (HPA) axis and the sympathetic–adrenal–medullary (SAM) axis resulting in immunosuppression. Pain is a factor that in and of itself may promote immunosuppression (Paige & Ben Eliyahoo, 1997). Stress is a second factor that has a deleterious effect on immune system functioning, and stress reduction has been shown to promote immune system functioning and improved prognoses in disease processes (Sali, 1997). Hypnosis has been used extensively in pain control and stress management as well as in indirectly addressing the immune system enhancement and disease processes. Bressler (2004) pointed out that most people do imagery all the time primarily by worrying.

Through the use of hypnosis, stress and pain, which are two significant variables influencing immune functioning, can be controlled. Specific to this chapter, superhero imagery within hypnosis can be directly and indirectly applied. Because psychoneuroimmunology can be represented by directional triad of psyche, neurology, and immunology, hypnosis can be introduced at the point of intervention where it can operate on any one of these variables. For example, superhero imagery can be introduced through the psyche to strengthen indirectly the immune system or to attack disease processes via imagery associated with healing—imagine Pac-Man scouring the lungs, cleaning up cancer cells and carcinogens such as tar and nicotine. Another example might be Superman freezing or burning out destructive tumor cells. Along similar lines, Atom Ant can shrink to molecular levels and repair damaged parts of the body.

Of course, the use of healing imagery is nothing new and authors have written about this technique for many years (Erickson, Rossi, & Rossi, 1976; Rossi, 1993). The restorative powers of the body can be enhanced through imagery. One healing technique I have found helpful is a derivation on the technique presented by Erickson, Rossi, and Rossi (1976) in *Hypnotic Realities*.

Case Study

From a psychoneuroimmunological perspective, the use of superhero imagery to fight cancer dates back to Pac-Man, a video game character of the

1970s who munched his way through the body chewing up cancer cells. Superheroes offer a focusing device for children and adults. Their images can be easily called on as a means of either inducing or maintaining a trance. A simple "yes set" suggestion such as "as you rest there with your eyes closed ... I wonder if you can imagine a picture of Superman? Can you see his red cape? ... the big S on his chest? ... Good ... Now as you see Superman, can you imagine using one of his wonderful superpowers of flying through the sky? ... I wonder if he will fly to the right first or to the left? ... Which way is he flying? ... Good." Superman often fights villains. As you see Superman fly, I wonder which villain he will come upon ... What happens when he meets this villain? ... Can you see the villain? ... [Notice I avoid the word "supervillain. We don't want to empower the disease.] Good. How does Superman defeat the villain? ... Which of his superpowers does he use? ... Good ... He uses his heat vision and what happens? ... It shrinks ... Good ... Do you know how it shrinks? ... Good ... You're shrinking it by burning it up."

This is a much-abbreviated version of a 45-minute session with a college-aged young man who, in addition to standard medical care, requested hypnosis to shrink a tumor. In this case, he was not Superman but rather, Superman provided the treatment. In this process, patients are led to seek an inner healer or hero to help them promote their healing but, above all, to trust their unconscious mind to find a healing method.

An alternative approach is to focus on the patient's presenting symptomology as a "royal road to their unconscious." By again focusing on their psychosomatics (i.e., "he makes me sick") or their somatopsychic manifestations (i.e., "movements, muscle tension"), the patient is led into an altered state of awareness. The concept is as stated earlier, to achieve focused internally directed experiential learning (FIDEL). For example, patients may come in discussing various stressors that ultimately affect their physical well-being and health. The patient is encouraged to converse about the stressors until a psychosomatic phrase or somatopsychic manifestation is observed. The patient is then encouraged (led) to perhaps repeat "he makes me sick" over and over again while noticing any other images, thoughts, or sensations that arise. If the patient reports, for example, that she can feel the pain, she is led into the visceral experience, if other associations arise, she is encouraged to focus on those. In so doing, the hypnotherapist works backward from the negative self-hypnotic statements to deeper and deeper levels of distress. Once there, the hypnotherapist can begin to see whether the patient can draw on phraseology, imagery, or sensations of a more positive or restorative nature. During these processes, superhero imagery can be introduced to assist the patient in dealing with those experiences and learn more adaptive responses.

A more symptom-specific approach is used when the patient presents an especially painful symptom such as a neck or back pain, which as noted earlier, may be immunosuppressing. The patient is asked to focus on the pain and visualize what it looks like to him. "Is it sharp or dull, constant or throbbing? ... Do any images come to mind?" A patient may use psychosomatics to describe it, such as "It looks like a rope (muscle) all knotted up." Via suggestion the patient is asked to alter the image "to unknot it." In another case, patients may then be encouraged to "wrap an area in healing bandages" or, in superhero imagery, to call on abilities to self heal. The classic superhero dialogue may go something like this: "Must ... get ... to ... switch ... must ... save ... the ... world." This type of superhero language can be called on to help patients turn on healing processes even when they feel unable to do so in their normal states. After visualizing the switch to be reached, patients can create a self image of turning on or off the switch to promote healing, shut off unwanted behaviors or shut off pain.

It is often not relevant that the imagery created is consistent with the actual physiological appearance of the condition. Few individuals actually know what a tumor looks like or the actual way in which blood vessels transport nutrients to cells. However, most people do have an internalized picture or representation of both healthy and unhealthy bodily states. For this patient, a mental representation was sufficient to create a picture of "heat vision" rays destroying a large whitish colored mass much in the way "laser surgery" would burn out or cut out the tumor. Obviously, one can imagine the surgeon performing the procedure as readily as Superman, but in some fashion might we not say that in that case we are merely substituting one set of superhero imagery for another.

The physiological process is still not clearly understood, but research has shown that the body does respond to hypnosis in positive ways with regard to remission of tumors. It is not an alternative to standard medical interventions, but is a definite adjunct. Improved immune system functioning and changes in T-helper and N-killer cells have been correlated with hypnosis. I have found that for some individuals, especially for children, hypnotic intervention via superhero imagery enables them to take control of the healing process more easily than recalling memories of interventions by medical professionals who may engender anxiety or fear in the patient. This is especially true when prior interaction with doctors or nurses entails memories of painful or invasive procedures that have, via the thalamus and amygdala, become associated to strong negative emotions.

Superheroes are usually associated with positive emotions whether in the form of calm relaxation as they are viewed on television, in the movies, or in print by the patient. Often positive feelings are internalized as they rescue characters with whom the viewer identifies. In effect, when we watch superheroes rescue or protect Joe or Jane Pedestrian on the street, we are more like him or her than the superhero. When we are ill, regression is not unusual, and we look to a greater power or healer for help. Superhero imagery allows for a positive controllable associational process. The patient, through hypnosis, is both the seeker and the provider of care.

The college student noted earlier was well aware that Superman was not truly healing him; rather, he understood that it was a technique to utilize the powerful healing abilities of his mind in a focused fashion. I often explain the connection of the thalamus, the amygdala, the anterior cingulate gyrus, and the prefrontal cortex as a way to teach adult patients how signals for dysfunction reach the brain and how they can be directed, interrupted, reevaluated, and returned to the body for healing purposes. By focusing on their own negative self-hypnotic communication, the patient can be guided to create superheroes to challenge and defeat the associations and emotions as well as the negative images they have created about their illness. Once patients understand how this occurs, they they welcome a wide range of healing images and for some (particularly children in pain), images of superheroes work well.

CAVEATS

Using superheroes in hypnosis with children seems an easy and useful tool and, indeed it is. Children embrace the opportunity to become superheroes in hypnosis because as one young client exclaimed, "it feels so real." However, we need to be careful and responsible about our use of hypnosis and posthypnotic suggestion to ensure that children do not attempt superhero feats (like flying) in ways that will place them in danger. Therefore, it is important that therapists who use these techniques are well trained in suggestion and posthypnotic suggestion, as well as in assessing for abreactions (negative and unwanted reactions while in or after trance). As Spider-Man learned, "with great power comes great responsibility."

Using superheroes with adults is no different. I believe it is the therapist's fear of looking foolish and not the patient's concerns that prevent many hypnotherapists from employing superheroes in hypnosis. I have found that while some adults may feel uncomfortable with this technique, the lightheartedness of incorporating their favorite superheroes from childhood often puts them at ease. Hypnosis has found its application with adults in not only pain management, psychoneuroimmunology, and trauma, but most notably in dealing with various forms of sexual dysfunction (Araoz, 1998; Araoz, Burte, & Goldin, 2001; Burte & Araoz, 1994). One of the interesting things about trance logic is that the physiology of the skill learned does not need to be the physiology of the symptom treated. What this means is that learning finger rigidity in hypnosis (a muscle tensing behavior) can be applied to improve functioning in erectile dysfunction (a blood-flow issue) and that learning to increase salivation can be used in treating hypolubrication disorders in women. Superhero imagery in trance logic takes on similar qualities. One need not understand the etiology of the superheroes' abilities for it to be applicable to treating a variety of sexual dysfunctions. I am sure that more than just a few adults have pondered what it was like for Lois Lane after she married Clark Kent or what it would be like to date Wonder Woman.

As we become adults the ability to alter physiological functioning via cognitive processes such as hypnosis becomes increasingly valuable. The use of superhero imagery can significantly enhance that process. Even the geriatric population were young once and had more prowess than they currently possess. The opportunity to return to youthful fantasies is both psychologically and physically empowering. Suggestions of increased powers, pain control, or functioning with anchors or superhero figures as queues associated with their prowess enable them to "return to those bygone days," building self-confidence and trust in the powerfulness of hypnosis and its ability to enable them to become "a man of steel, or a wonder woman." Just a few examples of the superhero traits I have incorporated with my patients have included:

- Johnny (the Human Torch) in Reynaud's syndrome: It can be useful when any part of the body needs warming (i.e., hand-warming techniques in treating headaches).
- The Silver Surfer (especially useful with teens and surfer-types on the barrier island beach town where I once lived) who would surf through the universe coming to the aid of others. Having once been a villain, this character can be used to address the ideas of changing one's self-definition and using coping skills for anger and remaining calm in difficult situations—he's "a very cool dude."
- The Hulk can be helpful for developing the ability to transform back to the meek David Banner, and in so doing, both experience anger and the management of emotions and images. A combination of hypnosis with rational emotive therapy is useful in visualizing and experiencing how what one tells themselves (beliefs) in a given situation (activating event) causes changes in ones behaviors and emotions (consequences).

- Superman, Supergirl, and Wonder Woman can be enlisted for myriad forms of pain control, anxiety, and sexual dysfunction issues.
- Supervillains such as Darth Vader can offer qualities we admire. Perhaps even "The Donald" (Trump) would see Darth as an ambitious apprentice who was able to successfully overcome numerous hurdles and handicaps in climbing the Empire's corporate ladder.

CONCLUSION

The use of superheroes in hypnosis represents an exciting and interesting approach to reach the inner self-defining concepts that patients carry within themselves. Since earliest times, hypnosis, imagery, storytelling techniques, and metaphors have been shown to be effective with a plethora of medical and psychological conditions in reducing human suffering. I have no doubt that some derivation of a superhero can be found in the inner psyche of all people. In this brief chapter, I hope to have introduced a new twist to an old storytelling tradition. I encourage all therapists with training in hypnosis to incorporate superhero identification, imagery, and experiences into their repertoire of hypnotherapeutic techniques and, for those not trained, to seek out reputable training in hypnosis and apply these imagery and experiential techniques with their patients.

REFERENCES

Anbar, R. D. (2000). Hypnosis, Theodore Roosevelt and the patient with cystic fibrosis. *Pediatrics*, *106*(20) 339–346.

Araoz, D. L. (1985). *The new hypnosis*. New York: Brunner/Mazel.

Araoz, D. L. (1998). *The new hypnosis in sex therapy*. Northvale, NJ: Jason Aronson.

Araoz, D. L., Burte, J. M., & Goldin, E. (2001). Sexual hypnotherapy for couples and family counselors. *Family Journal: Counseling and Therapy for Couples and Families*, *9*, 75–81.

Barber, J., & Adrian, C. (1982). Psychological approaches to the management of pain. New York: Brunner/Mazel.

Bassman, S. W., & Wester, W. C., II. (1992). Hypnosis, headache and pain control, an integrated approach. Columbus, OH: Psychology Publications.

Bressler, D. E. (2004). Clinical applications of interactive guided imagery for diagnosing and treating chronic pain. In R. Weiner, M. V. Boswell, & B. E. Cole (Eds.), *Pain management: A practical guide for clinicians* (7th ed.). Boca Raton, FL: CRC Press.

Burte, J. M. (1999). Introduction for creating a dissociative state. In S. Rosenberg (Ed.), *Course workbook*. New York: New York Society of Clinical Hypnosis.

Burte, J. M. (2002a). Hypnotherapeutic advances in pain management. In R. Weiner (Ed.), Pain management: A practical guide for clinicians (6th ed.). Boca Raton, FL: CRC Press.

Burte, J. M. (2002b). Psychoneuroimmunology. In R. Weiner (Ed.), *Pain management: A practical guide for clinicians* (6th ed.). Boca Raton, FL: CRC Press.

Burte, J. M. (2004). *Hypnotherapeutic advances in pain management*. In R. Weiner, M. V. Boswell, & B. E. Cole (Eds.), *Pain management: A practical guide for clinicians* (7th ed.). Boca Raton, FL: CRC Press.

Burte, J. M., & Araoz, D. L. (1994). Cognitive hypnotherapy with sexual disorders. *Journal of Cognitive Psychotherapy, 8*, 299–312.

Burte, J. M., Burte, W., & Araoz, D. L. (1994). Hypnosis in the treatment of back pain. *Australian Journal of Clinical Hypnotherapy and Hypnosis, 15*, 93–115.

Carlson, K. L., Broom, M., & Vessey, J. A. (2000). Using distraction to reduce reported pain, fear and behavioral distress in children and adolescents. A multi-site study. *Journal of the Society of Pediatric Nurses, 5*, 75–91.

Chapman, C. R., & Nakamura, Y. (1998). Hypnotic analgesia: A constructivist framework. *International Journal of Clinical and Experimental Hypnosis, 6*, 6–27.

Defochereux, T., Meurisse, M., Hamoir, E., Gollogly, L., Joris, J., & Faymonville, M. E. (1999). Hypnoanesthesia for endocrine cervical surgery: a statement of practice. *Journal of American Complementary Medicine, 5*, 509–520.

Erickson, M. H. (1966). The interspersal hypnotic technique for symptoms correction and pain control. *American Journal of Clinical Hypnosis, 8*, 198–209.

Erickson, M. H. (1986). Mind–body communication in hypnosis. In E. Rossi & M. Ryan (Eds.), *The seminars, workshops and lectures of Milton H. Erickson* (Vol. III). New York: Irvington.

Erickson, M., Rossi, E. L., Rossi, S. L. (1976). Hypnotic Realities: The induction of clinical hypnosis and forms of indirect suggestion. New York: Irvington.

Ewin, D. M. (1986). The effect of hypnosis and mental sets on major surgery and burns. *Psychiatric Annals, 16*, 115–118.

Foertsch, C. E., O'Hara, M. W., Stoddard, F. J., & Kealey, G. P. (1998). Treatment resistant pain and distress during pediatric burn dressing changes. *Journal of Burn Care and Rehabilitation, 19*, 219–224.

Fordyce, W. E. (1976). *Behavioral methods from chronic pain and illness*. St. Louis: Mosby.

Ginandes, C. S., & Rosenthal, D. L. (1999). Using hypnosis to accelerate the healing of bone fractures: A randomized controlled pilot study. *Alternative Therapies Health and Medicine, 5*, 67–75.

Gruzelier, J. (1998). A working model of neurophysiology of Hypnosis: A review of Evidence. *Contemporary Hypnosis, 15*, 3–19.

Havens, R. A., & Walters, C. (1989). Hypnotherapy scripts: A neo-Ericksonian approach to persuasive healing. New York: Brunner/Mazel.

Hilgard, E. R., & Hilgard, J. R. (1975). *Hypnosis in the relief of pain.* Los Altos, CA: Kaufman.

Hilgard, J. R., & LeBaron, S. (1982). Relief of anxiety and pain in children and adolescents with cancer: Quantitative measures and clinical observations. *International Journal of Clinical and Experimental Hypnosis, 30,* 417–442.

Howard, R. F. (2003). Current status of pain management in children. *JAMA, 290,* 2464–2469.

Mauer, M. H., Burnett, K. F., Ouelette, E. A., Ironson, G. H., & Dandes, H. M. (1999). Medical hypnosis and orthopaedic hand surgery: Pain perception, post operative recovery and therapeutic comfort. *International Journal of Clinical and Experimental Hypnosis, 47,* 144–161.

Melzack, R., & Wall, P. D. (1965). Pain mechanisms: A new theory. *Science, 150,* 971–979.

Melzack, R., & Wall, P. D. (1983). *The challenge of pain.* New York: Basic Books.

Meurisse, M., Hamoir, E., Defechereux, T., Gollogly, L., Derry, O., Postal, O., et al. (1999). Bilateral neck exploration under hypnosedation: A new standard of care in primary hyperparathyroidism. *Annals of Surgery, 229,* 401–408.

Mills, J. C., & Crowley, R. J. (1986). *Therapeutic metaphors for children and the child within.* New York: Brunner/Mazel.

Paige, G. G., & Ben-Eliyahu, S. (1997). The immune-suppressive nature of pain. *Seminars in Oncology Nursing, 13,* 10–15.

Patterson, D. R., & Jenson, M. R. P. (2003). Hypnosis and clinical pain. *Psychological Bulletin 129,* 495–521.

Patterson, D. R., & Ptacek, J. T. (1997). Baseline pain as a moderator of headache hypnotic analgesia for burn injury treatment. *Journal of Consulting and Clinical Psychology, 65,* 60–67.

Rossi, E. L. (1993). The psychology of minds—body healing. *New concepts of therapeutic hypnosis.* New York: Norton.

Sali, A. (1997). Psychoneuroimmunology: Fact or Fiction. *Journal of the Family Physican, 26*(11), 1291–1299.

Sellick, S. M., & Zaza, C. (1998). Critical review of five non-pharmacologic strategies for managing cancer pain. *Cancer Prevention and Control, 2,* 7–14.

Sternbach, R. A. (1978). Clinical aspects of pain. In R.A. Steinbach (Ed.), *The psychology of pain.* New York: Raven Press.

Turk, D. C., & Holzman, A. D. (1986). Chronic pain. Interfaces among physical, psychological and social parameters. In A. D. Holzman & D. C. Turk (Eds.), *Pain management. A handbook of psychological approaches.* New York: Pergamon.

Wright, B. R., & Drummond, P. D. (2000). Rapid induction analgesia for the alleviation of procedural pain during burn care. *Burns, 26,* 275–282.

Yang, E.V. & Glasser, R. (2000). Stress induced immunomodulation: Impact on immune defenses against infectious disease. *Biomedicine and Pharmacotherapy, 54*(5), 245–250.

Yapko, M. L. (2003). *Trancework* (3rd ed.). New York: Brunner-Routledge.

CHAPTER FIFTEEN

Heroes Who Learn to Love Their Monsters: How Fantasy Film Characters Can Inspire the Journey of Individuation for Gay and Lesbian Clients in Psychotherapy

Roger Kaufman

In The Lord of the Rings film trilogy, the brave hobbit named Frodo Baggins, questing in partnership with his loyal companion, Samwise Gamgee, can only destroy the evil Ring if he develops empathy for the tortured and deformed creature called Gollum (Jackson, 2001, 2002, 2003). Meanwhile, in the original Star Wars trilogy, it is Luke Skywalker's reborn love for his true father underneath the black helmet that redeems Darth Vader (Kershner, 1980; Lucas, 1977; Marquand, 1983). And at the beginning of the film *Alien*, Lieutenant Ellen Ripley braces herself for an anticipated encounter with her vicious, reptilian extraterrestrial nemesis, only to find instead a filthy, frantic, and traumatized human girl named Newt (Cameron, 1986). This evocative theme of the hero's compassion for the grotesque and wounded leading toward accomplishment of great goals closely parallels the heroic journey on which, ideally, every client

293

in a course of psychodynamic psychotherapy embarks: an initial fright-
ful encounter with the material of the unconscious in "shadow" form;
a growing ability to understand and value the disturbing, numinous imagery of the psyche; and the eventual progress toward the achievement of
integrated psychological wholeness.

On the pages that follow, I would like to highlight the value of using
heroic themes from fantasy and science fiction films when working in a
gay-centered psychoanalytic way with adult gay and lesbian clients, whose
valiant life journeys in the face of familial and societal homophobia and
heterosexism deserve mirroring on the epic scale of such sagas as Star Wars
and the Lord of the Rings. The ideas presented here are also potentially
relevant, with some adjustments, for work with adults and adolescents of
all sexual orientations.

In the latter part of this chapter, I describe a course of weekly psychotherapy with a gay male client who has benefited from looking at
fantasy film characters in a gay perspective, but first, I set the stage by
articulating my theoretical orientation, highlighting significant homosexual archetypes, clarifying my use of terms, and summarizing the path of
development that many gay people in our culture experience from birth
to adulthood. I then describe how the heroic journeys of Ripley, Luke,
and Frodo can be seen to parallel the life experiences and inner dramas
of gay men and lesbians.

In a book about the use of superhero imagery and fantasy in psychotherapy, it may initially seem odd that I be discussing such relatively
"earthy" characters. Yet a consideration of the distinctive traits of these
heroes and others like them, as I describe further subsequently, do match
closely with the attributes of the typical superhero. Furthermore, I have
intentionally chosen characters of nebulous overt sexuality who can rea-
sonably be experienced as "gay" without too much translating by the
viewer, in contrast with the many classic superheroes such as Superman
and Spider-Man who are explicitly portrayed as heterosexual, albeit often
frustrated in love.

Danny Fingeroth (2005), a veteran writer and editor of superhero
comic books, identified these basic qualities of the superhero: "strength
of character," a "system of positive values," "a determination to, no matter what, *protect* those values," and the possession of "skills and abilities
normal humans do not" (p. 17). He added that "one thing a superhero
will usually *not* do, at least permanently, is die" (p. 18). Following this description, it can be seen that in his effort to destroy the Ring of the villain
Sauron, Frodo displays all of these virtues and skills, including resilient
goodness in the face of seductive evil, and the ability to become invisible
when necessary. Additionally, he has an elfin cape that provides effective camouflage from enemies, a magic sword that warns of approaching

trouble, and an enchanted light that shows the way in dark passages. Most important, Frodo's main accomplishment is truly of superheroic stature: he saves an entire civilization from utter devastation. At the end of his journey, he does not die but sails off to a peaceful land of immortality. Likewise, Luke Skywalker successfully resists the temptation of great evil, and his many special abilities include razor-sharp reflexes, telekinesis, and telepathy. He also manages to save an entire galaxy from tyranny through his heroic actions. Meanwhile, Lieutenant Ripley valiantly battles a truly formidable alien by relying on her own immense courage, ingenuity, and stamina. It takes numerous death-defying encounters through the course of three films before she finally sacrifices her own life for the sake of humanity, only to be resurrected through cloning for yet another breath-taking adventure.

In my experience as a psychotherapist, I have found that many gay men and lesbians can recognize and find support for their own distinct life experiences in the adventures of these heroic characters and others like them. To provide context for how I work with these themes in the room with my clients, I now briefly describe my theoretical orientation.

A SOULFUL, ARCHETYPAL APPROACH TO GAY-AFFIRMATIVE PSYCHOTHERAPY

My method of conducting psychotherapy with gay and lesbian clients, as well as my own personal journey as a gay man, has been most directly inspired by the gay-centered psychoanalytic theories proposed by psychologist Mitch Walker (1976, 1991, 1994, 1997a, 1997b, 1999). His groundbreaking work in elucidating homosexual archetypes and developing the practice of gay-centered inner work has sparked the creation of an integrative modality known as contemporary Uranian psychoanalysis that is currently in the process of refinement by a small community of psychotherapists in Los Angeles. This flexible discipline synthesizes insights from Freudian psychoanalysis, object relations, Jungian psychology, and gay-affirmative psychotherapy, among other approaches, to achieve the most effective and meaningful possible treatment for gay men and lesbians, with possible implications for clients of all gender identities and sexual orientations. The term *Uranian* comes originally from *Aphrodite Urania,* the ancient Greek goddess who was described by the philosopher Plato (trans. 1994) in his *Symposium* as the champion of "celestial" same-sex love. In that same text, Plato suggested that, in contrast with heterosexual love's biological progeny, same-sex romantic love leads to the birth of immortal "children," by which he meant the creative achievements of poets, artists, and inventors (p. 53).

By asserting an essential salutary meaning and purpose for homosexual love, Plato inspired many of history's most prominent gay visionaries, including the German lawyer and writer Karl Heinrich Ulrichs (1864–1880/1994), who was the first modern person in Western civilization to come out publicly in 1867 and who wrote 12 unprecedented treatises on what he called "Uranian love." Likewise, the turn-of-the-century English writer Edward Carpenter (1987) wrote of the distinctive "Uranian temperament" in asserting the validity of a homosexual identity. Among other early proponents of same-sex romance, the American poet Walt Whitman wrote about the distinct "adhesive" love between comrades, and Harry Hay (1987), who cofounded the first gay rights organization in the United States in 1950, inspired the modern gay liberation movement by describing homosexuals as "a separate people whose time has come" (p. 279).

Walker (1976) has cultivated the germinal ideas of these homosexual pioneers by embracing a Jungian understanding of the vast unconscious psyche, which has made it possible for him to articulate the archetypal roots of homosexual love and modern gay identity. He has elucidated the archetype of the *double,* a same-sex "twin" complex in the psyche of all people, which has the equivalent valence as the *anima* in men or the *animus* in women and which can be seen as providing the archetypal underpinning for ego identity as well as "brotherly" and "sisterly" love. Walker (1991) further explored how libido, understood in Jungian terms as a comprehensive life force energy, can constellate in a person as a distinct pattern of *homosexual libido.* Homosexual romantic desire, and the gay identity that develops around it, can be seen to arise when a person's double complex is charged by homosexual libido, causing it to function in the psyche as what Jungians call the *soul-figure,* the internal personification of the ideal beloved who is projected out onto another person when falling in love, and who drives the journey of individuation through the internal and external drama of romance. This process can be greatly facilitated and deepened when this double soul-figure complex is apprehended consciously in one's own inner world. In this understanding, homosexual love has a distinctive quality of *libidinal twinship mutuality* that functions in gay romantic relationships but also inside the mind, possibly of all individuals, as supporting a conscious "romantic" relationship between the ego and the unconscious psyche, leading toward what Jung (1935/1966) called self-realization, or the experience of psychological wholeness.

By locating the roots of same-sex romantic love and modern gay personhood in the fecund depths of the unconscious, Walker has shown the significant place that homosexual archetypes can be seen to have in the pantheon of the psyche. This profound understanding of gay identity differs in many "soulful" ways from the so-called postmodern trend in gay-affirmative psychotherapy, which has been in large part inspired by the work of the French theorist Michel Foucault (1978), who argued that modern gay identity is a linguistic "construction" of "discourse" driven by insidious power dynamics throughout society, the primary effect of which is to control individuals and limit their idiosyncratic self-expression. In this same vein, psychoanalysts Bertram Cohler and Robert Galatzer-Levy (2000) warned that psychotherapists must be careful not to impose a "master narrative" of a favorite ideal pattern of gay identity or life-span development (or both) on their clients (p. 29). This postmodern perspective is intended to be supportive of the many variations of sexuality experienced by different individuals, including the possibility of gender and/or orientation "fluidity" either in the present moment or over the course of the lifespan. However, I would argue that it is equally important that concepts of sexual fluidity not be turned into a new kind of master narrative that gets imposed on those individuals who *do* have the felt experience of a stable, abiding sexual orientation that serves as an integral, even central, part of their personal identity. As Nimmons (2002) pointed out, this highly intellectual debate is by and large ignored by the millions of gay men and lesbians who happily and consistently self-identify as gay. For these individuals, as I hope to show here, developing an understanding of their sexual identity in archetypal terms can substantively support healthy ego development and the process of self-actualization. Along these lines, my use of words such as *gay, lesbian,* and *homosexual* are not meant as the constricting, categorizing labels that many postmodernists fear (Broido, 2000; Cohler & Galatzer-Levy, 2000), but rather as highly positive, self-determining ways of communicating and celebrating the conscious achievement of a distinct, immensely valuable kind of individuality organized psychologically around the experience of romantic same-sex desire.

In this chapter, I describe the challenges of developing a healthy gay or lesbian identity in the contemporary world by employing the overarching term *heteronormativity* to describe the pervasive "presumption and assumption that all human experience is unquestionably and automatically heterosexual" (Yep, 2000, p. 168). This oppressive attitude can be seen as deeply embedded throughout all levels of individual, familial, and societal life. I also use the similar term *heterosexism* to describe the preference for heterosexuality that is both overtly and covertly expressed by individuals and institutions at the expense of all sexual minorities. In addition, the word *homophobia* is used here to describe the feelings of revulsion, fear, hatred, or moralistic judgment that individuals may

experience in relation to gay men and lesbians, as well as toward homosexual sex and gay romantic love.

THE GAY HERO'S JOURNEY: PROCESS
OF INDIVIDUATION

Jung (1952/1956) described the hero as one "who passes from joy to sorrow, from sorrow to joy, and, like the sun, now stands high at the zenith
and now is plunged into darkest night, only to rise again in new splen-
dour" (p. 171). This is an apt description for the life-span development
of gay men and lesbians, who in countless real-world examples display
great personal resilience in the face of substantial obstacles, primarily in
the form of villainous familial and societal homophobia and heterosexism. Although there are notable differences of experience between lesbians
and gay men—as well as between homosexual White people and homosexual people of color—I have tried in the following paragraphs to offer
a basic-enough description that could be relevant for all.

The archetypal view of homosexuality supported in this chapter suggests an inborn pattern of meaning and libidinal intentionality that influences a gay or lesbian child's development from the beginning of life,
becoming gradually more prominent during the shift from the preoedipal
(0–4 years) to the oedipal (4–6 years) stages of development (Isay, 1989;
Sadownick, 2002; Walker, 1991).

In their earliest years, gay and lesbian children are just as dependent on the crucially formative relationship with their primary caregiver,
usually the mother, as are other children. The mother's ability to provide a warm, stable, mirroring, and authentically empathetic "holding"
environment is critical for basic ego development and a healthy sense of
self (Mahler, Pine, & Bergman, 1975; A. Miller, 1981; Winnicott, 1971).
Because of the prevalence of narcissistic wounding in so many parents
in our culture resulting from their own lack of childhood mirroring, this
task virtually always has complications, resulting in narcissistic injury
to the child (A. Miller, 1981, 1990). This delicate mirroring process can
be seriously complicated in the case of the gay or lesbian child by the
mother's heteronormative stance, where the heterosexuality of her child
is assumed. In the very moment when she thinks she is compassionately
mirroring her child's growing sense of self, body, and future as heterosexual, she is actually imposing her emotional and cultural view onto the
child's developing homosexual subjectivity. For example, a mother might
say to her infant son or daughter, "Someday, you will get married and
have children just like I did." In this way, societal heterosexism is trans-
mitted into the homosexual child's developing psyche from the earliest

years through the mother and eventually through similar patterns with the father.

Many gay men and lesbians in psychotherapy report that they have "always" felt different from other children of the same gender, with distinct memories of being somehow "alien" beginning as early as age 3 or 4 (Blum & Pfetzing, 1997; Derby, 1994; Isay, 1989). Of course, most people have few memories of anything earlier than this age, so that sense of difference may in fact be experienced or demonstrated substantially younger. A personal example is that I have a photo of myself from age 2 "doing drag," my small feet in my mother's much-larger high heels and carrying her pocketbook on my arm. This socially unacceptable "gender-atypical" behavior is common for gay and lesbian children. For example, most of my gay male clients in psychotherapy have reported to me that they were more emotionally sensitive and more creative than other boys, often wishing to avoid violent contact sports, and feeling very comfortable in friendships with girls during a period (latency) when other boys were still hateful toward them. Many lesbians report being "tomboys" as children, with their own gender-atypical behaviors.

These qualities of "difference," whether subtle or overt, provoke a variety of negative responses from parents, siblings, teachers, peers, and others in the gay or lesbian child's life (Blum & Pfetzing, 1997). Whether it is covert disapproval, outright rejection, or cruel abuse, those who cannot appreciate the unique qualities of homosexual children repeatedly traumatize them. Such hatred is introjected by the child into the sense of self, usually as an aspect of the internal parental imagoes. Emotionally, this internalized homophobia, combined with preoedipal narcissistic wounding, is experienced as what Bradshaw (1988) has called "toxic shame," the kind of pervasive self-loathing that burns all the way to the core of being, an "internal bleeding" of the psyche where "the self becomes an object of its own contempt" (p. 10).

An alternative childhood pattern that some gay male clients have described to me is that they felt different from other boys *inside,* but successfully "passed" on the outside by consciously suppressing their natural emotional and creative sensitivity for fear of familial and peer disapproval. In my clinical experience, this pattern often appears to have even more severe ramifications later in life, when the constant suppression of emotion has become automatic and entrenched.

As they reach the age of 4 or 5, gay children can be seen to enter into a predominant oedipal dynamic with their parents that is the reverse of what heterosexual children experience. In this understanding, gay boys fall in love with their fathers and develop a rivalry and identification with their mothers (Isay, 1989; Sadownick, 2002; Walker, 1997a), whereas lesbian girls fall in love in a newly oedipal sense with their mothers, generating a rivalry and identification with their fathers. The healthy resolution of the oedipal dynamic, which leads to the solidification of ego identity, requires that, in the case of gay boys, the father *gently* frustrate his son's desire to consummate the relationship. This is much too difficult for most fathers in our homophobic culture to navigate successfully. They most often respond to their son's advances with withdrawal, ridicule, shaming verbal attacks, or physical abuse. At the same time, mothers of gay boys, who unconsciously or consciously anticipate their son's erotic interest in them, may reject the son who affectionally turns toward the father, or, as often happens, may emotionally dominate him and become overprotective of him, especially if the father is abandoning. An analogous scenario plays out for lesbian girls, with the unique dynamic that both their preoedipal and oedipal cathexis is with the mother, making successful "separation and individuation," as Mahler et al. (1975) called it, have its own particular complications.

As gay and lesbian children enter their school years, they must continue to negotiate overt or covert homophobia at home while also frequently contending with ridicule, jeers, or violent assaults from their peers. At this stage, the child is often consciously aware of his or her difference from other children but does not have sufficient language, understanding, or support to be able to develop a positive identity that honors it. Instead, he or she may begin to "connect this differentness with something forbidden, terrible, unthinkable" (Blum & Pfetzing, 1997, p. 421).

The process of gay identity development, in which the homosexual person transforms this negative experience of differentness into a positive sense of self, has been articulated by many theorists, including Cass (1979, 1984), Plummer (1975), and Troiden (1979). Walker (1997b) summarizes the Cass model with minor variations as comprising of the following identity stages: *sensitization, confusion, comparison, tolerance, acceptance, pride,* and *synthesis.* These stages suggest a challenging path that takes the homosexual person from an initial state of sexual fantasy or exploration, through a difficult internal conflict between internal urges and societal expectations, to a gradual acceptance of self as homosexual and the integration of sexual orientation into a healthy, mature ego identity.

Thus, a gay or lesbian person's journey from infancy to adulthood is a series of painful erasures, traumatic obstacles, challenging initiations, and, it is hoped, vital steps forward toward self-regard and a meaningful life as gay. Surely, the coalescing of a stable gay or lesbian identity is a substantial, even heroic, psychological achievement. It can be conceived as only the midpoint, however, in the process of individuation as articulated by Jung (1935/1966) of becoming psychologically differentiated and self-aware (also see Edinger, 1972). In synch with this Jungian view of adult development, Walker (1991, 1997b, 1999) articulated a further stage of gay individuation, called *coming out inside* in which the gay person develops conscious relationship with his or her unconscious psyche. The first encounter with the psyche is usually in form of the *shadow complex,* understood in this context as the most shameful, violent, and infantile parts of the self remaining from childhood trauma, which are often personified in the psyche as a monstrously enraged infant or devastated, shameful young child. For the gay or lesbian person, who, like virtually all others in our society, has developed an "exterior" *false self* (Winnicott, 1971), these "deformed," split-off parts of the infantile self actually have a *true self* quality to them, especially in that they are more emotionally authentic than the "as-if" false-self personality. Through the Jungian technique of *active imagination* (Johnson, 1985), a gay or lesbian person can develop a conscious relationship with this wounded child-self of the psyche by enacting an ongoing imaginal dialogue or conversation with him or her. Eventually, a person can learn to defend this true self figure from the internalized feeling-laden images of the negative, attacking aspects of the parents, what in Jungian terms are known as the shadow sides of the *mother complex* and the *father complex.* This process of developing introverted self-awareness and self-advocacy is particularly important for gay men and lesbians whose subjectivity was erased in childhood and requires a paradoxical experience in which, to develop authentic self-esteem, the individual must learn to love and care for the infantile true self in all of its most grotesquely crushed and malformed aspects.

As these basic complexes from childhood and their archetypal resonances get differentiated in the mind, a gay or lesbian person can begin to develop a conscious experience of an inner lover, the double soul-figure of the unconscious most often personified as an ideal romantic figure of the same sex. Walker describes this experience for gay men as "having a special, erotic, twin 'brother' who is felt to be the 'source of inspiration'" inside the psyche (Walker, 1991, p. 62). He is "a powerful helper, full of magic to aid in an individual's struggles," and he may appear "with an aura of beauty, youth and perfection or near-perfection" (Walker, 1976, p. 168). Alternatively, in a variation known as the *youth-adult,* the double may appear in the guise of an older same-sex figure, where the ego identity "may gain loving guidance and stimulation to self-growth" (p. 172). Conscious partnership with this soul-figure can be seen to provide a firm ground for the full actualization of a gay or lesbian person's life potential, including the achievement of loving relationships and the development of an ever-deeper connection with the archetypal psyche, which can inspire new levels of personal creativity in all its myriad forms.

This brief and schematic summary of the process of gay individuation does not describe the many idiosyncrasies of development experienced by each individual but is intended to provide a rough roadmap for psychotherapists working with gay men and lesbians. Some of these themes are illustrated with examples from fantasy and science fiction films that follows.

USING FANTASY FILMS TO AMPLIFY HOMOSEXUAL ARCHETYPES AND THE JOURNEY OF INDIVIDUATION

In general, Hollywood blockbuster films are not known for their positive treatment of gay and lesbian characters. Yet with an appreciation of archetypes such as the double, along with some capacity for symbolic thinking, many films from the fantasy and science fiction genres can be fruitfully experienced in a gay way. In many cases, the archetypal resonances are stronger in these heroically epic films than in "gay genre" films that feature explicitly gay characters, where the plot and visual dynamism is almost always limited in scope. The films discussed here also seem to me to be more relevant for gay and lesbian clients in psychotherapy than more obvious "superhero" films, which are often drenched in overt heterosexual references and portray a vigorously heteronormative world. For example, *Spider-Man* opens with a voiceover narration by Peter Parker, aka Spider-Man, saying, "This story, like any other story worth telling, is all about a girl . . . the girl next door" (Raimi, 2002). The entire film and its sequel, *Spider-Man 2* (Raimi, 2004), are dominated by the mundane modern-day vicissitudes of heterosexual courtship. Furthermore, the plotlines of most superhero films involve the protagonist saving the "good" everyday, modern world from the "bad" villains. Their heroism is mostly limited to destroying their enemies and supporting the status quo. Although the fantasy films I discuss also highlight the differences between good and evil, there is an attempt by heroes like Ripley, Luke, and Frodo to achieve a more nuanced integration of the "shadow," leading toward a substantial transformation of character, and often, of the entire society portrayed.

In previous chapters (Kaufman, 2002, 2003, 2006), I have offered detailed arguments for how gay archetypal themes appear to be, regardless of the filmmakers' stated intent, an inherent symbolic aspect of The Lord of the Rings trilogy and the Star Wars saga. However, for the purposes of this discussion, the operative question is not if a film is *inherently* gay, but if it can be *appreciated* in a way that is mirroring and meaningful for gay men and lesbians. The films discussed here are some of the most relevant examples, but there are many other movies that can be enjoyed in a similar manner.

How can therapists effectively introduce mythic themes from films into their actual work with clients? Before taking this step, I believe that the therapist should first privilege a client's own personal imagery, especially as it comes from dreams, memories, feelings, and creative efforts such as writing or drawing. But often there are situations in the therapy in which a particular film character or image might provide an effective way to (a) educate the client about the process of dynamic psychotherapy and psychological growth, (b) mirror the client's life experiences, (c) validate the client's encounter with his or her own unconscious material, (d) inspire the client in seeking his or her full potential, or (e) a combination of these. This process works most easily if a client has already seen the film being referenced, but alternatively, when appropriate, the therapist can invite the client to watch a particular film at home if the clinician feels such a directive will not be too burdensome for the client in a way that might disrupt the therapeutic alliance.

I would suggest that effective psychoanalytic psychotherapy is an initiatory process in its own right, requiring the client to descend into his or her own unconscious underworld of painful trauma for successful treatment. In the midst of this process, it can be useful to offer accessible stories that both mirror the descent and show the future possibility for the clouds to break and the sun to shine again. As described here, the ordeals of Ripley, Luke, and Frodo are emblematic of this hero's journey, with specific meaningful resonances for lesbians and gay men.

The Alien Quadrilogy: The Struggle With the Terrible Mother

Whether they are gay, straight, or bisexual, all clients in psychoanalytic psychotherapy must come to terms with their original relationships with both parents. Because in almost all cases, the child's first relationship is with the mother, working through this primary affiliation becomes central in any long-term therapy process. Sometimes this work can appear to have a sexist quality to it, as if the mother gets solely "blamed" for all wounds of the child (J. Miller, 1986). Along these lines, from an adult perspective, it is easy to see how the forces of contemporary capitalistic patriarchal society oppress women, undermining their ability to authentically nurture their children while also putting them into the role of primary enforcer of dominant cultural attitudes. In therapeutic work, however, the focus must be on recovering and reconstructing the *actual emotional experience* that the client had as a *child* in relation to his or her mother (A. Miller, 1981, 1990). Because young children have no cognizance of larger societal forces, their only awareness is how their mother is actually treating them. Of course, even this awareness is limited at the conscious level, as large parts of the emotional experience of mother, especially in its traumatizing aspects, are too painful to bear and become split-off and pushed into the unconscious. The result is that the mother complex that develops in the psyche of young children—and especially in gay and lesbian children whose heteronormative mothers have overtly or covertly erased their budding sense of homosexual self—has a particularly demonic and toxic dark side. Jung (1952/1956) described the archetypal underpinning for this negative aspect of the mother complex as the "Terrible Mother."

The four-film Alien series (Scott, 1979; Cameron, 1986; Fincher, 1992; Jeunet, 1997) offers an unprecedented visceral depiction of the Terrible Mother in the form of a massively strong, viciously reptilian, extraterrestrial fiend with huge claws, multiple piercing sets of jaws, and steel-melting molecular acid for blood. The eggs she lays spawn spider-crab-like creatures that clamp onto the face of a human host, where they insert a small fetal version of the monster through the person's mouth into his or her torso that soon after births itself by ripping through the host's chest. It is the daunting task of Lieutenant Ellen Ripley, a tough young woman who is second in command on a far-range mining spaceship, to encounter and fight off repeatedly this relentless alien species. Throughout the four films there are minor references to Ripley having intimate relationships with men, but her overall image is one of fierce independence. What could be seen as her most overtly romantic relationship occurs with another woman, a young rebel named Annalee Call, in the fourth film, *Alien Resurrection*. Ripley's self-reliance, perseverance, and tremendous empathy for the defenseless make her an excellent role model for lesbians in the process of self-discovery. And with a little gender "translating," she is also a superb hero for gay men to appreciate.

It is Ripley's living nightmare in the second film, *Aliens*, that most strikingly illustrates primary themes of the individuation process for gay and lesbian clients in psychotherapy. Reluctantly returning to the alien planet where she barely survived her first terrifying encounter with the gruesome beast, Ripley is exploring a deserted colony when movement is detected by her military cohorts. The tension ratchets up as they all wonder, *is this to be our first encounter with the monster?* Instead, a disheveled and crazed human girl is spotted, and Ripley takes the lead to chase her through air ducts until she finally captures the girl. Ripley holds her tightly until her hysteria subsides and she relaxes in Ripley's arms. Through fits and starts, Ripley develops a bond with the girl, made mute from trauma, and manages to get her talking again. Ripley makes a promise to the girl, whose name is Newt, that she will not abandon her and will protect her from the destructive alien who has killed the girl's family and all the other people of her terraforming colony. Ripley and Newt form a secure youth–adult twin partnership of mutual support that endures throughout their shared journey. Unfortunately, at the climax of the film, Newt is snatched away by one of the aliens and brought to the central nest of the queen beast, where she is primed to become a host for one of the monster's many larvae. Terrified but undaunted, Ripley valiantly rescues Newt from the egg-laying behemoth and successfully battles her ferocious nemesis until finally victorious. It would be difficult to find a more apt metaphor for the epic challenge facing the gay or lesbian client in psychotherapy who must rescue his or her own abandoned child-self in the psyche and learn to defend on an ongoing basis the true self from the grasping, dominating, attacking aspect of the mother complex.

In the third film of the series, Ripley discovers that she has an alien fetus inside of her, and this is what compels her to sacrifice herself by falling into a pit of molten ore. But as shown in the fourth film of the series, still-surviving samples of her blood are used for a cloning technique that results in a "reborn" Ripley as well as a new alien fetus that is surgically removed and quickly grows into a full-grown extraterrestrial. Through this process, Ripley has actually taken on some of the qualities of the fiend, which then gives birth to a new half-human/half-alien hybrid. This complex imagery suggests that even the most monstrous parts of the psyche can eventually be integrated and possibly humanized. That process is incomplete at the end of *Alien Resurrection,* because the new hybrid is still too violent to be saved, but the fourth film does provide thematic imagery that can be seen as the development of lesbian love and identity out of that struggle. Through the course of that film, Ripley begins what can easily be appreciated as a lesbian romance with Call, a young principled female rebel posing as a thieving gangster who is determined to protect Earth from the dangerous aliens. It is eventually discovered that Call is an android, considered another kind of monster, and she is subjected to intense ridicule from other crew members, reminiscent of the jeers that gay and lesbian people have often suffered. Ripley defends her by saying, "No human being is that humane," referencing Call's devotion to her cause, and their affection for each other grows. Both Ripley in her clone existence and Call in her robotic construction are struggling to become "human," a process that serves as a mutual goal in their parallel journeys. The entire four-film series culminates in the two women standing together in the picture window of a spaceship, finally arriving at Mother Earth, which appears below them perhaps as a symbol of wholeness achieved through the process of differentiating out and then beginning to reintegrate both dark and light aspects of the archetypal feminine. Call asks, "What happens now?" and Ripley says, "I don't know, I'm a stranger here myself." The full flowering of individuated lesbian twinship love is unfamiliar territory, but now, finally, entirely possible.

Star Wars: Finding the True Father Through Abiding Same-Sex Partnerships

With its uniquely intense visual and aural complexity and texture, the six-film Star Wars saga (Kershner, 1980; Lucas, 1977, 1999, 2002, 2005; Marquand, 1983) can be appreciated in the aggregate as a symbolic evocation of the grandeur of the numinous unconscious human psyche and its epic internal dramas. Revealed through this kaleidoscopic sound and imagery is a vibrant galaxy where the primary mode of human relationship appears to be intimate, enduring same-sex partnerships, ranging from the affectionate, lifelong bond of Qui-Gon Jinn and Obi-Wan Kenobi to the loyal twinship of Queen Amidala and her bodyguard, Padmé, as shown in *Star Wars: Episode I—The Phantom Menace*. In a previous chapter (Kaufman, 2006), I have identified 28 same-sex "twin" partnerships throughout the six *Star Wars* films, all of which provide strongly evocative examples of the double archetype. As described earlier, the double serves as the love-inducing, individuation-inspiring soul-figure in the psyche of gay men and lesbians and can be seen to have similar possible benefits when cultivated in the minds of all people.

Central to the epic, as featured in *Episodes IV–VI*, is the initiatory odyssey of young Luke Skywalker, whose arduous individuation process is primarily spurred by supportive, transformative same-sex partnerships with Obi-Wan Kenobi, Han Solo, and Yoda. Luke's only minor flirtation with the opposite sex is with Princess Leia, who eventually turns out to be his twin sister.

The story of Luke training to become a Jedi Knight provides a meaningful analogy for the identity development process that gay men and lesbians experience. He starts out as just a kid on the farm but then discovers through his encounter with an older man, Obi-Wan "Ben" Kenobi, that he has an inborn potential to "learn the ways of the Force" and become a Jedi knight as his "true self" identity. The trouble is, by the time Luke is born, the eons-old Jedi Order has been outlawed and collapsed. Much of his training must come through his own trials and challenges. Likewise, gay men and lesbians respond to an inner "Force" of libidinal desire that spurs them to come out and individuate as gay despite the prohibitions of their parents and society, and they do this largely on their own, with few or no positive role models. It is hoped that a gay person will eventually meet his or her version of Obi-Wan Kenobi, in the form of a friend, teacher, or psychotherapist who can help validate and nurture the individual's budding gay identity.

Although he doesn't realize it until he's already far along in his journey, Luke has embarked on a quest to find and redeem his "true" father.
This mythic story line can be deeply evocative for gay men in particular who yearn for father-love but have been subtly or overtly rejected by
their biological fathers. A gay man who has been shamed, abandoned, or
abused by the man who raised him will constellate a hateful internal "dark
father," which is echoed in the name "Darth Vader," where "Vader" is the
Dutch word for "father." In the process of psychotherapy, a gay man may
be able to revisit the intensely passionate feelings and hurts from his own
oedipal drama to differentiate this Terrible Father and gain an internal
experience of a positive archetypal paternal presence that is nurturing and
loving of his gay identity.

Supported by his enduring partnerships with Obi-Wan and Yoda, but
also moving beyond their training, Luke grows in his ability to sense the
goodness buried deep in his imposing tyrannical adversary, Darth Vader.
In the climactic moment of the entire saga, Luke valiantly tosses aside his
light saber in a what can be seen as a homosexually creative moment of
what I have termed *phallic receptivity* (Kaufman, 2006). By putting aside
his aggression and refusing to fight, Luke successfully awakens compassion in Darth Vader, who is finally revealed just before dying to be Luke's
true father, Anakin Skywalker. If a gay man can in an analogous way
becomes receptive to the archetypal imagery of his own unconscious psyche, he may discover his own true loving archetypal "father" inside. This
theme is solidified at the end of the saga when Luke's soul-figures, Obi-
Wan and Yoda, appear to him in their ghostly form, now joined by the
ghost of his redeemed father, Anakin.

The Lord of the Rings: Celebration of the Double

Based on the original novel by J. R. R. Tolkien, Peter Jackson's popular
trilogy of *The Fellowship of the Ring*, *The Two Towers*, and *The Return
of the King* (Jackson, 2001, 2002, 2003) has satisfied countless filmgo-
ers of all genders and sexual orientations throughout the world, but it
has particularly strong resonances for gay men and, with a little gender
translating, can also be meaningful for lesbians. In the following section,
I describe an example of work with a client in weekly therapy that was
in progress during the theatrical release of the last two of these films, but
before doing that, I introduce some of the primary homosexual archetypal
themes that are so vividly portrayed in the trilogy.

The Lord of the Rings depicts the extended epic journey of individuation for a hobbit named Frodo. He is accompanied every step of the
way by his steadfast partner, Sam. As I have described in a previous article
(Kaufman, 2003), their pairing is perhaps one of the clearest examples of

the double archetype to appear in modern literature and film. Although it is somewhat toned down in the film version, Sam is clearly devoted to Frodo and repeatedly risks his life to save his comrade, even carrying him on his back for the final climactic hike up the side of Mount Doom. Furthermore, Sam and Frodo's primary pairing is evocatively echoed by myriad other same-sex partnerships. Frodo has transformative relationships with the would-be king, Aragorn, as well as the powerful wizard, Gandalf. There are also the everlasting same-sex pairs of hobbits Merry and Pippin, the dwarf Gimli and the elf Legolas, as well as, on the shadow side, Sauron and Saruman. In fact, of the nine original members of the Fellowship of the Ring, none are married or have children, and all spend their time in the close, intimate company of one another. In contrast to the countless Hollywood comedies, romantic dramas, and action pictures saturated with heterosexual imagery, it is a refreshing opportunity for gay men and lesbians to see a heroic three-film epic in which virtually all of the primary relationships are abiding, intimate same-sex bonds. When approached symbolically, these relationships can help a gay person to clarify imaginatively his or her own internal same-sex soul-figure.

Frodo does not possess the musculature of a typical superhero; in fact, as a hobbit he is only half the height of a grown man, but he has a superhuman ability to withstand the tempting influence of the evil Ring, and the unique insight to realize that he must befriend the grotesque creature named Gollum to find his way into the shadow realm of Mordor. Through breakthrough computer graphics, Gollum becomes fully alive on screen in a way that perhaps no fantasy creature ever has before. Almost 600 years old, Gollum actually appears as an overgrown, albeit emaciated, baby, virtually naked save for a tiny loincloth, full of raw, primitive emotion, simultaneously smashed and vital. This bizarre creature provides a ripe analogy for gay clients in psychotherapy who need to develop a relationship with their own devastated, inferior inner child. Just as Ripley bonds with the little girl named Newt in *Aliens*, so Frodo must make partnership with Gollum, who is an even more visceral image of the crushed infant-self in the psyche. Because Gollum has spent half a millennium hiding away in a dark cave, he serves as a powerful personification of the most painful childhood feelings of hurt—rage, toxic shame, and seething envy that were split off from the conscious personality in earliest childhood and sequestered in the dark corners of the unconscious. As seen in the case study that follows, Gollum provides a possible starting point for inner understanding for many gay men and lesbians whose internalized homophobia and self-hatred prevents them from initially identifying with a heroic character such as Frodo. *The Lord of the Rings* offers much additional imagery for gay people, some of which is highlighted in the following discussion.

CASE STUDY: A GAY MAN FINDS MIRRORING
IN *THE LORD OF THE RINGS*

When Derrick first came to my office in the summer of 2002, he presented as friendly, intellectually curious, and moderately depressed. A handsome, 28-year-old, gay White man who was working as a paralegal, he had moved to Los Angeles from a Midwestern state about 5 years earlier. Derrick was finding it difficult to make friends and tended to loose himself in long hours at work. He infrequently dated other men but had not yet made a satisfying, sustainable connection with anyone. (This discussion preserves the progression of an actual course of therapy but has been composited from several cases to protect the anonymity of individual clients.)

Derrick admitted to feeling painfully empty inside but otherwise had difficulty sensing or describing his own feelings. Instead, he would at certain moments describe feeling "shut-down" emotionally, loosing his ability to feel or think. This occurred especially when we began to talk about early childhood or when I asked him about his feelings toward me. In addition, Derrick was often nervous and fearful in a variety of different settings. Initially, he met the criteria for both dysthymic disorder and generalized anxiety disorder. He did not meet the full criteria for a personality disorder, but he clearly had narcissistic injuries that manifested predominantly in a depressive (rather than grandiose) pattern, and there were some borderline-level traits that might be called "holes" in his ego structure.

My initial treatment plan was focused on helping Derrick stabilize and increase his basic self-esteem so that he could set healthier limits on his work patterns and develop more satisfying friendships. My primary goal was to help Derrick become more interiorly focused and develop empathy for his own emotional experience. This would be achieved by (a) mirroring and validating Derrick's feelings; (b) highlighting the presence, as relevant, of unconscious feelings of toxic shame, hurt-rage, fear, and grief; (c) eliciting memories of early childhood in the relationship with his parents; (d) educating him about different basic complexes in the psyche; (e) describing the effect of internalized homophobia in his psyche; (f) identifying his defense mechanisms and feelings as they appeared in the transference relationship; and (g) educating him about an archetypal way of appreciating his gay identity.

First Phase of Derrick's Treatment

In our early sessions, Derrick gave me some details about his childhood relationship with his parents. As long as he could remember, his father had been overtly shaming of any behaviors in Derrick that were not distinctly masculine. He never consciously felt close with his father, who became more and more distant as Derrick grew up. In more recent years, his father had become visibly depressed and even more difficult to communicate with. Derrick did not have much trouble admitting disappointment and anger toward his father, but the situation with his mother was much more complicated. She had not been overtly derogatory toward Derrick's gender-atypical behavior, but she clearly held the heteronormative stance of her culturally conservative upbringing in the Deep South. Even though Derrick had come out to both parents when he was in college, there was no longer open discussion of it when he visited them. He was able to talk with his mother about it a little, but as far as he could tell, she never discussed it with his father, suggesting that she carried substantial shame about her son's homosexuality. He described his mother as emotionally "guarded," even "cold" in her demeanor, but more details of their dynamic were quite mysterious because he had difficulty remembering what it really felt like to be with her as a child. Often when I would probe his memories or feelings about her he would shut down emotionally. My sense was that Derrick harbored substantial hurt-rage toward his mother but became so overwhelmed with toxic shame around the taboo emotion that he had to dissociate from both feelings. I educated Derrick about the concept of toxic shame as an intense emotion that overwhelmed his ability to experience other feelings. I suggested that it had first developed in him because of a lack of basic positive mirroring by his mother, intensified by the homophobia he had internalized from both parents. These concepts resonated strongly with him, and he soon was able to name his frequent experience of this most corrosive emotion without prompting. Getting to the hurt-rage underneath was, however, still a big challenge.

Our sessions would often seem to get stuck when Derrick started to talk about his mother, and my various efforts to help him descend into deeper feelings were minimally effective. Likewise, my attempts to invite him to talk about any transference feelings in our relationship resulted in reports of feeling numb. I suggested to Derrick that this experience of emotional paralysis was probably how he responded to his mother when he was younger but that underneath this defense was a probably very hurt little boy full of painful feelings that she could not tolerate. Derrick appreciated the image but had difficulty achieving a felt experience of such an "inner person."

At this point in our work, Derrick came in one late December day quite excited about a movie he had just seen, *The Lord of the Rings: The Two Towers* (Jackson, 2002). He was bowled over by the dynamic visual intensity of the film, and in particular was impressed by the fantastical creature named Gollum.

I suggested to Derrick that perhaps Gollum was an image of his own wounded kid-self in the psyche, and his feelings for Gollum in the film were really the beginning of empathy for that part of himself. This was initially surprising to Derrick, but it began to make more sense to him as we explored the idea. I further described to Derrick how he might find a role model in the character of Frodo, and that he might continue to develop a relationship with this part of himself just as Frodo did with Gollum. I also explained to Derrick that Frodo's partnership with his loyal friend, Sam, could be seen as a gay romance, and that Frodo's ability to feel compassion for Gollum was perhaps born out of the steady support and fellowship he received from Sam. Derrick told me he thought that Sam was a "hottie," and I suggested in response that Sam might represent a kind of internal same-sex "muse" that spurred Derrick's psychological growth.

In the sessions that followed, Derrick would often be describing his feelings or behavior in various situations, and then he would say, "That's Gollum!" The theme of heroic Frodo feeling compassion for monstrous Gollum gave Derrick concrete imagery that he had not yet been able to access in his own unconscious. With the help of these symbolic themes, Derrick was beginning to differentiate out an authentic image of the devastated self found in the shadow-side of his psyche. It wasn't pretty, but it had a tangible, real resonance for him. Simultaneously, he found pleasure in the idea of seeing Frodo and Sam as a couple. His understanding here was still largely extroverted, experienced consciously as a longing for an "actual Sam" in his life, but it felt like a seed had been planted and that eventually Derrick might find his own double soul-figure inside the psyche along with the possibility of romance with another gay man.

Second Phase of Derrick's Treatment

Over the course of a year, Derrick ventured more frequently into the gay community, surprising himself by successfully developing new friendships and an active social life. On an interior level, Derrick was becoming quite sophisticated psychologically in terms of understanding early childhood dynamics and talking with his new friends about psychological concepts, especially learning how to name and work with "toxic shame." The direct references to Gollum, Frodo, and Sam subsided, but he did appear to have more empathy for his own internal experience. He seemed to have benefited from our work and was engaged in our sessions.

At about this time, Derrick started meeting other men for casual sex "hookups" through the Internet. This was almost an "adolescent" time for Derrick, and perhaps in part a natural outgrowth of his feeling more accepting of his body and himself as a sexually desirable man. He consistently reported maintaining "safer sex" practices, yet these liaisons sometimes involved the use of "crystal" (methamphetamine). A pattern developed where approximately once a month, he would get together with other men for sex and "partying," embarking on crystal binges that would last as long as 3 days. Afterward, he would "crash" painfully, feeling depressed, swearing to never do it again. But a month would go by, and he could not resist.

Derrick and I talked directly about the stresses that the crystal use was having on his body and mind, focusing on the highly addictive nature of the drug. There were also regular check-ins about safer sex practices. What had been subtly present all along in the transference now became obvious, where Derrick became the rebellious child, and I felt forced into the position of scolding parent. He began to oscillate between feeling angry with me and shutting down, as he had so often in the first year of our work together.

At this point, I realized that in my recent efforts to help Derrick my own anxiety had been rising during our sessions without my full awareness. Toxic shame about my abilities as a therapist had been provoked by Derrick's acting-out behavior, and I could feel unresolved infantile hurt-rage bubbling underneath my anxiety. Secretly, I had an inner voice that was yelling at Derrick, "How dare you have a setback and disprove my ability as a good therapist!" As Winnicott (1947/1975) pointed out, the psychotherapist must be conscious of his or her "hate" for the client, or else it gets acted out in the relationship. I began to appreciate that, through the phenomenon of projective identification (Cashdan, 1988; Klein, 1975), the client and I were reenacting aspects of his original childhood dynamic with his mother. I described for Derrick how I felt this was now happening between us, acknowledging how my own anxiety and hurt-rage may have been contributing to the reemergence of his shutting-down pattern, and even possibly his acting out around anonymous sex and crystal use. Derrick found my admission very helpful, although also scary, because it represented an increase in our intimacy and an admission of my fallibility.

By exploring our recent interactions with each other, Derrick and I were able to achieve a deeper understanding of what happened between him and his mother in his earliest years. Underneath her "guardedness," she was actually angry and anxious, just as I had been in our recent sessions. The client began to remember that she could actually be extremely mean sometimes, abruptly scolding him and his younger siblings. The client internalized her anxiety and hate but had to split this off from his conscious self to get the indulgences of the "good mommy." Now, in adulthood, it felt as if the internal "bad mommy" had resurfaced and taken over, most directly experienced as toxic shame. He resorted to anonymous sex and crystal as a substitute for the "good mommy."

As Derrick's insight around his childhood experiences grew, and as my ability to maintain awareness of my own feelings during the sessions increased, our rapport became newly secure, and his ability to stay engaged in the sessions improved.

Third Phase of Derrick's Treatment

Derrick's crystal use decreased but did not stop altogether. At this point, with my countertransference more "partnered" and Derrick's self-awareness growing, we were able together to explore more deeply the allure of the recreational sex and drug use. It wasn't only about a repetition compulsion seeking the soothing of the "good mommy," although that was an crucial aspect of it. There was also something deeply masculine about Derrick's sexual experiences, and he began to describe for me his phallic enthrallment with other gay men and the beauty of the male body.

Derrick and I began to discuss different ways that he could more healthfully celebrate his gay sexuality. I educated him more directly at this point about an archetypal, symbolic way of appreciating this burgeoning force within him. Together we were searching for satisfying images that would be substantial enough to encapsulate Derrick's rising homosexual desire.

This exploration lead to new conversations about themes we had discussed previously in *The Lord of the Rings*. Together, we revisited Frodo's heroic quest as it had been portrayed since our earlier conversations in the third installment of the Lord of the Rings film trilogy, *The Return of the King* (Jackson, 2003). We discussed Frodo's journey as a metaphor for Derrick's initiation into his full adult gay identity, intensified in recent years through the process of his work in psychotherapy. By tracking Frodo's continued descent into the shadow realm of Mordor and related aspects of the epic, Derrick found more meaningful parallels with his own life story. For example, the giant spider called Shelob that pierces Frodo and paralyzes him was an ideal metaphor for how Derrick's mother would "pierce" Derrick with her anger and render him numb. Similarly, Derrick could see in the despairing character of Denethor, steward of Gondor, a powerful metaphor for his relationship with his own deeply hopeless father. In a state of utter despair, Denethor attempts to die by throwing himself and his son, Faramir, on a burning pyre. In a similar way, Derrick felt his father's depression as drawing him into a deathly fire. The image further echoed how Derrick felt that he was being burned alive by his father's homophobia.

Derrick found the most positive and satisfying mirroring around his homosexual libido in the culminating scenes of the film trilogy. While massive battles are fought with stirring dynamism, Frodo's ardent partner, Sam, carries him up into the very core of the shadow-realm, the grand inner chamber of red-hot erupting Mt. Doom. Through a difficult struggle between Frodo, Sam, and Gollum, the evil Ring is finally destroyed. At this moment, the skyscraping tower of the villain Sauron shatters like glass, and the militant hordes suddenly disperse as the earth itself opens up and the massive Black Gate of Mordor collapses into the chasm. Now Mt. Doom with great orgasmic explosiveness releases the full force of its massive primordial molten rock into the air. Utterly surrounded by rivers of lava, Frodo and Sam ponder their ultimate death, only to be swooped up and saved by giant eagles under the command of the white wizard Gandalf in what can be appreciated as a potent reference to Zeus's homosexual abduction of Ganymede. Now the clouds really do lift and the sun shines again, in this instance on the coronation of Aragorn as the rightful beneficent King. As a huge crowd on top of the seven-tiered round white city of Minas Tirith celebrate his ascension, Aragorn strides over to greet the four heroic hobbits, Frodo, Sam, Merry, and Pippin. When they begin to bow down to him, he says emphatically, "My friends, you bow to no one," then he himself and everyone in the great throng bow down to the stouthearted nature of these four loyal comrades, a pair of two steadfast twinship pairs, the archetype of the double displayed doubly and celebrated in a heroic way perhaps never before seen on film. In these final moments of the epic, countless visual, musical, and thematic elements evoking homosexual twinship and the bursting energy of masculine phallic libido combine together in an inspiring, inspiriting, intoxicating climax.

Through this vibrant imagery, Derrick had found a memorable symbolic experience that deeply mirrored his love for other men and gave him a soul-level jolt of imaginative pleasure. I encouraged him to explore these same themes of libidinal twinship mutuality and homosexual eros in other films, focusing him on the visual imagination of the Star Wars saga, the Alien films, *E.T.: The Extra-Terrestrial* (Spielberg, 1982), *The Dark Crystal* (Henson & Oz, 1982), and *The NeverEnding Story* (Peterson, 1984), among others.

As this chapter is being written, Derrick has not used crystal in several months and is feeling more stable than ever before. He is enjoying more intimate friendships and is learning healthier ways to self-soothe and nurture himself. Furthermore, Derrick has a deeper experience of his own identity as homosexual. He has developed an interest in understanding the living psyche, especially as he is able to experience it through imaginative films and the heroic characters he identifies with in the process of viewing them. In this sense, he has taken on the role of Frodo in his own epic journey of gay individuation, his identity and sense of gay soul substantively strengthened. Derrick's struggle to develop an authentic and secure sense of self is by no means finished, as his wrestling with toxic shame has not ended and he still finds it difficult to fully express the depth of his own feelings. But overall, his satisfaction in life has grown substantially.

CONCLUSION: THE HEROIC POTENTIAL OF GAY AND LESBIAN CLIENTS

In this chapter, I have offered a description of the treacherous path that each gay or lesbian person must negotiate in a heteronormative world to honor the call of his or her homosexual libido and come out as gay despite the disapproval of parents, peers, and the larger society. From a broad evolutionary perspective, this honorable development of authentic gay personhood, even with the unavoidably deep scars from childhood trauma, is a huge historic achievement, comparable in its own way to the grandly heroic deeds of fantasy film characters such as Ellen Ripley, Luke Skywalker, and Frodo Baggins. Psychotherapists who practice in a gay-affirmative way are uniquely positioned to support and nurture this accomplishment in their gay and lesbian clients by offering them honest mirroring at the most gruesome, terrifying depths of the unconscious, as well as at the most satisfyingly meaningful heights of erotically alive, dynamically individuated self-acceptance and self-awareness.

For those who resonate with the themes, it is possible to integrate heroic film imagery into a course of psychoanalytically oriented gay-affirmative psychotherapy while also staying focused on the primary work of uncovering, validating, and working through the client's early childhood trauma. Eventually, many gay and lesbian clients can learn to take a heroic stance in their own mind to cultivate their individual subjectivity, and to neutralize the messages of hate and shame internalized from family, culture, religion, and government. Through these vitalizing practices, gay men and lesbians can model an urgently needed kind of internally centered, autonomously creative individuality that can be potentially inspiring for all people.

REFERENCES

Blum, A., & Pfetzing, V. (1997). The trauma of growing up gay. *Gender and Psychoanalysis, 2,* 427–442.

Bradshaw, J. (1988). *Healing the shame that binds you.* Deerfield Beach, FL: Health Communications.

Broido, E. (2000). Constructing identity: The nature and meaning of lesbian, gay, and bisexual identities. In R. Perez, K. DeBord, & K. Bieschke (Eds.), *Handbook of counseling and psychotherapy with lesbian, gay, and bisexual clients*. Washington, DC: American Psychological Association.

Cameron, J. (Director). (1986). *Aliens* [Motion picture]. United States: Twentieth Century Fox.

Carpenter, E. (1987). Selected insights. In M. Thompson (Ed.), *Gay spirit: Myth and meaning*. New York: St. Martin's.

Cashdan, S. (1988). *Object relations therapy: Using the relationship*. New York: Norton.

Cass, V. (1979). Homosexual identity formation: A theoretical model. *Journal of Homosexuality, 4*, 219–235.

Cass, V. (1984). Homosexual identity: A concept in need of definition. *Journal of Homosexuality, 9*, 105–126.

Cohler, B., & Galatzer-Levy, R. (2000). *The course of gay and lesbian lives: Social and psychoanalytic perspectives*. Chicago: University of Chicago Press.

Derby, D. (1994). Gay, lesbian, and bisexual youth. In T. DeCrescenzo (Ed.), *Helping gay and lesbian youth: New policies, new programs, new practice*. New York: Harrington Park Press.

Edinger, E. (1972). *Ego and archetype*. Boston: Shambhala.

Fincher, D. (Director). (1992). *Alien 3* [Motion picture]. United States: Twentieth Century Fox.

Fingeroth, D. (2004). *Superman on the couch: What superheroes really tell us about ourselves and our society*. New York: Continuum.

Foucault, M. (1978). *The history of sexuality—Volume I: An introduction*. New York: Vintage Books.

Hay, H. (1987). A separate people whose time has come. In M. Thompson (Ed.) *Gay spirit: Myth and meaning (279-291)*. New York: St. Martin's.

Henson, J., & Oz, F. (Directors). (1982). *The dark crystal*. [Motion picture]. United States: The Jim Henson Company.

Isay, R. (1989). *Being homosexual: Gay men and their development*. New York: Farrar, Straus & Giroux.

Jackson, P. (Director.) (2001). *The lord of the rings: The fellowship of the ring* [Motion picture]. United States: New Line Cinema.

Jackson, P. (Director.) (2002). *The lord of the rings: The two towers* [Motion picture]. United States: New Line Cinema.

Jackson, P. (Director.) (2003). *The lord of the rings: The return of the king* [Motion picture]. United States: New Line Cinema.

Jeunet, J. (Director). (1997). *Alien resurrection* [Motion picture]. United States: Twentieth Century Fox.

Johnson, R. (1985). (R. F. C. Hull, Trans.). *Inner work: Using dreams and active imagination for personal growth*. San Francisco: Harper San Francisco.

Jung, C. G. (1956). *Symbols of transformation*. Princeton, NJ: Princeton University Press. (Original work published 1952)

Jung, C. G. (1966). *Two chapters on analytical psychology* (2nd ed.). Princeton, NJ: Princeton University Press.

Kaufman, R. (2002, September–October). High camp in a galaxy far away. *Gay and Lesbian Review Worldwide, 33–35.*

Kaufman, R. (2003, July–August). *Lord of the Rings* taps a gay archetype. *Gay and Lesbian Review Worldwide, 31–33.*

Kaufman, R. (2006). How the *Star Wars* saga evokes the creative promise of homosexual love: A gay-centered psychological perspective. In M. W. Kapell & J. S. Lawrence (Eds.), *Finding the force of the Star Wars franchise: Fans, merchandise and critics* (pp. 131–156). New York: Peter Lang.

Kershner, I. (Director). (1980). *Star wars: Episode V—The empire strikes back* [Motion picture]. United States: Twentieth Century Fox.

Klein, M. (1975). *Envy and gratitude and other works 1946–1963.* New York: Free Press.

Lucas, G. (Writer/Director). (1977). *Star wars: Episode IV—A new hope* [Motion picture]. United States: Twentieth Century Fox.

Lucas, G. (Writer/Director). (1999). *Star wars: Episode I—The phantom menace* [Motion picture]. United States: Twentieth Century Fox.

Lucas, G. (Director). (2002). *Star wars: Episode II—Attack of the clones* [Motion picture]. United States: Twentieth Century Fox.

Lucas, G. (Writer/Director). (2005). *Star wars: Episode III—Revenge of the sith* [Motion picture]. United States: Twentieth Century Fox.

Mahler, M., Pine, F., & Bergman, A. (1975). *The psychological birth of the human infant.* New York: Basic Books.

Marquand, R. (Director). (1983). *Star wars: Episode VI—Return of the Jedi* [Motion picture]. United States: Twentieth Century Fox.

Miller, A. (1981). *The drama of the gifted child.* New York: Basic Books.

Miller, A. (1990). *Banished knowledge: Facing childhood injuries.* New York: Anchor Books.

Miller, J. (1986). *Toward a new psychology of women* (2nd ed.). Boston: Beacon Press.

Nimmons, D. (2002). *The soul beneath the skin: The unseen hearts and habits of gay men.* New York: St. Martin's Griffin.

Peterson, W. (Director). (1984). *The neverending story* [Motion picture]. United States: Warner Bros.

Plato. (1994). *Symposium* (R. Waterfield, Trans.). New York: Oxford University Press.

Plummer, K. (1975). *Sexual stigma: An interactionist account.* London: Routledge & Kegan Paul.

Raimi, S. (Director). (2002). *Spider-Man* [Motion picture]. United States: Columbia Pictures.

Raimi, S. (Director). (2004). *Spider-Man 2* [Motion picture]. United States: Columbia Pictures.

Sadownick, D. (2002). My father, my self: Coming out inside as the next stage of gay liberation. In B. Shenitz (Ed.), *The man I might become.* New York: Marlowe.

Scott, R. (Director). (1979). *Alien* [Motion picture]. United States: Twentieth Century Fox.

Spielberg, S. (Director). (1982). *E.T.: The extra-terrestrial* [Motion picture]. United States: Universal Pictures.

Troiden, R. (1979). Becoming homosexual: A model of gay identity acquisition. *Psychiatry, 42*, 362–373.

Ulrichs, K. (1994). *The riddle of "man-manly" love: The pioneering work on male homosexuality* (M. Lombardi-Nash, Trans.). Amherst, NY: Prometheus Books. (Original work published 1864–1880)

Walker, M. (1976). The double, an archetypal configuration. *Spring*, 165–175.

Walker, M. (1991). Jung and Homophobia. *Spring 51*, 55–70.

Walker, M. (1994). *Men loving men: A gay sex guide and consciousness book* (2nd ed.). San Francisco: Gay Sunshine Press.

Walker, M. (1997a). The Uranian complex: Father-son incest and the oedipal stage in gay men. *The Uranian soul: Studies in gay-centered Jungian psychology for a new era of gay liberation.* Unpublished manuscript.

Walker, M. (1997b). The Uranian coniunctio: A study of gay identity formation and the individuation model of C. G. Jung. *The Uranian soul: Studies in gay-centered Jungian psychology for a new era of gay liberation.* Unpublished manuscript.

Walker, M. (1999). *The revolutionary psychology of gay-centeredness in men.* Self-published.

Winnicott, D. (1971). *Playing and reality.* London: Routledge.

Winnicott, D. (1975). Hate in the coutertransference, *Through paediatrics to psychoanalysis: Collected papers.* London: Karnac Books. (Original work published in 1947)

Yep, G. (2002). From homophobia and heterosexism to heteronormativity: Toward the development of a model of queer interventions in the university classroom. *Journal of Lesbian Studies, 6*, 163–176.

Afterword

Bender's Legacy

Not too long ago, in a galaxy not particularly far away, a fierce battle was waged between powerful opponents: the Benderites and Werthamites. At stake was no less than the collective soul of childhood. At issue was whether comic books, and by association, superheroes, were a corrupting influence on children. Those on the side of Lauretta Bender believed that comic books and the superheroes they often depicted were a powerful vehicle for tapping into the inner lives of children, and in so doing, gave voice to hidden fantasies, repressed pain and unfulfilled longings. Those on the side of Fredric Wertham, believed that such fantasy, and the child's identification with both superheroes and supervillailns perverted and undermined healthy development, resulting in psychopathology and social deviance.

Fast-forward a half-century. Those glorious battlefields have long stood silent. The impassioned cries of war are but a faint echo. Whereas Wertham's moral vigilantism contributed to a greater awareness of our responsibility to protect children, his ideology has receded to the intellectual, academic, and clinical periphery. On the other hand, Bender's belief in the value of comics and superheroes to liberate, rather than imprison children, has continued to evolve, as evidenced in the essays contained in this volume.

To borrow a phrase, these essays "have boldly gone" where few clinicians have gone before—into the realm of popular culture, and, in particular, the genre of superheroes. These clinicians have playfully and creatively demonstrated that the icons of popular (children's) culture are far more than a banal manifestation of mass marketing, consumerism, and commercial greed. They are instead, as Bender rightfully suggested a mere 3 years after the introduction of Superman, a medium through which children and adults can communicate in a meaningful way both with themselves and each other.

There is a reason—or more likely many reasons—for the longevity and ubiquity of the superhero. I don't believe that Hollywood keeps churning out superhero movies simply for profit, although profit, of course, matters. I believe that superheroes, superhero movies, superhero television shows, superhero video games, superhero comic books, and superhero merchandise satisfy deep existential needs, at both the personal and societal levels, to be stronger than we are, to break through barriers both external and internal, to connect with others—to look, up in the sky!

Lawrence C. Rubin

Appendix

A Thumbnail Guide to the Use of Superheroes in Psychotherapy with Children, Adolescents and Adults[1]

Superhero/Supervillain	Origin Story (in Brief)	Special Power(s)	Weakness(es)	Unique Issues
Apocalypse (1986)	Born into Egyptian royalty, self-appointed "first mutant"	Super-strength, size/form-changing ability	Excess power burns away his body(bodies), requiring new hosts	Megalomania, superiority complex
Aquaman (1941)	Orphaned, bicultural	Strength, ability to command sea life, leader	Anger, bitter feelings	Identity—fish out of water, physical loss of hand
Archangel (1963)	Born into wealth and privilege, mutant	Flight, healing factor, strength, and sensory acuity	Wings are fragile	Reconciling "mutant" identity
Batman (1939)	Human, violently orphaned	Technology, science, zeal for justice	Mortality	Anger, vengeance, isolation, loss
Captain America (1941)	Super soldier serum, human	Perfect military mind and body	Mortality, limited in skills and powers	Power shield (a defense)
Captain Marvel (1940)	Orphaned, chosen by a wizard, Shazam, to be the world's mightiest man	Superstrength, flight, wisdom, invulnerability	Magic, too trusting and good-natured; not so wise when in boy form	Emotionally immature, naive/innocent
Catwoman (1940)	Victim/survivor/outsider	Agility, technology, animal-like powers	Delusional thinking that she is a feline	Internal conflicts between "right" and "wrong"
Daredevil (1940)	Blind from childhood, pro bono lawyer	Heightened senses, Olympic-level body	Blind, vulnerable to libidinal urges	Strives for justice, discouraged by injustice
Darth Vader (1977)	Human, immaculately conceived	Force powers, superior light-saber skills, telekinesis, telepathy	Trapped inside life-sustaining armor	Driven by "dark side," true heroism for "good" must be reawakened by son

322

Dr. Xavier (1963)	Paternal figure, the good son	Telekinesis, super mental abilities, leader-protector of X-Men	Paraplegic, limited mobility	Physical impairment (confined to wheelchair)
Fantastic Four (1961)	Human survivors of cosmic blast	Elasticity (Reed), Invisibility (Sue), Flame Power (Johnny), Strength (Ben); wisdom, family and team dynamic	Subdegree cold (Reed) Oxygen-deprivation (Johnny), unconscious mind control (Sue), no secret identities	Family conflicts-jealousy, martial conflict, power struggles
Flash (1940)	Human; chemical accident	Speed and time travel	Bad lover, destructible	Self-centered, hyperkinetic
Frodo Baggins (1954)	Hobbit, orphaned when parents drowned; made heir to Bilbo (distant relative)	Invisibility, magic sword, enchanted light, resilience against evil	Half-sized, weakened by burden of the One Ring	Goal accomplished through bonds with partner Sam and "shadow" figure Gollum.
Green Lantern (1940)	Human—magical Starheart fragment	Flight, creates and changes objects at will	Color yellow	Power ring
Han Solo (1977)	Human, orphan	Cunning, brave, daring	No superpowers, greed	Selfish antihero learns to care about others
The Hulk (1962)	Human, failed experiment by father	Great strength	Rage	Anger control, outsider

(continued)

A Thumbnail Guide to the Use of Superheroes in Psychotherapy with Children, Adolescents and Adults (*Continued*)

Superhero/Supervillain	Origin Story (in Brief)	Special Power(s)	Weakness(es)	Unique Issues
Iron Man (1963)	Genius engineer	Intellect, invulnerability (with shield), flight, weapons	Alcoholism, heart problems	Dependent on armor/machines to survive; heart condition
Lieutenant Ellen Ripley (1980)	Original birth unknown; reborn as clone after sacrificial suicide	Superhuman courage, ingenuity, and stamina after cloning; acid blood, self-healing capacity	Psychologically traumatized by encounters with aliens	Encounter with alien nemesis turns ordinary human into a hero
Luke Skywalker (1977)	Adopted, inherits Jedi skills from birth father	The Force—strength, will, telepathy, telekinesis	Incomplete, self-doubt, hate, rage	Internal struggle, must renounce violence and hate
Lex Luthor (1940)	Billionaire industrialist, deceased father, made bald by Superman	Supergenius intellect	Greed, megalomania, single-mindedness	Massive superiority complex
Martian Manhunter (1956)	Survivor/alien	Strength, wisdom, fairness, invisibility, shape shifting	Fire, mind control	Family trauma-loss of family and home acculturation issues—skin color versus real appearance
Magneto (1963)	Survivor of German death camps, mutant	Flight, master of control metal, flight, generate magnetic fields	Isolation from metal/metallic materials	Loathing/mistrust of humanity

Namor (1939)	Biracial, human, bicultural	Superstrength, flight, amphibious	Needs water for strength	Arrogant, willful, impatient, short-tempered
Nightcrawler (1965)	Son of X-Men terrorist	Strength, faith, teleportation, invisibility, agility, night vision	Despite amazing abilities, he is mortal	Isolated-marginalized, low self-esteem due to appearance, "hides" in shadows
Nightwing (1984); previously Robin, the Boy Wonder	Family killed, trained by Batman	Strength and agility, master combatant	Human, no superabilities	Self-esteem/identity issues, overshadowing parent figure (Batman)
Obi-wan Kenobi (1977)	Teacher, mentor	Force powers, excellent light-saber skills, telekinesis, telepathy	Too philosophical, faulty mentoring skills; lacks patience and ability to "contain"	Guilt over Anakin's turn to the "dark side"
PowerPuff Girls (1998)	Created in lab	Flight, strength, and tenacity	Childish; mischievous	Human foibles
Punisher (1974)	Lost family, ex-Marine, Vietnam War veteran/hero	Toughness, tenacity	Suffers from posttraumatic stress syndrome	Cannot forgive; vigilante-revenge obsessions
Scooby-Doo (1969)	Animal, adopted, human emotions	Supportive team, Inner-strength	Weakness for food	Easily distracted, fearful
The Silver Surfer (1966)	Semidivine being created by godlike Galactus	Energy blasts, near-invulnerability, great strength, surfboard (allows flight)	Detachment and introspection leaves him unaware; uses magic, mental manipulation	Question of identity and purpose, lacks understanding of good versus evil

(continued)

A Thumbnail Guide to the Use of Superheroes in Psychotherapy with Children, Adolescents and Adults (*Continued*)

Superhero/Supervillain	Origin Story (in Brief)	Special Power(s)	Weakness(es)	Unique Issues
Spider-Man (1962)	Human, orphaned, adopted, radioactive accident	Cunning, pseudoflight, strength, persistence	Adolescence, mortality	Loss, pseudo-maturity, losses in love
Star Trek heroes (1966)	Humans, aliens, and androids separated from home and families	Intelligence, bravery, compassion, technology, alien powers	Individual frailties and idiosyncrasies	Expression and repression of emotion and humanity
Supergirl (1962)	Orphaned, alien, survivor	Flight, strength, goodness	Kryptonite, magic	Immaturity
Superman (1938)	Orphaned, alien, adopted	Flight, strength, goodness	Kryptonite, magic	Outsider, identity concealed
Thor (1940)	God of thunder	Lightning powers, storms, superstrength, flight, near invulnerability	Arrogant, godlike	Cultural assimilation, question of personal identity
Wonder Woman (1942)	Born of Olympian gods, master race of women	Strength, wisdom, goodness	Physical vulnerability	Cultural assimilation, gender equality
Wolverine (1974)	Human; victimized by others	Strength, compassion, agility, steel claws	Paranoia	Easily angered; anger management issues; outsider

[1] Thanks to Daniel Leveille, Monique Wilson, John Shelton Lawrence, and the essayists in this volume for their contributions to this chart.

Index

123 Magic (book), 41

A

Achilles (hero), 124
Active Imagination (technique), 300
Adderall (medication), 61
Adlerian theory, 52-54
Adoption, 217-218; and triangle, 218
Aggression Nurturance (concept), 128
Alan Scott (character), 11; *See also* Green
    Lantern
Albert Malik (character), 77; *See also* Red
    Skull
Alien (films), 293, 303–305
Almond Board of California, *170*
Almost-Perfect Parenting (book), 41
American Professional Society on the
    Abuse of Children, 194
Ammann, Ruth, 71
Anakin Skywalker (character), 214–215,
    307; use in hypnosis, 281
Anger Log (technique), 92
Antiheroes (villains), 54
Applied Behavioral Analysis-Lovaas
    Therapy, 178
Aquaman (superhero), 12
Araoz, Daniel, 275, 276, 278, 289
Archetype, 74
Arena (*Star Trek* television episode),
    252
Aristotle (philosopher), 11
Armstrong, Lance (bicyclist), 154
Asperger, Hans, 172
Atom Ant (cartoon character), 285
Attachment disorder, 196–198

Atomic Ace: He's Just like My Dad (book),
    151; *See* Weigel, Jeff
Atomic Sock Monkey (game publisher); *See*
    Truth and Justice
Autism (autism spectrum disorders-ASD),
    172–175;
    features in, 175–176
Autism and Play (book), 176; *See* Beyer,
    Jannik and Gammeltoft, Lone
Autism Society of America, 174
Avengers, The (superheroes), 11, 146
Axline, Virginia, 181

B

Bale, Christian (actor), 124
Bambi (film), 118
Bandura, Albert, 148
Barclay, Commander (character), 252
Baron-Cohen, Simon, 178;
Barry Allen (character), 12; *See also* Flash
Bart Allen (character), 56–57; *See also*
    Impulse
Batman-aka Dark Knight, Caped Crusader
    (superhero), 9–12, 54, 57, 124,
    132–133, 137, 148, 197; as myth
    79–80
Batman Begins (film), 113
Batman the Movie (film), 106, 113
Beast, The (superhero), 228
Bender, Lauretta, xix–xxi, xxiii–xxv, 7, 17
Bettleheim, Bruno, 5–6, 23, 70, 173
Beverly Hills 90210 (television show),
    118
Beyer, Jannik, 176, 180
Bibliotherapy (technique), 53

Big Goodbye, The (*Star Trek* television episode), 259
Blade (superhero), 12
Borg, The (aliens), 260
Boy Code (book), 123; *See also* Pollack, William
Bradshaw, John, 299
Brain structures and emotion, 93–95
Bridge on the River Kwai, The (film), 118
Brodzinsky, David, 217
Bromfield, Richard, 180
Brothers (*Star Trek* television episode), 251, 262
Bruce Banner (character), 11, 89, 125; *See also* Hulk
Bruce Wayne (character), 11, 57, 105, 216; *See also* Batman
Bruner, Jerome, 5
Buenher, Caralyn, 151
Buffalo Creek Disaster, 108
Buzz Lightyear (character), 170
By Any Other Name (*Star Trek* television episode), 251

C

California Department of Developmental Services, 173
Call (character), 305
Campbell, Joseph, 9, 13, 16, 76, 229
Captain America, xxiii
Captain Hook (character), 208
Carpenter, Edward, 296
Cartoon Network, 50
Categorical diagnostics, 174
Catholic Legion of Decency, xx
Catwoman (superheroine), 51
Centers for Disease Control-CDC, 173
Chowchilla Incident, 107 111–112; *See also* Terr, Lenore
Chunky Dungeon (RPG), 235
Cinderella, 207
Clark Kent (character), 10, 57, 148, 216; *See also* Superman
Cliff Secord (character), 149; *See also* Rocketeer
Code of Chivalry, 235
Collective unconscious, 72–73
Comics Code Authority, The, xxvi
Committee on the Evaluation of Comic Books, xx

Complex; mother, father, shadow (concept), 301
Crow, The (antihero), 54

D

Daredevil (superhero), 12–13,124, 148, 156; the movie, 163
Dark Knight, 11; *See also* Batman
Darth Maul (character), 204
Darth Vader (character), xxvi, 290, 306
Datalore (*Star Trek* television episode), 251, 262
Data, Mr. (character), 244, 248, 251, 264
DC Comics, 136
Deana Troi, Counselor (character), 248
Death Guilt (concept), 108
Defenders, The (superheroes), 134
Denethor (character), 313
Descent (*Star Trek* television episode), 251
Diana Prince (character), 11; *See also* Wonder Woman
Diaz, Ruben, 126
Dick Grayson (character), 86; *See also* Robin
Dissociation, 274
Doctor Doom (antihero), 146
Donald Blake (character), 11; *See also* Thor
Dory (character), 170
Double Dragon (television show), 37
Double, the (concept), 296
Dragon Ball Z (cartoon), 25
Draw the Marvel Comics Super Heroes (book), 151,162
Dreikurs, Rudolf, 52
Dr. Strange (superhero), 135
DSM-Diagnostic and Statistics Manual (book), 172–174
Dungeons and Dragons (RPG), 227–228, 230, 232, 235
Dyer, Wayne, 280

E

Echoplaylia (concept), 176
Ego, 72–74
Elektra (superheroine), 14, 123
Elektra Nachios (character), 14; *See also* Elektra
Ellen Ripley, Lt. (character), 293, 295, 304
Elliotson, John, 272
Ellis, Albert, 98; *See also* Rational Emotive Therapy

Emotional Literacy (concept), 91–93
Erickson, Milton, 272, 283
Erikson, Erik, 4, 116, 219
E.T., the Extraterrestrial (film), 118

F

False Self (concept), 301
Fantastic Four, The (superheroes), 11–12, 131; the movie, 162
Fantasy, 4–6, 271; and metaphor, 6–7; and superhero, 7–9; and play, 69–70
Feiffer, Jules (journalist/cartoonist), 115, 129
FIDEL (hypnotic technique), 280, 286
Field of Dreams Program, 145: *See also* Onarga Academy
Finding Nemo (film), 170
Fingeroth, Danny, 126, 130, 134, 294
Flash (superhero), 12–13
Floor Games (book), 70, 231; *See* Wells, H.G.
Floor Time (technique), 179
Foucault, Michel, 297
Freud, Anna, 5, 106
Freud, Sigmund, 5, 106
Frodo Baggins (character), 293–294, 307–308, 311

G

Gammeltoft, Lone, 176, 180
Gandalf (character), 314
Genealogical Bewilderment (concept), 218
General Zod (antihero), 146
Ginott, Haim, 7
Gollum (character), 293, 308, 311
Goodwin, Barbara, 72
Great Comic Book Heroes, The (book); *See* Feiffer, Jules
Green Arrow (superhero), 156
Green Goblin, The (antihero), 78
Green Lantern (superhero), 11–12, 136
Green Ronan: *See* Mutants and Masterminds
Gurian, Michael, 140

H

Harry Potter (character), 162; the movie, 163
Hay, Harry, 296

He-Man (hero), 277
Henry Duncard (character*)*, 79–80; *See also* Ra Al Ghul
Hero (song), 165; *See* Superchic[k]
Hero Clicks (RPG), 231, 238
Hero Machine, The (hero creation software), 26–28
Heroscape (RPG), 228, 230
Hero's Journey 76–77
Heteronormativity (concept), 297
Heterosexism (concept), 297
History Box (technique), 205
Hobbit (character), 308
Holodeck, 252, 265
Hollow Pursuits (*Star Trek* television episode), 252
Homophobia (concept), 297
Hulk Syndrome (concept), 90–91
Hulk, The Incredible (character), xxvi, 11, 53, 124–125, 134–135, 284, 289; the movie, 163
Human Torch, the (superhero), 289
Hybrid (RPG), 228, 230
Hypnosis, 271–274; use of superheroes in, 272–274; and pain, 274–276; and neurocognition; and trauma, 278–280; and ego-strengthening, 282–283; and psychoneuroimmunology, 285
Hypnotic Realities (book), 283–285; *See* Erickson, Milton & Rossi, Ernest

I

I Borg (*Star Trek* television episode), 245
Impulse (superhero), 53, 56
Incredibles, The (superheroes), 161; the movie, 163
Infinite Crisis (comic book storyline), 133
Invisible Girl (superheroine), 51
IQ (intelligence quotient), 254
Iron Man (superhero), 10, 12, 156–157
Iron Winds (game publisher); *See* War Machine

J

Jackman, Hugh (actor), 134
James T. Kirk, Captain (character), 244, 251
Jay Garrick (character), 12; *See also* Flash
Jean Luc Picard, Captain (character), 244, 260–261

Jean Paul Valley (character), 80
Jewett, Robert, 8, 246
Joe Chill (character), 79
John Henry Irons (character), 62; *See also*
Steel
Joker, The (antihero), 146
Jonathan Crane, Dr. (character), 80; *See
also* Scarecrow
Jones, Gerard, xxiv, 126–127, 129
Joyce, James, 76
Jung, Carl, 15, 72–73, 75, 233, 296 , 298
Justice League of America, The
(superheroes), 11, 131
Justice Society of America (superheroes),
131

K

Kael, Pauline (journalist), 106, 114
Kahn (character), 248
Kalff, Dora, 70–71, 75, 231; and phases of
ego development, 75
Kane, Bob (cartoonist), 79, 106
Kanner, Leo, 172
Karma (concept), 146
Kathryn Janeway, Captain (character),
247, 251
Kefauver Senate hearings, xix, xxi, xxiv
*Killing monsters: Why children need
fantasy, superheroes
and make-believe* (book), 126; *See*
Jones, Gerard
Kirby, Jack (comic artist), xxiii, 125, 133
Klingons (aliens), 244
Koontz, Dean (author), 14
Kottman, Terry, 52
Krypton (fictitious planet), 9
Kryptonite (pieces of Krypton), 12

L

Labovitz-Boik, 72
Lady Shiva (character), 80
Landreth, Garry, 6–7
Lanyado, Monica, 181
Lawrence, John Shelton, 8, 246
League of Shadows, The (superheroes), 79
Lee, Ang (director), xxvi
Lee, Stan (cartoonist), 125, 133, 135
Leia Organa-Princess Leia (character), 215
Leonard McCoy, Dr. (character), 248
Levitz, Paul, 124
Limbic System, 195

Little Wars (book), 231–232; *See also*
Wells, H.G.
Live long and prosper (expression), 170
Lone Ranger (western hero), xxiii
Look, up in the sky! (expression), 169
Lord of the Rings (films), 293, 307–308;
See Tolkein, J. R. R.
Lourie, Reginald S., xx, xxiv
Lowenfeld, Margaret, 70, 231
Luke Skywalker (character), 9, 198, 203,
214–216, 293, 295, 306–307;
use in hypnosis, 281

M

Mad Pad (technique), 206
Make-Your-Own Comic Book (toy),
162
Man of Steel, see Superman
Marfan's Syndrome, 283
Marvel Comics, 126; and characters,
136
Marvel Hero Clicks (RPG), 228, 238
Mary Jane Watson (character), 78
Massively Multiplayered Online Role
Playing Game-MMORPG, 227
Matt Murdock (character), 12; *See also*
Daredevil
Maul (superhero), 228
May, Rollo, *16*
Menagerie, The (*Star Trek* television
episode), 251
Men of Tomorrow (book), *See* Jones,
Gerard
Metal Men (superheroes), 131
Metaphor, 6–7, 273
Meyer, Adolph, xxi
Mia Dearden (character), 156–157
Mighty Men and Monster Maker Kit, The
(toy), 58
Mindreading/mindblindness (concepts),
178; *See* Baron-Cohen, Simon
Mirroring games (technique), 206
Monomyth, 8, 76–77, 246; See also
Lawrence, John and Jewett,
Robert
Monsters and Mutants (RPG), 228
Morris, Tom and Mat, 132
Mr. Fantastic (superhero), 283–284
Mutants and Masterminds (RPG), 231
Mystery Men, The (film), 163
Myth, 76

N

National Adoption Clearinghouse, 217
National Comics Publications, xxiv
Nemesis (film), 243; *See also Star Trek*
Neuroscience, 195–196
New Hypnosis (book), 278; *See also* Araoz, Daniel
Newt (character), 304
Nexus Cornerstones (treatment ideals), 148: *See* Onarga Academy
Nietzsche, Freidrich, xxiii
Nip/Tuck (television show), 118
Norin Radd (character), 11; *See also* Silver Surfer
Norman Osborn (character), 78; *See also* Green Goblin

O

Oates, Joyce Carol, 108
Obi-Wan Kenobi (character), 215, 306
OLD-C (technique), 278
Omega Man (superhero), 156
Onarga Academy (treatment center), 143
Ororo Munroe (character), 14; *See also* Storm
Osborne, Norman (character), 78; *See also* Green Goblin

P

Pac Man (video game), 285–286
Padme Amidala (character), 215, 306
Partners in Play (book), 53; *See also* Kottman, Terry
Pathfinder (*Star Trek* television episode), 252
Pawnbroker, The (film), 108
PECS (technique), 179
Pervasive Developmental Disorder-PDD, 173;
 and PDD-NOS (not otherwise specified), 173–174
Peter Pan (character), 208
Peter Parker (character), 10, 12, 57, 148, 216; *See also* Spiderman
Phallic Receptivity (concept), 307
Piaget, Jean, 4, 23
Pipher, Mary, 123
Plato, 295–296

Pollock, William, 123, 128
Private Little War, A (*Star Trek* television episode), 251, 261
Powerpuff Girls, The (superheroines), 11
Prescriptive Play Therapy, 182; *See* Schaefer, Charles
Primal wound (concept), 217
Prince Adam (character), 277; *See also* He-Man
Psychosemantics, 278
Punisher, The (antihero), 54, 124

Q

Qui-Gon Jinn (character), 215, 306

R

Ra'as Al Ghul (character), 79
Race hatred (in comics), xxii
Rachel Dawes (character), 79
Rational Emotive Therapy, 98
Real Boys (book), 123; *See also* Pollack, William
Realm of Fear (*Star Trek* television episode), 252
Red Skull, The (antihero), 77
Reed Richards, 283–284; See also Mr. Fantastic
Reviving Ophelia (book), 123; *See* Pipher, Mary
Riddler, The (antihero), 146
Rimland, Bernard, 173
Robert Bruce Banner (character), 89; *See also* Hulk
Robbins, Tom, 46
Robin (superhero), 86
Rocketeer, The (superhero), 149
Rodenberry, Gene (director), 243; *See also Star Trek*
Rogers, Carl, 71
Rogers, Fred, 129
Role Playing Games-(RPGs), 227–228
Role-playing (technique), 58, 227
Romero, Cesar (actor), 117
Romita, John Sr. (cartoonist), 125
Romulans (aliens), 245
Rossi, Ernest, 283
RPGs-Role Playing Games, 227–228

S

Sabertooth (superhero), 239
Sailor Moon (superheroine), 11

Samwise Gamgee (character), 293,
    307–308, 311
Sanders, Bernard, xxi
Sandplay Therapy, 70
Sandplay Therapy (book), 72; See
    Goodwin, Barbara and Labovitz-Boik,
    Anna
Sauron (character), 294
Scarecrow, The (antihero), 79
Schaefer, Charles, 182–183; See
    Prescriptive Play Therapy
Schwartz, Julius (editor), 131
Scooby Doo (cartoon character), 284
Seduction of the Innocent (book), See
    Wertham, Fredric
Senator Palpatine, aka Darth Sidious/the
    Emperor (character), 216
Serena (character), 11; See also Sailor
    Moon
Shadow Complex (concept), 300
Shadow Run (RPG), 228
She Hulk (superheroine), 51
Shelob (fictitious animal), 313
She-Ra (hero), 277; See He-Man
Shmi (character), 215
Shore Leave (Star Trek television episode),
    251
Showalter, Barbra, 108
Silver Surfer (superhero), 11, 135, 289
Skeletor (character), 277
Skinner, B.F., 178
Sky High (film), 163
Slammers Ultimate Milkshakes,
    170
Smith, Helen Dr., 126
Social Stories (technique), 179
Soul figure (concept), 296
Spawn (antihero), 54
Speedy (superhero), 156
Spiderman (superhero), xxvi, 9, 12, 53, 58,
    155, 157, 197, 216, 228;
as myth 77–79; the movie, 163, 302
Spider-Man and Power Pack (book),161
Spock, Mr. (character), 70, 244, 248, 251,
    261, 264
Squiggle Game, The, 25–26: See also
    Winnicott, Donald
Star Trek(television show), 243; TOS (The
    Original Series), 243;
    TNG (The Next Generation), 243; VOY
    (Voyager), 243; DS9 (Deep

Space Nine) 243; ENT (Enterprise)
    243–244; captains and
    commanders, 247
Star Wars (film), 163, 213–216, 293,
    306–307
Star Wars Miniature Game (RPG), 238
Steel (film), 49
Storm (superhero), 9, 14, 51; See also
    X-Men
Story Maker 2.1, The (story creation
    software), 25–27
Submariner (superhero), 13, 135
Suicide Squad, The (superheroes), 147
Sulu, Ensign (character), 251
Superchic[k] (rock group), 165
Super Dog: Heart of a Boy (book), 151:
    See Buehner, Caralyn
Supergirl (superhero), 290
SuperHero Comic Book Maker (superhero
    creation software), 162
Superhero motif: origins, 9; costumes, 10;
    dual/secret identity, 10;
    families, 11; powers and flaws, 12;
    transformation, 13; play, 24
    science/magic, 14; villains, 15; and
    attachment disorder, 196–198;
    and Star Trek , 245–246
Superman (superhero), xxiii, 9–12, 146,
    216, 285, 290; the movie, 163

T

Tabletop Combat Games (RPG), 231
TEACCH (technique), 179
Technomythic (term), 14
Teen Titans (superheroes), 131
Temenos (concept), 71
Terrible Mother, the (concept), 304
Terr, Lenore, 107
Test anxiety, 262
Theory of mind (concept), 178
Thing, The (superhero), 124, 284
Thor (superhero), 11
Thunderbolts, The (superheroes), 147
Tillman, Pat (football player), 154
Toad, The (antihero), 138
To infinity and beyond (expression),
    170
Tolkein, J. R. R., 307
Tony Starks (character), see Iron Man
Toxic Shame (concept), 299; See Bradshaw,
    John

Toy Story (film), 170
T'Pol (character), 244
Trance logic, 277
Transcendent Child, The, 198
Transformation (in hypnosis), 276
Transitional object (concept), 171, 202; See Winnicott, Donald
Trauma, 195
Trouble with Tribbles, The (*Star Trek* television episode), 248
Truth and Justice (RPG), 228, 230

U

Übermensch (the Superman), *See* Neitzsche, Friedrich
Uhura, Officer (character), 248
Ulrichs, Karl Heinrich, 296
Uranian love/temperament, 296
Uranian Psychoanalysis, 295; *See also* Walker, Mitch

V

Vicki Vale (character), 113
Vertigo (film), 113
Vitamin C and Bioflavonoids: The Batman and Robin of Eye Health (book), 170; *See* White, Gina
Voodoo (superhero), 239
Vygotsky, Lev, 5–6

W

Walker, Mitch, 295–296
Warhammer (RPG), 227
Weigel, Jeff, 151

Wein, Len (cartoonist), 125
Wells, H.G., 70, 231
Wertham, Fredric, xix–xxiv, xxvi, 117; See *Seduction of the Innocent*
What Would Jesus Do?-WWJD (technique), 49
What Would Superman Do?-WWSD (technique), 49,
Whisper in the Ear (technique), 177
White, Gina, 170
Whitman, Walt, 296
Wing, Lorna, 172
Winnicott, Donald, 23, 25, 69, 171
Wizards of the West Coast (game publisher); *See* Dungeons and Dragons
Wolverine (superhero), 124–125, 133–134, 155, 239
Wonderland (book), 108; *See* Oates, Joyce Carol and Showalter, Elaine
Wonder Woman (superheroine), 10, 12, 290
Wonder Years, The (television show), 118
World of Warcraft (RPG), 230
World Technique, 70; *See* Kalff, Dora
Wrath of Kahn, The (*Star Trek* television episode), 248

X

Xavier, Francis Dr. (superhero), 133
X-Men, The (superheroes) 9, 11, 138, 216

Y

Youth-Adult (concept), 301

CPSIA information can be obtained at www.ICGtesting.com
Printed in the USA
BVOW06*2059080616

451309BV00002B/3/P